Clinica

Chemical Dependence

Edited by

Domenic A. Ciraulo, M.D.
Richard I. Shader, M.D.

*Departments of Pharmacology and Experimental Therapeutics
and Psychiatry
Tufts University School of Medicine
Boston, Massachusetts*

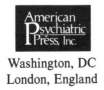

Washington, DC
London, England

Copyright © 1991 American Psychiatric Press, Inc.
ALL RIGHTS RESERVED
Manufactured in the United States of America on acid-free paper.
First Edition
94   93   92   91   4   3   2   1

American Psychiatric Press, Inc.
1400 K Street N.W., Washington, DC 20005

Library of Congress Cataloging-in-Publication Data

Clinical manual of chemical dependence / edited by Domenic A. Ciraulo, Richard I. Shader.—1st ed.
    p.   cm.
Includes bibliographical references.
Includes index.
ISBN 0-88048-280-X (alk. paper)
1. Alcoholism—Treatment. 2. Drug abuse—Treatment. I. Ciraulo, Domenic A. II. Shader, Richard I., 1935-   .
[DNLM: 1. Alcoholism—therapy. 2. Substance Dependence—therapy. WM 270 C6414]
RC565.C489   1991
616.86′06—dc20
DNLM/DLC
for Library of Congress   90-14511
                                                                              CIP

British Library Cataloguing in Publication Data

A CIP record is available from the British Library.

Contents

List of Tables   vii
List of Figures   viii
Contributors   ix
Preface   xiii
       Domenic A. Ciraulo, M.D.
       Richard I. Shader, M.D.

Chapter 1   **Alcoholism**   1
       Domenic A. Ciraulo, M.D.
       John A. Renner, Jr., M.D.

Chapter 2   **Opioids**   95
       Jerome H. Jaffe, M.D.
       Steven Epstein, M.D.
       Domenic A. Ciraulo, M.D.

Chapter 3   **Anxiolytics**   135
       Domenic A. Ciraulo, M.D.
       Brian F. Sands, M.D.
       Richard I. Shader, M.D.
       David J. Greenblatt, M.D.

Chapter 4   **Marijuana**   175
       Jack H. Mendelson, M.D.
       Nancy K. Mello, Ph.D.

Chapter 5   **Cocaine**   195
       Herb Roehrich, M.D.
       Mark S. Gold, M.D.

Chapter 6   **Stimulants**   233
       Donald C. Goff, M.D.
       Domenic A. Ciraulo, M.D.

Chapter 7	**Hallucinogens**	259
	Ulrich Tacke, M.D.	
	Michael H. Ebert, M.D.	
Chapter 8	**Phencyclidine**	279
	Edward F. Domino, M.D.	
Chapter 9	**Inhalants**	295
	Charles W. Sharp, Ph.D.	
	Luis Fornazzari, M.D.	
Chapter 10	**Tobacco**	321
	Reese T. Jones, M.D.	
Chapter 11	**Psychotherapy and Chemical Dependence**	345
	Lance M. Dodes, M.D.	
	Edward J. Khantzian, M.D.	
Chapter 12	**Alcoholics Anonymous**	359
	Margaret Bean-Bayog, M.D.	
Chapter 13	**Relapse Prevention**	377
	Genell G. Sandberg, Ph.D.	
	G. Alan Marlatt, Ph.D.	
	Index	401

List of Tables

Table 1-1. DSM-III-R diagnostic criteria for psychoactive substance dependence

Table 1-2. DSM-III-R diagnostic criteria for psychoactive substance abuse

Table 1-3. Markers in high-risk studies

Table 1-4. Ethanol elimination facts

Table 1-5. Symptoms of alcohol withdrawal syndrome

Table 1-6. Nutritional supplementation in alcoholics

Table 1-7. Benzodiazepine protocols for alcohol detoxification

Table 1-8. DSM-III Axis I diagnoses of 88 alcoholics requiring psychiatric admission

Table 2-1. Signs and symptoms of opiate withdrawal

Table 2-2. Protocol for administration of clonidine (dose mg/day)

Table 3-1. Approximate benzodiazepine dose equivalency

Table 3-2. Sedative-hypnotic dose equivalency (equal to 30 mg phenobarbital)

Table 3-3. Nonbarbiturate sedative-hypnotic agents: dosage and duration associated with withdrawal symptoms

Table 3-4. Trends in percentage of persons reporting sedative/ tranquilizer use in past year: 1974–1985, selected years

Table 3-5. Barbiturates and selected other drugs mentioned most frequently in emergency rooms in 1985

Table 3-6. Barbiturates and selected other drugs mentioned most frequently by medical examiners in 1985

Table 3-7. Barbiturates

Table 3-8. Short-acting barbiturates: brand and street names

Table 3-9. Signs and symptoms of barbiturate withdrawal

Table 3-10. Guidelines for barbiturate detoxification

Table 4-1. Trend in estimated prevalence of marijuana use among three age groups, 1972–1985, selected years

Table 4-2. Trend in estimated prevalence of marijuana use among high school senior classes, 1975–1985

Table 5-1. A comparison of proposed cocaine withdrawal syndromes

Table 5-2. A comparison of treatments for cocaine abstinence symptoms

Table 5-3. Suggested treatment regimen of oral bromocriptine in acute cocaine withdrawal

Table 6-1. Major stimulants: trade and street names

Table 6-2. Major stimulants: half-life and dose range

Table 6-3. Anorectics

Table 6-4. Common sources of caffeine

Table 7-1.   Major groups of hallucinogens
Table 7-2.   Street names of hallucinogens
Table 7-3.   DSM-III-R diagnostic criteria for hallucinogen hallucinosis
Table 7-4.   Symptoms of anticholinergic intoxication
Table 8-1.   Street names for phencyclidine
Table 8-2.   Clinical spectrum of acute phencyclidine intoxication
Table 8-3.   Possible biochemical and behavioral mechanisms underlying phencyclidine psychosis
Table 8-4.   Pharmacokinetic parameters of ^{3}H-phencyclidine given 1.3 $\mu g/kg$ iv in normal volunteers: comparison of two- and three-compartment models
Table 12-1.   The Twelve Steps of Alcoholics Anonymous

List of Figures

Figure 8-1.   Some Abused Phencyclidine Derivatives
Figure 13-1.   Cognitive-behavioral Model of the Relapse Process
Figure 13-2.   Relapse Prevention: Specific Intervention Strategies
Figure 13-3.   Relapse Prevention: Global Self-Control Strategies

Contributors

Margaret Bean-Bayog, M.D.
Department of Psychiatry
Harvard Medical School
Cambridge Hospital
Cambridge, Massachusetts

Domenic A. Ciraulo, M.D.
Departments of Pharmacology and Experimental Therapeutics and
  Psychiatry
Tufts University School of Medicine
Boston, Massachusetts

Lance M. Dodes, M.D.
Department of Psychiatry
Mount Auburn Hospital
Harvard Medical School
Cambridge, Massachusetts

Edward F. Domino, M.D.
Department of Pharmacology
University of Michigan
Ann Arbor, Michigan

Michael H. Ebert, M.D.
Department of Psychiatry
Vanderbilt University School of Medicine
Nashville, Tennessee

Steven Epstein, M.D.
Department of Psychiatry
Georgetown University School of Medicine
Washington, D.C.

Luis Fornazzari, M.D.
Clarke Institute of Psychiatry
Toronto, Ontario, Canada

Donald C. Goff, M.D.
Department of Psychiatry
Harvard Medical School
Erich Lindemann Mental Health Center
Boston, Massachusetts

Mark S. Gold, M.D.
Director of Research
Fair Oaks Hospital
Summit, New Jersey
Delray Beach, Florida

David J. Greenblatt, M.D.
Departments of Pharmacology and Experimental Research,
    Psychiatry, and Medicine
Tufts University School of Medicine
Boston, Massachusetts

Jerome H. Jaffe, M.D.
Associate Director
Office for Treatment Improvement
Alcohol, Drug Abuse, and Mental Health Administration
Rockville, Maryland

Reese T. Jones, M.D.
Department of Psychiatry
University of California, San Francisco
San Francisco, California

Edward J. Khantzian, M.D.
Harvard Medical School
Cambridge Hospital
Cambridge, Massachusetts
Danvers State Hospital
Hathorne, Massachusetts

G. Alan Marlatt, Ph.D.
Department of Psychology
University of Washington
Seattle, Washington

Nancy K. Mello, Ph.D.
Alcohol and Drug Abuse Research Center
Harvard Medical School
McLean Hospital
Belmont, Massachusetts

Jack H. Mendelson, M.D.
Alcohol and Drug Abuse Research Center
Harvard Medical School
McLean Hospital
Belmont, Massachusetts

John A. Renner, Jr., M.D.
Department of Psychiatry
Department of Veterans Affairs Outpatient Clinic
Tufts University School of Medicine
Boston, Massachusetts

Herb Roehrich, M.D.
Department of Psychiatry
St. Catherine's Hospital
Kenosha, Wisconsin

Genell G. Sandberg, Ph.D.
Parkview Psychological Services
Sioux City, Iowa

Brian F. Sands, M.D.
Department of Psychiatry
Department of Veterans Affairs Outpatient Clinic
Tufts University School of Medicine
Boston, Massachusetts

Richard I. Shader, M.D.
Departments of Pharmacology and Experimental Therapeutics and
  Psychiatry
Tufts University School of Medicine
Boston, Massachusetts

Charles W. Sharp, Ph.D.
Division of Preclinical Research
National Institute on Drug Abuse
Rockville, Maryland

Ulrich Tacke, M.D.
Department of Pharmacology
University of Kuopio
Finland

Preface

The intent of this manual is to provide a concise overview of the treatment of alcoholism and substance abuse. It is written both as an introduction for clinicians who may be new to the field and for those experienced clinicians who require a reference to assist in the diagnosis and treatment of patients with alcoholism and substance abuse. The first 10 chapters focus on a specific substance, drug, or class of drugs and address clinical pharmacology, differential diagnosis, detoxification, medical consequences, and long-term treatment of alcoholism and drug abuse. The last three chapters provide overviews of commonly used therapeutic modalities: psychodynamic psychotherapy, Alcoholics Anonymous, and relapse prevention. Although other modalities certainly could have been included, we limited our selection to those with the most clinical relevance for the generalist. We also hope that by limiting the selection we preserved conciseness. For each chapter we asked experienced scientist-clinicians to contribute an up-to-date and authoritative synthesis of their area. Variation in the proportions of basic and clinical pharmacology, treatment recommendations, and political tone occurs among these contributions. This was a deliberate choice by the editors, because we wanted this volume to reflect the existing spectrum of attitudes and data. We have tried to give exposure to several different viewpoints, some of which may not necessarily represent the personal views of the editors.

We would like to thank the contributors to this volume who took the time out of their busy schedules to support this project. We also would like to thank Dr. Carol Nadelson and the staff at the American Psychiatric Press, Inc., for help in planning and guiding the project. Most of all we would like to thank our families for their understanding and support.

Chapter 1

Alcoholism

Domenic A. Ciraulo, M.D.
John A. Renner, Jr., M.D.

PREVALENCE

Since the end of prohibition there has been a steady increase in the
number of Americans who drink alcoholic beverages. In 1938, only
58% of the population were drinkers. This increased to 64% in 1969
and to 71% in 1978; today more than 100 million Americans drink.
The major increases in the last two decades have been among women
and teenagers. Among young adults, drinking has become almost uni-
versal. In 1985, 51.5% of Americans between the ages of 12 and 17,
87.2% of those between 18 and 25, and 73.6% of those 26 and older
reported using alcohol in the past year (National Institute on Drug
Abuse 1988). There has been a shift away from the consumption of
hard liquor and a greater increase in the consumption of beer and
wine (Moser 1980).

As the number of drinkers has increased, so has the number of
alcoholics. Current estimates suggest that more than 10 million
Americans experience problems because of their drinking; of this
group, approximately 6 million are probably alcoholic. Among the 6
million alcoholic Americans, only 3% fit the stereotype of the skid
row drunk; the remainder are to be found among every race, age
group, and social class. Even more striking is the number of Americans who report alcohol-related problems in the immediate family.
This has increased from 12% in 1962 to 33% in 1982 (Fox 1983).
There is no way of knowing whether this indicates a real increase or
simply a greater willingness to acknowledge the problem. The most
comprehensive survey to date, released in 1984 by the National Insti-

1

tute of Mental Health, reported that alcohol abuse and/or dependence was the most common psychiatric disorder in adult males in the United States, affecting between 8.2% and 10.4% of the population (Myers et al. 1984). The problem must also be seen in a broader context. Alcohol-related deaths are the third ranking cause of death in the United States, after cancer and heart disease. Alcohol- and drug-related problems account for more than 20% of all emergency room visits. Alcoholism and psychiatric problems complicated by alcoholism are related to 35–50% of all admissions to public psychiatric hospitals (Strauss et al. 1985). The rate of successful suicide is much higher in alcoholics than in comparable nonalcoholic groups (Kessel and Grossman 1961; Jaffe and Ciraulo 1986).

It is clear that alcohol abuse and alcohol dependence are major public health problems impacting on one-third of all American families. It has been estimated that more than 50% of all patients undergoing psychiatric treatment in this country are alcohol abusers or have mental disorders that are significantly complicated by their use of alcohol. No psychiatrist can avoid working with such patients, nor can any psychiatrist justify a lack of familiarity with the treatment of these disorders.

DIAGNOSIS

Diagnostic Systems

Recent changes in DSM-III-R (American Psychiatric Association 1987) reflect an ongoing debate over the best diagnostic approach to substance abuse problems. Psychiatrists have yet to agree on the etiology of alcoholism; it is not surprising that diagnosis remains imprecise. Some of this confusion stems from our society's long-standing ambivalence about drug abuse and those who suffer from it. The founders of American psychiatry, including Benjamin Rush, accepted alcoholism and the alcoholic as legitimate medical problems (Rush 1785). During the 19th century, a major change in social attitudes led to the growth of the temperance movement and the eventual adoption of prohibition (Musto 1973). With alcoholics branded as sinners or criminals and legally banned from many medical facilities, it is hardly surprising that medicine and psychiatry ignored the condition.

It was not until the 1930s that clinicians again began to direct serious attention to this problem. The first modern attempt at a diagnostic system was the work of Jellinek, the social worker who established the Yale Center for Alcohol Studies. In his seminal work, *The Disease Concept of Alcoholism*, Jellinek (1960) made the case that alcoholism was a medical illness and not a moral or criminal problem. He felt that it was a progressive disease that inevitably led to a total loss of control over drinking and that had a fatal outcome. He described an invariable progression through stages that begins with occasional relief drinking; leads through blackouts, violent behavior, and avoidance of friends; and ends with cycles of obsessive continuous drinking.

Jellinek proposed five diagnostic "species":

- alpha: a purely psychological continual dependence on the effect of alcohol to relieve bodily or emotional pain; there is no progression, no loss of control, or an inability to abstain
- beta: heavy social group drinking with physical complications (such as cirrhosis) but no dependence
- gamma: drinkers with physical dependence (tolerance and withdrawal symptoms); a chronic, progressive disease, leading to loss of control
- delta: heavy daily drinkers with physical dependence, but no loss of control or other symptoms
- epsilon: binge or periodic drinkers

The gamma category was regarded by Jellinek as the common form of alcoholism in the United States; the delta form was prevalent in France. Only these two species of alcoholism were considered to be true disease states (Jellinek 1952). Modern research has questioned both the concept of inevitable progression and the specific stages described by Jellinek (Vaillant 1983), and there is general agreement that his five categories are not mutually exclusive, as he had suggested. Problem drinkers often shift from one to the another, with most eventually ending up as gamma alcoholics.

Some of the earliest diagnostic conflicts centered around the distinctions between social drinking, heavy drinking, alcohol abuse, and alcoholism. These conflicts have never been fully resolved. Chafetz (1975) settled on the concept of problem drinking as a practical alternative formulation with considerable clinical utility. He described problem drinking (or alcoholism) as a chronic behavior disorder manifested by an undue preoccupation with alcohol and its use to the detriment of physical and mental health, by loss of control when drinking is begun, and by a self-destructive attitude in dealing with personal relationships and life situations.

A different approach was taken by the British psychiatrist, Griffith Edwards. Edwards (1976) described the syndrome of alcohol dependence as a gradual progression from social drinking on to abuse and physical dependence. The sequence of steps is as follows:

1. narrowing of the drinking repertoire
2. salience of alcohol-seeking behavior
3. increased tolerance to alcohol
4. repeated withdrawal symptoms
5. avoidance of withdrawal symptoms by further drinking
6. rapid reinstatement of the syndrome after abstinence

Many of Edwards observations were incorporated in DSM-III-R. It should be noted, however, that the syndrome described by Edwards is accurate for only a subset of alcoholics. Many of the most severe alcoholics follow a different course, often marked by loss of control from the time of their first drinking experience.

DSM-III-R retains the categories of alcohol abuse and alcohol dependence included in DSM-III (American Psychiatric Association 1980), despite the desire of some clinicians to eliminate what was felt to be an artificial and often arbitrary distinction. In a useful effort to maintain consistency between these diagnostic categories and the standard system utilized in DSM-III, the category of psychoactive substance dependence (Table 1-1) was established and structured so as to give the clinician a wide degree of flexibility in diagnosis by including many descriptive items that are pertinent to a broad range of drugs and to a wide group of individual drug and alcohol abusers. It permits a more precise diagnosis, without forcing the clinician to make the sometimes artificial distinction between abuse and dependence. Although the category of alcohol abuse is maintained, it is now possible to make a diagnosis of alcohol dependence even in the absence of tolerance or physical dependence. The DSM-III-R criteria for psychoactive substance abuse are given in Table 1-2.

The major value of the DSM-III-R system is its power in describing the nature and severity of clinical symptoms. However, it does little to clarify issues of etiology or prognosis. There is compelling evidence that alcohol dependence is not a single entity and, in fact, may include two or more distinct diseases (e.g., familial alcoholism or reactive alcoholism) with totally different etiology, course, severity, and prognosis. Until a consensus is reached on the exact eti-

Table 1-1. DSM-III-R diagnostic criteria for psychoactive substance dependence

A. At least three of the following:
  (1) substance often taken in larger amounts or over a longer period than the person intended
  (2) persistent desire or one or more unsuccessful efforts to cut down or control substance use
  (3) a great deal of time spent in activities necessary to get the substance (e.g., theft), taking the substance (e.g., chain smoking), or recovering from its effects
  (4) frequent intoxication or withdrawal symptoms when expected to fulfill major role obligations at work, school, or home (e.g., does not go to work because hung over, goes to school or work "high," intoxicated while taking care of his or her children), or when substance use is physically hazardous (e.g., drives when intoxicated)
  (5) important social, occupational, or recreational activities given up or reduced because of substance use
  (6) continued substance use despite knowledge of having a persistent or recurrent social, psychological, or physical problem that is caused or exacerbated by the use of the substance (e.g., keeps using heroin despite family arguments about it, cocaine-induced depression, or having an ulcer made worse by drinking)
  (7) marked tolerance: need for markedly increased amounts of the substance (i.e., at least a 50% increase) in order to achieve intoxication or desired effect, or markedly diminished effect with continued use of the same amount
Note: The following items may not apply to cannabis, hallucinogens, or phencyclidine (PCP):
  (8) characteristic withdrawal symptoms (see specific withdrawal syndromes under Psychoactive Substance-induced Organic Mental Disorders)
  (9) substance often taken to relieve or avoid withdrawal symptoms
B. Some symptoms of the disturbance have persisted for at least one month, or have occurred repeatedly over a longer period of time.

Source. Reprinted with permission from American Psychiatric Association (1987).

ology of alcoholism(s), there will never be a fully satisfactory diagnostic system.

Clinical Approaches to Diagnosis

Despite the clarity of the symptoms in advanced alcohol dependence, it can be quite difficult to recognize early cases. The patient's denial or conscious efforts to mislead the clinician often present many prac-

Table 1-2. DSM-III-R diagnostic criteria for psychoactive substance abuse

A. A maladaptive pattern of psychoactive substance use indicated by at least one of the following:
   (1) continued use despite knowledge of having a persistent or recurrent social, occupational, psychological, or physical problem that is caused or exacerbated by use of the psychoactive substance
   (2) recurrent use in situations in which use is physically hazardous (e.g., driving while intoxicated)
B. Some symptoms of the disturbance have persisted for at least one month, or have occurred repeatedly over a longer period of time.
C. Never met the criteria for Psychoactive Substance Dependence for this substance.

Source. Reprinted with permission from American Psychiatric Association (1987).

tical problems in diagnosis. Psychiatrists should have a high index of suspicion when evaluating any patient, particularly those diagnosed as antisocial or borderline. Every psychiatric history should include a comprehensive history of drug use and a review of the family history for alcoholism or other drug abuse. The incidence of alcohol abuse can run as high as 60% in some inpatient settings, particularly in urban public institutions. It is also helpful to be alert to indirect signs that are highly suggestive of alcohol problems. These include a history of multiple automobile accidents, frequent injuries and fights, unexplained job losses, and marital problems. One of the most useful alcoholism screening tools is the CAGE system. CAGE is a mnemonic developed by Ewing and Rouse (1970) for a series of four questions that can be easily included in a clinical interview without arousing either the patient's antagonism or denial:

C — Have you ever felt you should CUT down on your drinking?
A — Have people ANNOYED you by criticizing your drinking?
G — Have you ever felt bad or GUILTY about your drinking?
E — Have you ever had a drink first thing in the morning to steady your nerves or get rid of a hangover (EYE OPENER)?

These questions have been extensively validated in a wide group of inpatient and outpatient settings and have proven highly reliable in detecting patients with alcohol problems. If a patient answers yes to two or three of these questions, an accurate diagnosis of alcoholism can be made in 89% of the patients interviewed (Mayfield et al. 1974).

If there is any suspicion of an alcohol problem, it is extremely helpful to review the situation with the family. Successful treatment usually requires that the family be involved in the process. This is particularly important if the patient continues to deny the problem. When a patient is cooperative, but the exact extent of the drinking is unclear, it is helpful to ask the patient to collect a detailed drinking history for 1 week. The patient should be directed to keep a daily log of all drinking events, including type of beverage, quantity consumed, and the circumstances of use. This technique can be very useful for patients with less pathologic forms of denial (Hanna 1979).

Whenever there is any question of possible intoxication or confusion regarding a patient's use of alcohol or drugs, it is helpful to obtain a blood alcohol level (BAL) and to screen for other drugs of abuse. A BAL over 0.15% in the presence of minimal intoxication is evidence of physiologic dependence. For research and clinical purposes, a number of simple paper and pencil tests have been developed to screen for alcoholism. The Johns Hopkins Alcohol Screening Test (Stone et al. 1965) uses 20 standard questions; this was further refined in the 24-question Michigan Alcoholism Screening Test (MAST) (Selzer 1971), which also exists in a shorter version called the SMAST. Another commonly used test is the MacAndrew Alcoholism Scale (MacAndrew 1965), a 49-item subscale of the standard Minnesota Multiphasic Personality Inventory (MMPI) (Hathaway and McKinley 1943). These tests are generally useful as screening devices for research, but none equals the practical clinical value of the CAGE system. Ultimately, the clinician's most useful diagnostic tool is a high level of concern that all psychiatric patients are at risk for alcohol abuse and should be carefully evaluated for this problem. There remains a tendency for middle- and upper-class women and others not meeting stereotypes of the alcoholic to be underdiagnosed by primary care physicians.

Biological Markers

Biological markers (Salaspuro 1986) of alcoholism are laboratory tests that are able to identify alcoholic patients. Such markers may help to identify alcoholics in medical and emergency room populations or in screening of large populations. To be of practical utility, such tests must show good specificity and sensitivity and be inexpensive and available in typical hospital or clinic laboratories.

Liver enzymes.   Serum gamma-glutamyl transferase (GGT) is a membrane-bound enzyme found in the sinusoidal membranes of the liver cell. It is elevated in alcoholics before the noticeable development of liver disease and correlates with the quantity of alcohol consumed. It normalizes after 4–5 weeks of abstinence and will increase again about 2 weeks after relapse. GGT is elevated in 34–85% of alcoholics or heavy drinkers. It may also be elevated in liver disease, obesity, diabetes, pancreatitis, acute renal insufficiency, severe trauma, and type IV hyperlipidemia; by drugs that induce the liver microsomes; and with a high-carbohydrate diet. It is higher in the elderly, in smokers, and in pregnant women. Men have higher levels than women.

Serum aspartate aminotransferase (ASAT) and alanine aminotransferase (ALAT).   Increased serum ASAT and ALAT are nonspecific markers of hepatic injury. A ratio of ASAT/ALAT greater than 2 is suggestive of alcoholic liver disease (Diehl et al. 1984; Ishii et al. 1979; Matloff et al. 1980; Nalpas et al. 1984; Panteghini et al. 1983; Rej 1978).

ASAT exists as two isoenzymes: one mitochondrial and the other cytosolic. The mean mitochondrial ASAT/total ASAT is four times higher in alcoholics than in patients with viral hepatitis (Nalpas et al. 1984).

Mean corpuscular volume.   Mean corpuscular volume is elevated in 31–96% of alcoholics. Other causes of increased mean corpuscular volume include deficiencies of vitamin B_{12} and folate, reticulocytosis, menopause, and treatment with antiepileptic drugs. Mean corpuscular volume may be higher in the elderly and smokers. One advantage of mean corpuscular volume as a marker is that it is readily available and inexpensive.

Erythrocyte enzymes.   The activity of erythrocyte aldehyde dehydrogenase is lower in chronic alcoholics than in controls, but the test has unacceptable specificity and sensitivity for clinical use.

Erythrocyte delta-aminolevulinic acid dehydratase is decreased after acute or chronic ethanol consumption, but does not have high enough sensitivity to be of clinical value. Cupro zinc superoxide dismutase of erythrocyte lysates is increased in black alcoholics compared to black or white controls, but specificity is too low to be a useful marker of alcoholism (Salaspuro 1986).

Blood acetate and ethanol. Ethanol is metabolized to acetaldehyde, which is converted to acetate in the liver. While ethanol is present in the body, chronic alcoholics and heavy drinkers have higher levels of acetate than nonalcoholic volunteers or occasional drinkers (Korri et al. 1985).

The measurement of blood ethanol concentration is not a useful marker in itself. One possible exception would be high levels (150 mg%) without evidence of intoxication or extremely high levels (300 mg%), as suggested by the National Council on Alcoholism Criteria Committee (1972).

Acetaldehyde adducts. Acetaldehyde forms adducts with hemoglobin and levels are higher in chronic alcoholics (Hoberman and Chiodo 1982; Stevens et al. 1981). The clinical significance of acetaldehyde adducts is an area of active research.

Immunoglobulin. Elevation of IgA and the IgA/IgG ratio has been used to distinguish alcoholic liver damage from other forms of liver disease (Iturriaga et al. 1977).

Beta-hexosaminidase. Levels of beta-hexosaminidase, a lysosomal glycosidase, are increased following 10 days of ethanol (60 g/day); GGT is not (Isaksson et al. 1985). Chronic alcoholics also have elevated levels of beta-hexosaminidase (Hultber et al. 1980).

AANB-to-leucine ratio. AANB decreases during acute ethanol administration (Shaw et al. 1976) and in protein malnutrition (Shaw and Lieber 1978), but is increased following chronic alcohol (Shaw and Lieber 1977). Plasma AANB-to-leucine ratio is increased in chronic alcoholics, but its low sensitivity and specificity limit its clinical value (Chick et al. 1982; Dienstag et al. 1978; Herrington et al. 1981; Jones et al. 1981; Morgan et al. 1977; Shaw et al. 1976, 1979).

HDL cholesterol.   HDL cholesterol is elevated by chronic ethanol, exercise, and enzyme-inducing drugs (Barboriak et al. 1980; Belfrage et al. 1977; Castelli et al. 1977; Danielsson et al. 1978; Devenji et al. 1981; Hartung et al. 1983). HDL phospholipids and apolipropoteins A-I and A-II may be increased by alcohol consumption (Puchois et al. 1984). By combining GGT and A-II, 72.9% of heavy drinkers were detected; only 59% were detected with GGT alone (Puchois et al. 1984).

Platelet MAO.   Although most studies have reported lower platelet MAO activity in alcoholics (Alexopoulos et al. 1981; Major and Murphy 1978; Sullivan and Stanfield 1978; Wiberg et al. 1977), some have not (Tabakoff et al. 1988). One study found no differences in baseline activity, but found that inhibition of MAO by ethanol was significantly higher in the platelets of alcoholics than in controls (Tabakoff et al. 1988). They also found that the basal activity of adenylate cyclase was the same in alcoholics and controls, but activity was lower in platelets of alcoholics after stimulation with guanine nucleotide, cesium fluoride, or prostaglandin E_1.

Adenosine receptors.   Basal and adenosine receptor-stimulated cyclic AMP levels were reduced 75% in lymphocytes from alcoholic subjects as compared with controls (Diamond et al. 1987).

Phosphatidylethanol synthesis.   Lymphocytes from male alcoholics with family histories of alcoholism have a significantly greater capacity to synthesize phosphatidylethanol, a unique metabolite of ethanol, than do nonalcoholic controls (Mueller 1988). Phospholipase D, which mediates this synthesis, may have altered activity in familial alcoholics.

Discriminant function analysis.   Various combinations of markers have been determined by discriminant function analysis to classify alcoholic patients better than single markers (Chalmers et al. 1981; Dolinsky and Schnitt 1988; Ryback et al. 1980, 1982).

Related Clinical Syndromes

DSM-III-R defines a number of other disorders commonly associated with alcoholism. The most common is alcohol intoxication. This diagnosis requires "maladaptive" behavioral changes following alcohol ingestion such as aggressiveness, emotional lability, or depression. This is to be distinguished from alcohol idiosyncratic intoxication, a relatively rare disorder that is manifested by markedly aggressive behavior following the ingestion of amounts of alcohol that are usually insufficient to produce intoxication. In this condition, the behavior is quite atypical of the person when sober and is followed by amnesia for the event.

Alcohol withdrawal delirium (delirium tremens or DTs) is evidence of physiologic dependence and is seen only after 5 to 10 years of heavy drinking. It follows the termination of drinking or a marked drop in BAL and requires a delirium, tremor, marked autonomic hyperactivity, and the absence of any other physical or mental cause for a delirium. Characteristically, the patient experiences vivid visual hallucinations.

Alcohol hallucinosis also occurs most frequently after the cessation of drinking in an alcohol-dependent person. However, there is no delirium or significant autonomic hyperactivity, and the hallucinations are usually auditory and paranoid in character. This condition usually clears in a few weeks, but it can become chronic. Unlike schizophrenia, the onset is later in life, and there is no family history or premorbid personality suggestive of schizophrenia.

The alcohol amnestic disorder (Korsakoff's syndrome) is due to thiamine deficiency and is seen primarily in chronic alcoholics. It usually begins after an acute episode of Wernicke's encephalopathy (confusion, ataxia, nystagmus, and peripheral neuropathies) and is marked by severe memory impairment. Patients may confabulate to mask their memory problems; there are no other cognitive deficits.

Impairment of judgment and learning capabilities has been demonstrated in many heavy drinkers. As this condition progresses, it may evolve into dementia associated with alcoholism, a dementia with both severe memory deficits and other signs of more general cognitive deterioration.

ETIOLOGY

Speculations about the etiology of alcohol abuse date back to biblical times. It has long been observed that alcoholism tends to run in families. However, the problem has alternately been seen as a moral aberration or weakness, as the toxic effect of a powerful drug, or as some type of physical illness. As modern medicine and psychiatry evolved over the last two centuries, our view of this problem has often reflected attitudes prevalent in the general society. It is of interest that Benjamin Rush treated alcoholics and saw them as patients worthy of care. However, by the end of the 19th century, the Prohibition movement had gained ascendancy, and alcohol abusers were generally seen as sinners, if not as criminals. They were banned from most American hospitals and were consigned to jails. These attitudes still impact on our judgment and feelings about individuals who abuse alcohol and other drugs. This significantly delayed scientific inquiry into the etiology and treatment of this condition. Although many of the key figures in the history of psychiatry have commented on the problem of alcoholism, it is only within the last 30 years that rigorous scientific attention has been directed to the subject.

Psychological Theories

Clinicians have often noted a connection between alcoholism and depression, anxiety, antisocial personality, and "oral" personality traits. There was a recurrent assumption that these psychological difficulties "caused" the alcoholism. Although numerous studies have documented the fact that these problems often coexist with alcoholism, it has been impossible to prove that any specific symptom or psychological disorder causes the illness.

Clinical and psychometric studies, primarily using the MMPI, have failed to document a unique "alcoholic personality." Nor has it been possible to identify a typical prealcoholic personality or any specific preexisting "oral" personality traits. The studies in this area have been extensively reviewed by Sutherland et al. (1950) and Syme (1957) and more recently by Pattison (1984). These studies have rejected the notion of any predisposing characterological variables. In general, alcoholics have been found to share the same conflicts, the same personality traits, and the same developmental problems found in nonalcoholic control populations.

Despite the absence of evidence for a specific alcoholic personality, there have been two interesting findings on MMPI studies that compared populations before and after the development of alcoholism. Prealcoholics have elevated psychopathic deviate scores and elevated hypomania scores. Psychopathic deviate elevations are not as high as those seen in psychopathic individuals, but the elevations persist after sobriety (Cox 1979). Active alcoholics also have consistently elevated depression scores, but these remit after sobriety. Alcoholics have also been shown to have a state of hypophoria (mild depressed feelings) that persists for extended periods after sobriety (Haertzen et al. 1980). These persistent symptoms will not be identified using the MMPI or the Self-Rating Depression Scale (Zung 1974), but can be measured by the Haertzen et al. (1980) Psychopathic State Inventory (Jaffe and Ciraulo 1986). The meaning of this hypophoria is unclear; it remains to be demonstrated if it antedates the alcoholism and if it continues indefinitely after sobriety. The diagnosis of major depression is not warranted in these cases; Jaffe and Ciraulo (1986) recommended against the routine use of antidepressant medication in such patients. Single doses of some benzodiazepines, such as diazepam and alprazolam, rapidly reverse mild dysphoria in abstinent alcoholics, which may contribute to abuse liability in this population but may also hold promise for treatment of dysphoria in these patients. Other nonprospective trait studies have demonstrated that alcoholics are more neurotic than control subjects. Although alcoholics can be shown to be anxious, hysterical, hypochondriacal, and ambivalent, there is no proof that these traits existed prior to the development of the alcoholism (Donovan 1986). Some prospective studies have shown evidence for a mild behavior disorder in prealcoholic males (Hoffman et al. 1974). However, the meaning of these findings is still unclear. After looking at some of these issues from the perspective of the genetics of psychiatric disorders, Cloninger et al. (1979) suggested that alcoholism, depression, and sociopathy have strong genetic predispositions and that they often run in the same families and may appear in the same individuals, but that they are separate etiologically and clinically (see below).

Recent work has focused on temperament as a guide to discovering an etiologic link between personality and alcoholism. Contemporary psychology has identified six primary dimensions of human temperament makeup: activity level, attention span and persistence, emotionality, soothability, reaction to food, and sociability. Numerous studies have demonstrated that prealcoholics, as well as males at high risk for alcoholism, show significant deviations in all six dimensions. These findings are consistent with a dysfunction of neural systems lying along the frontal-midbrain neuroaxis. This work suggests both a psychological and a neurobiological marker that may identify the prealcoholic and may prove invaluable as a link between the neuroanatomy and the behavior that predisposes to this condition (Tarter et al. 1985b).

One of the few other consistent findings in studies of alcoholics is that they are field dependent. The concept of field dependence and field independence refers to a cognitive style that is a stable individual trait reflective of the way people experience themselves in relationship to their environment. Field-dependent persons see themselves as less differentiated from their environment; they rely on external cues rather than internal cues to orient themselves in space. This trait is also associated with greater interpersonal dependency. Alcoholics continue to be field dependent with sobriety, although this trait diminishes gradually with prolonged abstinence (Witkin et al. 1959).

In one of the rare prospective studies that has looked at the development of alcoholism and other emotional disorders, Vaillant (1983) showed that problems in childhood predisposed to various adult personality difficulties, but not to alcoholism. In his sample of male college students, he noted that depression, anxiety, and other symptoms tended to appear after the individual lost control of his or her drinking and tended to improve if control of the drinking was reestablished. These studies have strongly supported Vaillant's hypothesis that alcoholism is the cause of psychiatric difficulties and not vice versa.

At present there is only one psychiatric condition that shows evidence that it might represent a specific predisposition to alcoholism. Goodwin et al. (1975) suggested that attention-deficit disorder in childhood is associated with the future development of alcoholism. Schuckit et al. (1987) could not establish this link in their study of males at high risk of becoming alcoholic. The question, however, is still open to further study.

Psychoanalytic Theories

Early analysts had little interest in alcoholism. The last two decades, however, have produced many papers and often conflicting theories on the psychodynamics of alcoholism (addiction). Although no analytic study to date has established a common alcoholic personality, there have been some areas of consensus, with a general agreement that 1) alcoholics have common deficits in personality structure; 2) similar problems are present in abusers of alcohol and all other drugs; and 3) the problems are preoedipal in nature.

Classical psychoanalytic theory. Freud (1985) saw alcoholism as symptomatic of unconscious instinctual conflicts, with drinking as a substitute for sexual gratification. Infantile masturbation was Freud's "model" addiction, compelling as a source of instinctual gratification and also guilt inducing. He emphasized the primitive pleasurable aspects of drinking and the reduction of unconscious sexual drives through indulgence in such hedonistic activities. Alcoholics were thought to have conflicts over repressed homosexual impulses, which were then expressed with less guilt during the drunken state. Abraham (1908) was the first to consolidate these theories into the notion of the "oral-dependent" personality. The theory was further advanced by Rado (1933), who used the term *pharmacothymia*. He shifted the focus from the pleasurable effect of the drug and saw this as a purely psychological disorder caused by a psychosexual fixation. Another famous element of this theory was the notion that the bottle was an unconscious symbolic representation of the mother's breast. It is of interest how this focus on forbidden sexual indulgence parallels the moral–sin model espoused by the Prohibitionists of the same era. Despite their theoretical interest in these problems, the early analysts actually did little clinical work with this population. Because of the presumed preoedipal nature of the pathology, traditional psychoanalysts felt that these patients were untreatable. Accordingly, they had little practical experience working with alcoholics.

In the late 1930s and the 1940s, psychoanalysis began to look in more detail at alcoholics and other patients with preoedipal structural problems. The work of Robert Knight (1937, 1938) at the Menninger Clinic produced a classic description of the passive-dependent (alcoholic) personality. He also described a family constellation of an overly indulgent, overaffectionate mother and an inconsistent, cold, and rejecting father that produced an oral, dependent alcoholic son, who constantly demands affection and feels enraged when rejected. Knight suggested that because of his passivity and immaturity, the alcoholic male feels inferior and doubts his masculinity. The drinking becomes a way both to satisfy his demands for oral gratification and to assert his masculinity. At the same time, he can act out his defiance against his parents and masochistically indulge in self-destructive behavior that reduces his feelings of guilt. Knight saw alcoholism as a psychogenic symptom, not as a disease entity. He felt there was an underlying personality disorder, although there was no one specific type of neurotic conflict. His work with alcoholic patients led directly to his initial description of the individual with borderline personality disorder.

As with many of these analytic retrospective constructs, Knight's etiologic model (1937) has been impossible to verify using more scientific prospective techniques. Without questioning the validity of the analyst's clinical observations, it has become apparent that these personality constructs are not unique to the alcoholic, nor do they predispose to future alcoholism. For example, oral-erotic breast symbolism has been found to be far more common in schizophrenic patients and in other diagnostic groups than in alcoholics (Pattison 1984).

Psychoanalytic structural theory.   Based on Knight's (1937) initial observations, Kernberg (1975) and Kohut (1971) saw alcoholism as an attempt to correct a structural self-object flaw in the personality. Kernberg suggested that the borderline patient used alcohol in a symbolic way as a "transitional object," to compensate for flaws generated by difficulties in the mother-child relationship. He postulated that a developmental fixation occurred between 15 and 36 months of age. Kohut used similar theoretical constructs to explain how an individual with a narcissistic personality disorder used alcohol not as a substitute for a loved object, but as a replacement for a defect in the psychological structure. The major problem with these formulations is that there are no scientific data that this type of character pathology is present in any significant number of alcoholics, either before or after the development of the illness.

Psychoanalytic ego psychology.   These theories were the first to be developed by contemporary analysts who had worked with alcoholics and addicts as a primary focus in their clinical practice. Khantzian (1982) and Mack (1981) proposed that there are deficits in basic ego operations necessary to maintain what they termed "self-care functions." They described problems with affect regulation, the maintenance of self-object stability, reality testing, and judgment. Krystal (1979) identified additional problems with anhedonia, alexithymia, and severe ambivalence.

Of most importance to this group is their contention that addiction is a regressive process, that a flawed ego regresses under the influence of alcohol from a higher level of original functioning. They do not suggest that there is any type of structural fixation. Khantzian (1974) stressed the notion that the addict often turns to a particular drug because of its ability to compensate for very specific defects in affect control. For example, a person feeling overwhelmed by rage might prefer opiates because of the specific sedative effects, especially the capacity to reduce aggressive drives. Amphetamines are preferred by some individuals because they give a stronger sense of self-esteem and power; this is clearly desirable for depressed persons or those who wish to feel more active and competent in the face of a hostile environment (Frosch and Milkman 1977). Despite the initial, often salutary effect of the drug, the long-term outcome of the addictive process is a fairly predictable deterioration in ego functions leading to a uniform pattern of character pathology.

This theory is consistent with the pattern of regression observed in longitudinal studies and the observation that sober alcoholics often regain higher levels of ego functioning. These observations also argue strongly against any uniform pattern of structural fixation. The major problem with this theoretical construct is that some alcoholics show no evidence of any regression and that the common pattern of psychodynamics is not found in all alcoholics. As noted before, empirical studies continue to show a wide variety of personality types among alcoholics.

Pharmacodynamic psychology. In an even more complete rejection of the notion that alcoholics have some type of preexisting character pathology, Bean (1981) and Vaillant (1981) argued that there is no common premorbid alcoholic personality or character. The common psychodynamic patterns often observed in alcoholics are the direct pharmacologic effect of the alcohol on previously normal ego functions, combined with ineffective neurotic responses to these deficits. Vaillant's longitudinal studies (1983) documented such patterns of ego regression following the development of addiction. However, this work does not account for the obvious premorbid structural deficits in some alcoholics, nor for the evidence that some alcoholics maintain a high level of functioning with little or no evidence of regression.

Sociological Theories

Sociological factors have long been thought to have a powerful influence in both the development and treatment of alcoholism. Although it is often impossible to unravel the complex interactions between the chemical effect of the alcohol, intrapsychic factors, group dynamics, and broader sociocultural influences, the obvious success of the Alcoholics Anonymous (AA) program suggests that therapists must pay more careful attention to the sociological forces that impact on the individual alcoholic. Cross-cultural studies have identified five sociological conditions that are present in societies that have low incidences of alcohol abuse and alcoholism:

1. Group drinking is usually associated with religious or ritualistic celebrations and is differentiated from drunkenness.
2. Drinking usually occurs in association with eating.
3. Drinking usually occurs during multigenerational, often family or community events, involving both men and women.
4. Alcohol is not seen as a medicinal drug, and drinking is not approved as a mechanism for the individual to use to cope with anxiety or personal problems.
5. Violence or overt sexual behavior while drinking is strongly disapproved, and behavioral controls are enforced by the group; there is no status associated with drunkenness, nor is it part of any male or female puberty rites.

Anthropologists have suggested that the industrial revolution caused major changes in the rituals associated with alcohol use and led to marked increases in alcoholism, particularly in more "advanced" cultures. Factory work often separated men from their families and separated drinking activities from religious or family-oriented activities. Controlled or moderate drinking changed to uncontrolled drinking often associated with violence and sexual acting out (Zinberg 1981).

Bales (1946) identified three factors that he felt determined a society's incidence of alcohol use: 1) the amount of inner stress and anxiety in the culture; 2) whether the society provides alternatives besides alcohol as a means of relieving these stresses; and 3) the society's continuing attitudes toward alcohol and drunkenness. Many sociologists have applied these observations to European and American subcultures and have frequently compared the Irish and the Jews because of their marked difference in the incidence of alcoholism. Jewish drinking practices reflect the five factors associated with a low incidence of alcoholism. Alcohol use most commonly occurs at ritual feasts with men and women of different generations in attendance.

Drunkenness and violence are discouraged. In contrast, Irish drinking often excludes women and encourages heavy consumption and drunkenness as a sign of masculinity (Bales 1962). The Irish culture is also seen as sexually repressive, with few other outlets for stress besides drinking. In one of the more fascinating cross-cultural studies, Jessor (1970) traced the evolution of drinking patterns among young Italian males, comparing groups in rural Italy with cousins who had moved to Rome or Boston. Since all three groups shared the same genetic roots, it could be assumed that differences in drinking behavior reflected changes in cultural variables. He found that the actual amount of alcohol consumed was equal in all three groups, but that there were more than three times as many episodes of drunkenness in the Boston group. In both groups in Italy, there was no association between drunkenness and personality factors such as alienation and frustration. The opposite was true in the Boston group. The Italian groups continued to use alcohol primarily for dietary needs, whereas the Italian-American men had adopted more American attitudes and practices, were drinking to excess, and were using alcohol to cope with feelings of alienation and frustration.

Biological Theories

Several converging lines of evidence support the general idea that a predisposition to alcoholism, or at least to subtypes of alcoholism, are genetically transmitted.

Twin studies. Twin studies assume that monozygotes have identical genetic makeup whereas dizygotic twins have similar but not identical genetic material. Any genetically determined trait, therefore, should be more common in monozygotic twin pairs than dizygotic twins (i.e., have a higher concordance rate in monozygotics). An early Swedish study examined 174 male twin pairs where one twin had been registered with a Swedish temperance board for drunken conduct and found a 54% concordance rate for alcoholism among monozygotic twins and a 28% rate for dizygotic twins (Kaij 1960). It also found that more severe alcoholics were more likely to have an alcoholic twin. In contrast, a Finnish study found no evidence for a genetic component to addictive symptoms, arrests for drunkenness, or other social complications but did find frequency and amount of drinking were more concordant among monozygotic twins, including concordance of abstinence (Partanen et al. 1966). A subsequent study of 1,500 twin pairs in Sweden again found monozygotic twins more concordant regarding the quantity of alcohol consumed, but that social and economic factors largely determined drinking consequences (Jonsson and Nilsson 1968). More recently, a Finnish study of 879 monozygotic and 1,940 dizygotic twins found a genetic influence in frequency (days drinking per month), quantity per month, density (drinking more than five beers, a bottle of wine, or half a bottle of distilled spirits at least once per month), but not in the frequency of alcohol-induced loss of consciousness (Kaprio et al. 1987). Another study examined 13,000 twin pairs and found excessive drinking higher in monozygotic than dyzygotic twins. The effect was more pronounced among women (Cederlof et al. 1977).

Thus the weight of the evidence from twin studies supports the concept that the quantity of alcohol consumed may have a genetic determinant, but that many other factors influence the consequences of drinking.

Adoption studies. An early study by Roe (1944) concluded that there was no apparent hereditary influence in the development of alcoholism. Roe studied 49 foster children: 27 with a biological parent who was heavy drinker and 22 control subjects without a parental history of alcoholism. Use of alcohol did not vary significantly between groups, nor did problems resulting from alcohol. Goodwin (1976) criticized this study, based on its small sample size, the large number of women (who at that time were at low risk for alcoholism), inadequate matching of probands with controls, and use of the criteria "heavy drinking" rather than alcoholism.

More recent adoption studies support a genetic component to alcoholism. Schuckit et al. (1972) studied 164 half-siblings of whom 32 were alcoholic; 62% of alcoholic siblings had an alcoholic biological parent compared with only 20% of nonalcoholic siblings who had an alcoholic biological parent. These data suggest that the presence of alcoholism in a biological parent (not the foster parent) determines vulnerability of the half-sibling to alcoholism.

The Danish adoption studies examined children of alcoholics raised by either their alcoholic biological parents or nonalcoholic foster parents (Goodwin 1979; Goodwin et al. 1973). Sons of alcoholics were approximately four times more likely to be alcoholic themselves, whether raised by their alcoholic parent or nonalcoholic foster parent, suggesting a genetic predisposition. With women, however, a higher rate of alcoholism was found in all adopted groups compared with nonadopted controls; 30% of daughters raised by alcoholics had received treatment for depression by age 32 compared to approximately 5% of controls. Thus for women adoption alone may increase the risk of alcoholism, while living with an alcoholic may predispose to depression.

Bohman (1978) studied 862 men and 913 women of known paternity who were adopted at an early age by nonrelatives (average age of separation, 4 months; average age of adoption, 8 months). Bohman et al. (1981) reported that in this cohort alcohol abuse was significantly greater in adopted-out sons of alcoholic biological fathers than adopted-out sons of nonalcoholic parents. Twice as many sons of alcoholic mothers were themselves alcoholic compared with sons of nonalcoholic parents. For daughters of alcoholic mothers, alcohol abuse was three times as common as for controls. Daughters of alcoholic fathers showed no increase in alcohol abuse over controls. If biological fathers were subdivided into fathers with mild abuse and no criminality versus more severe paternal alcoholism or criminality, the daughters of the former had a twofold increase in alcohol abuse over controls, whereas the latter showed no difference. Alcohol abuse in adoptive parents was not associated with greater risk for alcoholism; however, adoptive fathers with unskilled occupations provided a milieu associated with greater risk of alcohol abuse for both sons and daughters.

Based on the aforementioned study, Cloninger (1987) hypothesized the existence of two types of alcoholism. Type 1 typically has its onset after age 25 and is characterized by "loss of control" or binge drinking. It is associated with traits characteristic of individuals with passive-dependent or anxious personalities. These are defined as

> high reward-dependence (that is, one who is eager to help others, emotionally dependent, warmly sympathetic, sentimental, sensitive to social cues, and persistent), high harm avoidance (that is, one who is cautious, apprehensive, pessimistic, inhibited, shy, and susceptible to fatigue), and low novelty seeking (that is, one who is rigid, reflective, loyal, orderly, and attentive to details). (p. 411)

Both men and women may develop type 1 alcoholism, but hospital treatment samples of men are more likely to be type 2. Women who develop type 1 typically have a later onset, more rapid progression, and psychiatric and medical complications. Type 1 is characteristic of male relatives of alcoholic women. Type 2 alcoholism is characterized by persistent alcohol-seeking behaviors or an inability to abstain. Personality traits are those that are characteristic of antisocial personality disorder:

> high novelty seeking (that is, one who is impulsive, exploratory, excitable, disorderly, and distractable), low harm avoidance (that is, one who is confident, relaxed, optimistic, uninhibited, carefree and energetic), and low reward dependence (that is, one who is socially detached, emotionally cool, practical, tough-minded, and independently self-willed). (p. 411)

The type 2 syndrome was found in male relatives of alcoholic men and typically had its onset prior to age 25 and was characterized by arrests for driving while intoxicated and auto accidents, fighting when drunk, and multiple hospital treatments for alcoholism.

These two types of alcoholism are viewed by Cloninger (1987, p. 411) as "polar extremes of personality traits that vary continously" and should not be viewed as discrete disease entities because alcoholics typically share features of each. Furthermore, the applicability of the model to alcoholics in the United States remains unknown.

Genetic components of ethanol pharmacokinetics. Goldstein (1983) provided a discussion of the genetic components of ethanol pharamacokinetics. Very strong evidence exists that ethanol metabolism is genetically determined. One study of 14 twin pairs found that ethanol elimination rates had a "heritability value" of 0.98; that is, the rates were almost completely genetic in origin (Vesell et al. 1971). Another study of 14 twin pairs in Finland found a value of 0.80 for ethanol elimination and 0.60–0.80 for the acetaldehyde content of venous blood (Forsander and Eriksson 1974). Another study of 40 twin pairs found a value of 0.46 (Kopun and Propping 1977).

Studies of ethnic differences in elimination rate are contradictory. One study found that American Indians and Eskimos metabolize ethanol more slowly than Caucasians, perhaps explaining higher incidences of alcoholism in these populations (Fenna et al. 1971). Another study, however, found opposite results (Reed et al. 1976). Definite evidence does exist, however, that some Asians (Japanese, Taiwanese, and Koreans) experience a distinctive adverse reaction to ethanol, which includes flushing and nausea. The flushing reaction begins within minutes of ingesting alcohol, peaks at about 30 minutes, and subsides by 60–90 minutes (Wolff 1972). Between 47% and 85% of Asians experience flushing, compared with 3% to 29% of Occidentals (Chan 1986; Ewing et al. 1974; N Miller et al. 1988; Seto et al. 1978). In one study of 78 Asians given an ethanol challenge (one beer for the Asians, two for the Caucasians), 83% of the Asians flushed, whereas only 6% of the Caucasian controls did (Wolff 1972). Asian infants flush when exposed to ethanol, ruling out environmental factors. Since American Indians also flush when exposed to ethanol (Wolff 1973), and the rate of alcoholism in American Indians is much higher than for Asians, the flushing reaction may not entirely explain low alcoholism rates among Asian populations.

Early studies indicated that 85% of Asians had a variant of alcohol dehydrogenase (known as "atypical"), which is very active at physiologic levels of pH (Stamatoyanopoulos et al. 1975) and could be responsible for the flush reaction. Shortly after ingestion of ethanol, liver alcohol dehydrogenase may be the rate-limiting step of ethanol metabolism because there is an overabundance of nicotinamide adenine dinucleotide (NAD). The "atypical" form of alcohol dehydrogenase found in Asians may then produce a rush of acetaldehyde, explaining the flushing reaction (Goldstein 1983).

It has been found, however, that the mitochondrial, low K_m form of aldehyde dehydrogenase that is responsible for the oxidation of acetaldehyde is inactive in flushers, which impairs acetaldehyde metabolism, leading to higher levels (Agarwal et al. 1981). Absence of this enzyme occurs in 42% of Japanese nonalcoholics, but in only 2% of Japanese alcoholics, suggesting that the flush reaction may indeed protect against alcoholism (Harada et al. 1985).

A combination of histamine receptor antagonists, diphenhydramine (an H_1 antagonist) and cimetidine (an H_2 antagonist), blocked the flushing response and the hypotensive response to ethanol in Asians (N Miller et al. 1988). Skin temperature and pulse changes were not affected by drug treatment. Although one study attributed the diminished flush response to lowered BALs (Sheppard et al. 1970), a larger study found that antihistamines had no effect on BALs (N Miller et al. 1988). The more likely mechanism is the blocked action of histamine in the central nervous system and/or peripheral vasculature. Aspirin may also block the flush reaction (N Miller et al. 1988), perhaps by decreasing prostaglandin-induced histamine release.

Animal studies.   Goldstein (1983) reviewed the biological theories of alcoholism based on animal studies. Rates of voluntary ethanol consumption differ greatly between inbred strains of mice, suggesting a genetic component to ethanol preference in animals. Those favoring ethanol have higher aldehyde dehydrogenase activity than nondrinking strains and correspondingly lower blood acetaldehyde levels during ethanol intoxication (Eriksson 1973), suggesting high levels of acetaldehyde produce ethanol aversion. Studies on inbred rat strains show those favoring ethanol are less sensitive to acute effects of intoxication (Riley et al. 1976). Mice who are sensitive to the effects of alcohol or other hypnotics may have altered functioning of the gamma-aminobutyric acid (GABA) system, and in vivo receptor binding has indicated increased benzodiazepine receptor number, but not increased affinity in cortex and hippocampus (L Miller et al. 1988). Studies have also shown interspecies differences in alcohol preference (e.g., hamsters favor ethanol over water, and guinea pigs avoid it) (Arvola and Forsander 1961).

High-risk studies.   With much evidence suggesting a genetic influence in the development of alcoholism, several investigations have attempted to identify those factors that may predispose children or young adults to alcoholism. While the so-called high-risk research strategy varies among centers, it usually involves studying various biological and psychological characteristics in sons and daughters of alcoholics and comparing them with children of nonalcoholics. A number of interesting findings resulting from these studies are outlined in Table 1-3.

Genetic markers.   Attempts have been made to link occurrence of alcoholism with occurrence of a physical trait known to be genetically determined (a genetic marker). An association might support genetic transmission of alcoholism. Goodwin (1985) discussed the work done in this area.

Three studies found that alcoholics of blood group A do not secrete ABH substances in their saliva (Swinson and Madden 1973). There is also less strong evidence that alcoholics are predominantly from blood group A (Swinson 1983). Genes for the MNS blood group and esterase-D may be located close to those genes that determine alcoholism (Hill et al. 1988; Tanna et al. 1988). One study found that the A1 allele of the dopamine D_2 receptor gene was common in alco-

Table 1-3. Markers in high-risk studies

Markers	References
Reaction to ethanol	
1. SOA have less intense subjective feelings than controls despite similar blood alcohol concentration.	Schuckit (1984a, 1984b, 1985)
2. SOA have less body sway after ethanol challenge (static ataxia) than controls.	Schuckit (1985)
3. SOA have lower cortisol ACTH and prolactin levels after ethanol challenge compared to controls.	Schuckit et al. (1988)
Psychological factors	
1. Higher scores on MMPI hysteria, hypochondriasis, depression, and lie scales than controls. High novelty seeking and low harm avoidance were strongly predictive of early alcohol abuse.	Tarter et al. (1985b) Cloninger et al. (1988)
2. No increase in hyperactivity over controls in some studies; impulsivity noted in others.	Knop (1985)
3. Many studies show no neuropsychological test differences, although one study of high-risk pregnancies showed lower vocabulary scores on Wechsler Adult Intelligence Scale (Wechsler 1981) and more errors on Porteus (1933) maze and Halstead-Reitan (Reitan 1979) categories in SOA compared with controls. Childhood behavior indicated they were more explosive and had lower verbal proficiency. More SOA subjects had to repeat a grade, take special classes, or see a psychologist than controls. Another study showed lower scores on reading comprehension, auditory attention span for words and objects, various memory tests, trail-making tests A and B, and the Halstead-Reitan aphasia subtest.	Drejer et al. (1985) Knop et al. (1984) Tarter et al (1985a) M Hesselbrock et al. (1985)

(continued)

Table 1-3. Markers in high-risk studies —*continued*

Markers	References
Electroencephalographic	
1. SOA have excess high frequency activity. After ethanol they showed greater increases in slow alpha energy than controls, suggesting a borderline abnormal electroencephalogram, normalized by ethanol.	Gabrielli et al. (1982) Pollock et al. (1983)
2. Ethanol-induced reduction of P300 was greater in subjects with a family history positive for alcoholism than for family-history-negative subjects. P300 waves are larger in normal controls compared to SOA aged 7–13 years. At baseline and after ethanol challenge, P300 latency was similar for family-history-positive subjects and family-history-negative subjects, but the former group returned to baseline more quickly after challenge, suggesting P300 amplitude and, to a lesser extent, latency were affected by alcohol more for family-history-positive subjects than family-history-negative subjects, but only when task used was difficult. Some studies have found no differences.	Elmasian et al. (1982) Volavka et al. (1985) Begleiter et al. (1984)
Platelet MAO activity	
The activity of MAO may be lower in alcoholics and first-degree relatives. MAO-B is lower in alcoholics during withdrawal but normalizes by 5 weeks.	Sullivan et al. (1979) Giller and Hall (1983) Giller et al. (1984)
Thyrotropin response to protirelin	
SOA had higher basal thyrotropin levels and, after protirelin challenge, had higher peak thyrotropin levels and thyrotropin areas under the curve than did control boys. Daughters of alcoholics showed no differences from controls.	Moss et al. (1987)

Note. SOA = sons of alcoholics. ACTH = adrenocorticotropic hormone. MMPI = Minnesota Multiphasic Personality Inventory. MAO = monoamine oxidase.

holics, but not in nonalcoholics (Blum et al. 1990), and the investigators suggested a gene that is located on the q22-q23 region of chromosome 11 may lead to susceptibility to at least one form of alcoholism. Another study, however, was unable to replicate that finding (Bolos et al. 1990).

Capacity to taste phenylthiocarbamide, an autosomal dominant trait, may be higher in alcoholics, although the results are conflicting (Peeples 1985; Swinson 1983). Color blindness among alcoholics is well documented; however, the condition seems to be caused by nutritional deficits or by direct toxic effects of ethanol (Cruz-Coke 1964). Two studies found that female relatives of alcoholics have higher rates of color blindness, suggesting transmission by a recessive sex-linked gene (Cruz-Coke and Varela 1966; Varela et al. 1969). However, a study of sons of sons of alcoholics and sons of daughters of alcoholics found no difference between the groups, making a sex-linked recessive gene unlikely (Kaij and Dock 1975). This study did find that 43% of the grandsons of alcoholics were having drinking problems, suggesting that a dominant gene exists.

THE PHARMACOLOGY OF ETHANOL

Much of this discussion of the pharmacology of ethanol is based on works by Goldstein (1983, 1989).

Absorption and Distribution

Ethanol is absorbed from both the stomach and duodenum. When food is consumed with alcohol, it dilutes the ethanol concentration in the stomach and delays passage into the duodenum, slowing absorption and decreasing subjective effects. Food delays and lowers peak blood ethanol concentration but also lowers total amount of ethanol reaching the systemic circulation. Ethanol absorption is fastest when the stomach empties quickly, as in the fasting state, but high concentration alcoholic beverages such as distilled spirits may cause pylorospasm and delay emptying.

Ethanol distributes rapidly, with concentrations in the body water 10 times higher than in body fat. Those tissues with the greatest blood supply equilibrate most rapidly with arterial blood circulation. Shortly after ingestion, brain ethanol concentration is higher than venous concentration.

Approximately 5–10% of ethanol is excreted unchanged in the breath and urine. The blood-to-breath ratio of ethanol is 2,100 to 1, an important relationship that permits blood alcohol determination from expired air (see Table 1-4).

Metabolism

There are three different enzyme systems capable of oxidizing ethanol: liver alcohol dehydrogenase, catalase, and the microsomal ethanol-oxidizing system. Gastric alcohol dehydrogenase also metabolizes ethanol, and lower levels of this enzyme in women may account for higher blood ethanol concentrations in women than in men given equivalent amounts of alcohol (Frezza et al. 1990). By far the most important enzyme is liver alcohol dehydrogenase (LAD), which requires NAD as a coenzyme. The major rate-limiting step of ethanol oxidation by LAD is the concentration of the coenzyme NAD. Because ethanol is consumed in such high doses, metabolism requires that the liver must continuously regenerate NAD from NADH (the reduced form of NAD). This, in turn, relies on a number of NAD-dependent dehydrogenases and their substrates. Fasting impedes ethanol elimination, perhaps by reducing the dietary supply of these substrates or by decreasing the amount of LAD in the liver. This explains, in part, why drinking while dieting may increase the duration of intoxication. Metabolism is also limited by substrate inhibition.

As a result of ethanol oxidation, the lactate-pyruvate ratio increases, which may explain why alcoholics who originally drank to relieve anxiety experience an increase in panic attacks with chronic drinking.

Table 1-4.   Ethanol elimination facts

- For a 70-kg man, the mean rate of metabolism is 8 g or 10 ml of absolute ethanol per hour. A "drink" usually contains 15–20 ml alcohol.
- A cocktail with 2 ounces of 86 proof bourbon contains 26 g of ethanol.
- There are approximately equal amounts of ethanol in
     12-ounce can of beer (4.5% ethanol by volume)
     4-ounce glass of wine (12%)
     1.2 ounces of whiskey (45%)
- Metabolism of various drinks by normal drinkers (g/hour)
     pure alcohol   7
     whiskey   8
     dessert wines   9
     table wine   12
     beer   9–11

LAD exists in different forms. Current terminology identifies three classes (I–III) of isoenzymes with several different subtypes. Different molecular forms vary considerably in their kinetic properties, which may partially explain why there are large interindividual differences in the rate of ethanol metabolism. LAD also has clinical relevance because some agents being studied as agents to sober up patients act on this system. Fructose, for example, can regenerate NAD during its reduction to sorbitol or by its metabolism to glyceraldehyde, which is a substrate for alcohol dehydrogenase.

LAD also has clinical significance in the metabolism of methanol and ethylene glycol, two drugs with toxic metabolites. Methanol is oxidized by LAD to formaldehyde, which damages the retina and can cause blindness. Ethylene glycol is metabolized by LAD to oxalic acid, which has renal toxicity. The toxic effects of both methanol and ethylene glycol can be reduced by ethanol administration, which inhibits their metabolism by competing for the oxidizing enzymes and allows elimination of the intact parent compounds.

Catalase is a liver enzyme that uses hydrogen peroxide to oxidize other substances. In vivo, the catalase system does not play a significant role in ethanol metabolism, probably because the quantities of hydrogen peroxide available are insufficient for ethanol metabolism. Despite the fact that catalase inhibition does not impair ethanol metabolism, ascorbic acid (vitamin C) pretreatment (5 g/day for 2 weeks) enhances blood ethanol clearance, presumably through its ability to supply peroxide for the catalase system; yet the ability of vitamin C to reduce ethanol-induced motor impairment is not a pharmacokinetic effect, but probably represents a receptor site action.

The microsomal ethanol oxidizing system is another mechanism of ethanol metabolism. It is similar to the mixed function oxidase system that metabolizes drugs and other toxins. It is probably not identical to it, because it is not inhibited by SKF 525A, whereas the other system is. The microsomal ethanol oxidizing system may be important at high blood ethanol concentrations and after chronic ethanol consumption.

Acetaldehyde

Acetaldehyde is the first metabolic product of ethanol. Several hepatic enzymes, aldehyde oxidases, and dehydrogenases metabolize acetaldehyde to acetate. The most important enzyme is a low-K_m mitochondrial aldehyde dehydrogenase. If ethanol is being metabolized at the same time, acetate cannot be further metabolized by the liver due to the abnormal redox balance. In this case, acetate is metabolized by other tissues such as skeletal muscle, where it is converted to carbon dioxide.

The role of acetaldehyde in inducing intoxication or being responsible for reinforcing effects is controversial. On the one hand, behavioral signs of intoxication parallel ethanol blood levels but not acetaldehyde levels, especially during the ascending limb of the ethanol concentration versus time curve. Acetaldehyde levels remain high even during the period when signs of intoxication are diminishing. Furthermore, pyrazole, which inhibits alcohol dehydrogenase, does not block or diminish intoxication, which one would predict if acetaldehyde were responsible for intoxication. On the other hand, evidence has shown that acetaldehyde may be reinforcing in animals, suggesting that central and peripheral acetaldehyde may have different effects (Smith et al. 1985).

In addition to a direct effect, acetaldehyde may form condensation products called tetrahydroisoquinolines (TIQs). Tetrahydropapaveroline (THP) is the condensation product of imipramine and its own aldehyde, 3,4-dihydroxyphenylacetaldehyde (DHPA), which is formed from dopamine by MAO. In an in vitro brain homogenate model, addition of ethanol or acetaldehyde increases the formation of THP from dopamine and 3,4-DHPA. THP has drawn interest because it occurs in the opium poppy, and some authorities have suggested that there may be a common mechanism underlying alcohol and opiate dependence, although this remains highly speculative.

Acetaldehyde can nonenzymatically condense with catecholamine to form TIQs and with indoleamines to form beta-carbolines. Salsolinol is the condensation product of dopamine and acetaldehyde. Salsolinol has been detected in brain tissue of animals after ethanol was administered with a drug that inhibits TIQ metabolism, and it has also been found in the urine of alcoholics on hospital admission. An interesting study reported that salsolinol and THP, when infused in the cerebral ventricles of rats, increases ethanol consumption (Meyers and Melchior 1977). Some studies have been unable to replicate these findings.

Alcohol and Biomembranes

One theory of alcohol's biological effect is based on the drug's effect on biomembranes. Ethanol makes membranes more fluid, perhaps by increasing the amount of lipid that is in a fluid rather than a gel state. This, in turn, may affect the function of membrane proteins. These changes may be a mechanism for intoxication. Chronic ethanol administration may lead to membrane adaption (tolerance), the mechanism of which may be enhanced membrane rigidity through an increase in the cholesterol content.

Neurotransmitter and Neuroreceptor Effects

Ethanol has effects on several different neurotransmitter and neuroreceptor systems (Bannister and Losowsky 1986; Goldstein 1983; Hoffman and Tabakoff 1985).

Adrenergic systems. Chronic ethanol increases the rate of synthesis of norepinephrine and increases its release. This results in postsynaptic receptor subsensitivity as evidenced by both a decrease in cyclic adenosine monophosphate (AMP) response to norepinephrine and decreased binding. During ethanol withdrawal, there appears to be continuously increased synthesis of norepinephrine, with release normalizing as receptors move from a subsensitive to supersensitive state. In humans, cerebrospinal fluid (CSF) norepinephrine and 3-methoxy-4-hydroxyphenylglycol (MHPG) are elevated in withdrawing alcoholics and return to normal range over several days. It has been suggested that the alpha$_2$-receptors in the locus coeruleus (which inhibit sympathetic outflow and decrease blood pressure) are damaged by chronic alcohol. Chronic ethanol reduces beta-receptors in rat heart and whole mouse or rat brain (Banerjee et al. 1978). Beta-receptor changes are primarily at beta$_2$-receptors (Rabin et al. 1980).

GABA. Increases, decreases, and no changes in GABA have been found after acute ethanol administration. A consistent finding is reduced brain GABA after chronic alcohol. Plasma GABA levels are lower in abstinent alcoholics compared to nonalcoholics (Coffman and Petty 1985) and CSF GABA appears to be lower in alcoholics who have seizures during withdrawal compared to those who do not (Goldman et al. 1981). GABA agonists decrease symptoms of ethanol withdrawal, whereas GABA antagonists produce pharmacodynamic effects resembling an ethanol abstinence syndrome. Ethanol potentiates GABA inhibition in animal models.

Ethanol, barbiturates, and benzodiazepines stimulate GABA receptor-mediated chloride uptake in brain vesicles of experimental animals, a mechanism that may be responsible for some aspects of intoxication. The GABA-A receptor complex has four sites: 1) a benzodiazepine-sensitive site; 2) a GABA-sensitive site; 3) a picrotoxin site, which is proconvulsant by blocking the receptor and the inhibitory action of GABA; and 4) a barbiturate-sensitive site. Chronic ethanol reduces both the number and the affinity of central type benzodiazepine-GABA receptor sites. A benzodiazepine partial inverse agonist, RO15-4513, has been shown to antagonize some of the effects of ethanol, but its proconvulsant and anxiogenic properties limit its clinical potential (Lister and Nutt 1988). Furthermore, the fact that certain effects of ethanol (e.g., hypothermia, motor stimulation, and social and aggressive behavior) are not blocked implies that not all of ethanol's effects are mediated by the benzodiazepine-GABA receptor.

Opiate systems.   Several areas of investigation have linked ethanol and opioids. Similarities between the two have been noted with respect to acute effects, tolerance, and antagonism by naltrexone.

Cross-tolerance between ethanol and morphine has been found in analgesic and hypothermic effects (Kalant 1985). Although initial reports suggested that naloxone reversed coma induced by ethanol, later studies were unable to replicate this finding (Kalant 1985). It may, however, block some behavioral effects, subcortical seizure activity, and hypothermia induced by ethanol (Boggan et al. 1979; Brick and Horowitz 1983; McCarty and Ewing 1983; Shippenberg and Altshuler 1985; Sinclair et al. 1982; Triana et al. 1980). Both morphine and naloxone reduce ethanol preference in rodents (Altshuler and Shippenberg 1982; Altshuler et al. 1980; Myers and Critcher 1982; Sinclair et al. 1982). Furthermore, administration of nalorphine, an antagonist, to alcoholics can produce symptoms of withdrawal (Markley and Mezey 1978).

Studies of the effects of ethanol on opiate receptors have produced contradictory findings. In general, acute ethanol decreases binding of enkephalins to delta-receptors, while it increases beta-endorphin levels and binding to mu-receptors. Chronic ethanol decreases beta-endorphin levels and binding to the mu-receptor (although some studies have found an increase in the number of mu-receptors) and an increase in binding to the delta-receptor (Bannister and Losowsky 1986; Kalant 1985).

Serotonin.   Ethanol shifts serotonin (5-hydroxytryptamine [5-

HT] metabolism from production of 5-hydroxyindoleacetic acid (5-HIAA) to 5-hydroxyindoleacetaldehyde and 5-hydroxytryptophol, which may enhance the actions of ethanol. Although some evidence suggests chronic ethanol depletes serotonin, other studies show no change or increase in brain levels.

More consistent, however, are the data that alterations in the serotonergic system affect ethanol consumption in animals and in humans. In animals, increases in central serotonergic function decrease ethanol consumption. Selective serotonergic uptake inhibitors, such as citalopram, fluoxetine, quipazine, and zimelidine, decrease ethanol preference in animals. Fenfluramine, which causes release of serotonin into the synaptic cleft, and 5-hydroxytryptophan (5-HTP), the immediate precursor of serotonin, have similar effects.

Conversely, serotonin depletion by parachlorophenylalanine, which inhibits tryptophan hydroxylase, or by the selective neurotoxin 5,6-dihydroxytryptamine results in an increase in ethanol consumption.

Antidepressants that do not specifically affect serotonin, such as amitriptyline, doxepin, and despiramine, do not alter ethanol intake in animal models.

In human studies, zimelidine treatment decreased the amount of alcohol consumed and increased the number of days abstinent in men who were heavy drinkers (Naranjo 1985). This effect was independent of antidepressant activity. Zimelidine is no longer marketed, however, because of an unacceptably high risk (1 in 7,000) of Guillain-Barré syndrome.

With the subsequent release of fluoxetine, this drug is in wide clinical use in alcoholics and problem drinkers. In our hands, fluoxetine has been useful in reducing craving for alcohol, promoting abstinence, and reducing quantity of ethanol consumed. While early clinical experience is very encouraging, we are currently awaiting the results of several controlled clinical trials. Some alcoholics have experienced concomitant reductions in cravings for cigarettes, cocaine, and food while taking fluoxetine. At the time of this writing, other serotonergic agents that may decrease alcohol consumption in humans (e.g., citalopram) are not available for clinical use in the United States.

Dopamine. Conflicting data are reported for the effects of ethanol on the dopamine system. Dopamine turnover may be affected by both acute and chronic ethanol, but no changes were found in total brain dopamine content in one study (Hunt and Majchronwicz 1974). In animal models, acute ethanol in low doses (less than 2 g/kg) inhibits activity within the dopamine system, whereas higher doses stimulate activity. These effects may differ, depending on the species and brain region studied. During chronic exposure, there appears to be tolerance to the effects of ethanol on dopamine metabolism. An interesting human study found that apomorphine increased some measures of intoxication in male moderate drinkers, suggesting that dopamine may play a role in the intoxicating effects of ethanol (Alkana et al. 1982). No consistent changes in CSF homovanillic acid, a dopamine metabolite, were found in alcoholics given ethanol (Major et al. 1977; Orenberg et al. 1976a). Ethanol did not affect labeled haloperidol or spiroperidol binding (Hunt et al. 1979). Although some studies have shown an increase in sensitivity to dopamine in rats chronically administered ethanol (Engel and Liljequist 1976; Liljequist 1978), others have reported a reduction in dopamine-stimulated adenylate cyclase activity (Hoffman and Tabakoff 1977; Tabakoff and Hoffman 1979).

Acetylcholine.   Acute ethanol decreases cholinergic activity, whereas chronic exposure produces changes consistent with behavioral tolerance (Hunt et al. 1979; Tabakoff et al. 1979). There is increased sensitivity to electrical stimulation or potassium-induced depolarization and decreased sensitivity to inhibition by ethanol (Hoffman and Tabakoff 1985). There was no change in quinuclidinyl benzilate binding to muscarinic receptors in striatal tissue from mice withdrawn from chronic ethanol (Hunt et al. 1979; Tabakoff et al. 1979), but quinuclidinyl benzilate binding in the cortex and hippocampus was increased. In humans, older alcoholics may have lower numbers of muscarinic receptors in the hippocampus than controls (Nordberg et al. 1983). Decreased muscarinic receptor density but not affinity in the frontal cortex of alcoholics has been reported (Freund and Ballinger 1988). Acute ethanol did not affect [^{3}H] nicotine binding in rats, but exposure for 5 months was associated with an increase in the number of nicotinic binding sites in the hypothalamus and thalamus and a decrease in the hippocampus (Yoshida et al. 1982).

Glutamate.   In rats, acute ethanol decreased cortical and cerebellar glutamate levels, whereas with chronic exposure they were increased in the cortex, hippocampus, and substantia nigra (Sytinsky et al. 1975). At ethanol concentrations of less than 50 mM, binding of glutamate was enhanced, whereas higher concentrations decreased binding (Michaelis et al. 1978). Because glutamate is an excitatory neurotransmitter, some have suggested the change in the glutamate system is an adaption to the depressant effects of ethanol (Michaelis et al. 1983).

Calcium. Calcium plays a critical role in neurotransmitter function and may play a role in the hypnotic effects of ethanol (Yamamoto and Harris 1983). Low concentrations of ethanol increase calcium uptake or binding in mouse brain preparations (Harris 1979). In animals chronically exposed to ethanol, this effect is reduced. In contrast to an early report (Towle and Sze 1981), neither calmodulin levels nor its relative distribution as either membrane bound or cytosolic appears to be affected by ethanol (Luthin and Tabakoff 1984). As with neurotransmitters, there may be regional differences within the brain with respect to ethanol-induced calcium alterations.

Receptor-effector coupling. More recently, postsynaptic effects of ethanol have been studied (Tabakoff and Hoffman 1987). Species and brain regions differ in alterations of cyclic nucleotides in response to ethanol. Cyclic AMP levels in the cortex and cerebellum fall after acute exposure to ethanol in animals, whereas after chronic exposure in animals increased cyclic AMP levels are found (Shen et al. 1977). In humans, when alcoholics were administered 3g/kg of ethanol, CSF levels of cyclic AMP decreased (Orenberg et al. 1976b); in alcoholics with delirium tremens, CSF cyclic AMP was reduced (Zimmer et al. 1982). Both acute and chronic ethanol exposure decrease cyclic guanosine monophosphate in brains of animals (Church and Feller 1979; Dodson and Johnson 1979; Ferko et al. 1982; Hunt et al. 1977; Volicer and Hurter 1977), but CSF cyclic guanosine monophosphate is increased during delirium tremens (Zimmer et al. 1982). Adenylate cyclase activity in cortex, cerebellum, and striatum is increased by ethanol (Hoffman and Tabakoff 1982; Hruska and Silbergeld 1980; Israel et al. 1982; Rabin and Molinoff 1981; von Hungen and Baxter 1982). The mechanism by which ethanol increases adenylate cyclase activity may be through enhancement of the interaction between the G/F protein (a guanine nucleotide binding protein) and the catalytic unit of adenylate cyclase (Hoffman and Tabakoff 1985). Ethanol may also influence the interaction of the G/F protein and the receptor and may directly affect the catalytic unit of adenylate cyclase.

ALCOHOL WITHDRAWAL SYNDROME

Abrupt termination of chronic drinking may result in a withdrawal syndrome, which appears hours after the last drink and lasts 5–7 days (Greenblatt and Shader 1975) (Table 1-5).

Initially, the patient experiences anxiety, tremulousness, sleep disturbance, and mild gastrointestinal upset. The condition may worsen, producing irritability and agitation, sweating, fever, tachycardia, elevated blood pressure, nausea, and vomiting. If it progresses, the patient may become confused, disoriented, and delusional and may experience vivid hallucinations. This constellation of severe symptoms is commonly referred to as delirium tremens. Seizures, temperatures over 104° F (40° C), malnutrition, and fluid and electrolyte disturbances increase the risk of developing delirium tremens. Due to improved medical care, the mortality rate for delirium tremens has dropped over the last 20 years from 20% to 1%.

Grand mal seizures, commonly referred to as "rum fits," are also possible. These most often occur 7–48 hours into abstinence, although some believe the danger peaks 31–48 hours into abstinence (Sellers and Kalant 1975). Any seizures occurring after 48 hours are probably caused by other dependencies, cranial injury, or metabolic disturbances.

Criteria for Hospitalization of Alcoholics for Detoxification

Detoxification from alcohol may be done in an outpatient setting, a nonmedical residential facility, or a medical or psychiatric hospital ward.

Hospital admission for detoxification is indicated:

1. When severe withdrawal symptoms are present. These include severe tremulousness, hallucinosis, confusion, clouding of sensorium, fever, or seizures. In the presence of *any* of these symptoms, we recommend inpatient detoxification.
2. When there are serious medical sequelae of alcoholism that require evaluation and/or treatment. These include but are not limited to, dehydration, malnutrition, gastrointestinal bleeding, pan-

Table 1-5. Symptoms of alcohol withdrawal syndrome

Time abstinent (hours)	Symptom	Duration/progression
6–24	Nervousness Irritability Agitation Anorexia Tremors Conjunctival infection Elevated blood pressure Prone to startle Sweating Flushed face Tachycardia Hyperreflexia Fever Insomnia/sleep disturbance Nausea leading to vomiting Mild disorientation Nystagmus Illusions Hallucinations (visual and mixed visual-auditory)	48–72 hours' duration May progress to more severe symptoms 5% progress to delirium tremens

(continued)

Table 1-5. Symptoms of alcohol withdrawal syndrome—*continued*

Time abstinent (hours)	Symptom	Duration/progression
7–48	Grand mal seizures (2–6, "rum fits") Distractible Suggestible	Peaks 36 hours after onset, 30% develop delirium tremens
73–96	Delirium tremens: Confusion Disorientation Delusions Vivid hallucinations Agitation Tremors Insomnia Fever Sweating Tachycardia Mydriasis	24–72 hours duration, 1% mortality

creatitis, severe liver disease, respiratory infection or failure, clouded sensorium, loss of consciousness, serious head trauma, Korsakoff's syndrome, or other serious medical consequences.

3. When there is any medical illness that, by itself, would require inpatient treatment.
4. When there is any acute medical illness that would complicate detoxification (e.g., poorly controlled diabetes mellitus, or preexisting seizure disorder).
5. When there is any acute psychiatric illness that would complicate detoxification.
6. When there is polysubstance abuse that requires detoxification from other drugs in addition to alcohol.
7. When the patient has been unable to detoxify as an outpatient.

Some authorities recommend that BAL be used in conjunction with clinical symptoms to guide the clinical decision to hospitalize for detoxification (Feldman et al. 1975). Under this protocol, patients with a BAL over 0.10 are medically observed and monitored with sequential BALs until it drops below 0.10. A patient with minimal withdrawal symptoms and a BAL between 0 and 0.10 is not considered to be in medical danger and is suitable for entry into a rehabilitation program. For patients with severe withdrawal symptoms, regardless of BAL, hospitalization is indicated. We would caution against relying on the BAL in alcoholics who are using sedative-hypnotics or antianxiety agents, because these drugs may alter the time course and severity of the alcohol abstinence syndrome.

Nursing Care

Basic to the inpatient treatment of the alcohol withdrawal syndrome is appropriate nursing care. Patients are admitted to quiet, private rooms, and sensory stimuli are reduced. Interpersonal contacts during the withdrawal are limited to nurses, physicians, and counselors trained to use techniques such as reassurance and reality orientation to reduce anxiety. Initially, visitors are not allowed. Several programs successfully use these techniques to treat mild withdrawal without medication in nonmedical residential settings (Whitfield et al. 1978). This approach is indicated only in cases of mild dependence, when there is no history of withdrawal complications or medical or psychiatric illness.

Nutritional Treatment

Alcoholism may lead to chronic nutritional and vitamin deficiencies resulting in Wernicke's encephalopathy, Korsakoff's syndrome (alcohol amnestic disorder), megaloblastic anemia, peripheral neuropathy, and prolonged prothrombin time, all of which require evaluation and treatment during the hospital stay (Table 1-6).

Pharmacologic Treatment

Although appropriate nursing care can be effective treatment of mild withdrawal, pharmacologic therapy is indicated in moderate to severe cases. Most of the discussion that follows is based on work by Jaffe and Ciraulo (1985) and Ciraulo and Ciraulo (1988).

The sedative, muscle relaxing, anxiolytic, and anticonvulsant effects of benzodiazepines make them the agents of choice treating the symptoms of alcohol withdrawal. The clinical protocols used on our service are presented in Table 1-7.

The pharmacokinetics of individual drugs necessitate careful planning of a patient's drug therapy. The long-acting benzodiazepines are diazepam, chlordiazepoxide, clorazepate, halazepam (Paxipam), and prazepam (Centrax). They are converted to the active metabolite desmethyldiazepam. The elimination half-life of desmethyldiazepam is 50–100 hours. Diazepam, chlordiazepoxide, halazepam, and prazepam are converted to desmethyldiazepam by demethylation in the liver. Clorazepate is a prodrug hydrolyzed to desmethyldiazepam in the stomach.

These drugs share the advantage of being self-tapering under the effects of cumulative active metabolites. With the notable exception of diazepam, the parent compounds do not produce euphoric responses and present lower liability for abuse than most barbiturates.

Their disadvantages include drug and metabolite accumulation in the elderly or in patients with cirrhosis. In these cases, confusion, sedation, or ataxia may occur.

A further difficulty lies in the route of administration. Diazepam and chlordiazepoxide absorption is erratic when the drugs are injected intramuscularly in the gluteal area. Oral or intravenous administration is the preferred method, although diazepam is reliably absorbed from intramuscular injection in the deltoid.

Short-acting benzodiazepines are also effective. Lorazepam is preferred because a parenteral formulation exists for rapid and reli-

Table 1-6. Nutritional supplementation in alcoholics

Symptoms of deficiency state	Etiology	Treatment	Comments
Wernicke's encephalopathy, Korsakoff's Syndrome (alcohol amnestic syndrome)	Thiamine deficiency	Thiamine 50–100 mg im or iv daily for 3 days (often with oral multivitamins)	
Megaloblastic anemia or peripheral neuropathy	Folate deficiency	1–5 mg folic acid po or im	
Lethargy, arrhythmias, decreased seizure threshold, weakness	Magnesium depletion	Magnesium sulfate 1–2 g iv as a 50% solution every 6 hours or 0.5–2 mEq magnesium per kg body weight over 24 hours	Anticonvulsant dose is 1–5 im as 25–50% solution up to 6 times per day iv. Dose is 1–4 g as a 10–20% solution administered at a rate not to exceed 1.5 mL of a 10% solution per minute. Does not appear to be effective prophylactic agent against alcohol withdrawal seizures. May cause respiratory depression, decreased cardiac conduction, and cardiac arrest. Calcium gluconate (10–20 ml of 10% solution iv) should be available to reverse heart block and respiratory depression.

(continued)

Table 1-6. Nutritional supplementation in alcoholics—*continued*

Symptoms of deficiency state	Etiology	Treatment	Comments
Weakness, fatigue, cardiac arrhythmias	Hypokalemia	Potassium 100 mEq/day	Monitor renal function during potassium replacement
Anorexia, weakness, lethargy, bone pain, tremor, cardiomyopathy, hemolysis, respiratory failure	Hypophosphatemia	Hospital diet sufficient to replace	If patient is not eating, supplementation may be required. Serum levels below 1 mg% may lead to symptoms.
Anxiety, irritability, dizziness, sweating	Hypoglycemia		If iv glucose administration is required, it may further deplete thiamine and precipitate Wernicke's encephalopathy.
Dehydration		Routine use of parenteral fluid not justified	Follow daily weights, using specific gravity and urinary sodium to assist in monitoring hydration.
Sideroblastic anemia	Altered pyridoxine metabolism		Withdrawal of alcohol leads to reticulocytosis and disappearance of ringed sideroblasts within 3–10 days. Pyridoxine replacement is not helpful because pyridoxine metabolism is altered by ethanol.

Night blindness	Zinc deficiency	Zinc replacement	Zinc is a cofactor for vitamin A dehydrogenase, which is required for conversion of retinol to retinal.
Abnormal dark adaptation and hypogonadism	Vitamin A deficiency	Vitamin A replacement	Ethanol increases hepatotoxicity of vitamin A.
Aseptic necrosis, fractures, decreased bone density	Vitamin D deficiency	Vitamin D replacement	
Excessive bleeding	Vitamin K deficiency	Vitamin K replacement	Serious hepatic injury is present if 10 mg of vitamin A for 3 days does not reduce a prolonged prothrombin time.

Table 1-7.   Benzodiazepine protocols for alcohol detoxification

Benzodiazepine	Oral dose	Intravenous dose
Long-acting		
Chlordiazepoxide	Initial 50–100-mg oral dose. Repeat every 1–2 hours until patient is mildly sedated.	In severe cases only, 12.5 mg/minute slow infusion.
Diazepam	Initial 10–20-mg oral dose. Repeat every 1–2 hours until patient is mildly sedated.	In severe cases only, 2.5 mg/minute by slow infusion.

Drug taper: Long-acting benzodiazepines are sometimes self-tapering if high enough initial doses are used (e.g., a minimum of 60 mg of diazepam over first 24–36 hours). In many cases, tapering over 3–6 days or longer is necessary. If gradual tapering is chosen, single daily doses are preferable to divided doses.

Short-acting		
Lorazepam	Initial 2–4-mg oral dose. Repeat every 1–2 hours until patient is mildly sedated. Divide total 24-hour dose into four times daily dose to stabilize and taper.	0.5 mg/minute by slow infusion.
Oxazepam	Initial 30–60-mg oral dose. Repeat every 1–2 hours until patient is mildly sedated. Divide total 24-hour dose into a four times daily dose to stabilize and taper.	Not available.

Drug taper: Short-acting benzodiazepines must be tapered over 4–8 days or longer. Individual doses are decreased; do not omit any of the four daily doses.

able absorption, but oxazepam is also acceptable. Oxazepam has less euphorigenic effect than diazepam. These short-acting agents are especially useful in detoxification of elderly or cirrhotic patients because these drugs are metabolized to the glucuronide, which is highly water soluble and rapidly eliminated by the kidney.

Beta-blockers. Propranolol is less effective for alcohol detoxification than are the benzodiazepines, and beta-blockers are rarely indicated as sole therapy. At doses of 10 mg every 6 hours, it may reduce hyperadrenergic symptoms of withdrawal such as tremor, tachycardia, elevated blood pressure, and diaphoresis; at 40 mg every 6 hours, it decreases arrhythmias (Gross 1982; Zilm et al. 1975). It is most effectively used on those patients at risk for cardiovascular impairment from hyperadrenergic symptoms. Even so, propranolol will not prevent seizures and is contraindicated for asthmatics, insulin-dependent diabetics, and those with congestive heart failure. Most importantly, it may mask symptoms of serious withdrawal. It may also be associated with toxic confusional states (Jacob et al. 1983). Atenolol has also been effective in mild cases of withdrawal and may reduce the amount of benzodiazepine required. One study found that the addition of atenolol (50–100 mg) to a benzodiazepine regimen reduced length of hospital stay (4 versus 5 days) and reduced the amount of benzodiazepine administered compared with placebo (Kraus et al. 1985). Among those patients with withdrawal symptoms at baseline, vital signs normalized more rapidly in the atenolol group. Although behavorial improvement was also noted in the atenolol group, atenolol patients with behavioral disturbances at baseline also received higher doses of benzodiazepines. Some treatment centers now routinely prescribe atenolol, in combination with a benzodiazepine, as part of their detoxification protocol. Because lower benzodiazepine doses are used, patients often experience less sedation and cognitive impairment than with standard protocols, which permits early involvement in self-help and educational groups.

Lithium. Lithium may reduce some symptoms of withdrawal, but it does not have a therapeutic role. When administered for 3 days prior to stopping alcohol (300 mg 3 times per day), anxiety is reduced and sleep improves. It does not, however, reduce tachycardia, blood pressure, or tremors. Furthermore, lithium has been shown to potentiate withdrawal symptoms in alcohol-dependent rats when given in high doses (Ho and Tsai 1976).

Chlormethiazole. Chlormethiazole is a short-acting sedative-hypnotic with anticonvulsant effects. It is a derivative of the thiazol moiety of thiamine. Although not available in the United States, it is popular in Europe. While its onset is rapid, its effects are of short duration, and cases exist of abuse and overdose. Typical doses are three capsules or tablets (each containing 192 mg of chlormethiazole base) every 6 hours for 2 days, followed by two capsules every 6 hours for the next 4 days. Treatment typically lasts no longer than 9 days.

Chloral hydrate. Chloral hydrate is a sedative-hypnotic that is an effective pharmacologic agent for withdrawal but rarely used since the introduction of benzodiazepines. It can be irritating to the mucous membranes, causing abdominal discomfort and gastrointestinal distress (nausea, vomiting, and flatulence). In toxic doses, it may cause gastric necrosis. Central nervous system side effects include ataxia, light-headedness, nightmares, and occasionally disorientation and paranoia. Chloral hydrate also interacts with anticoagulants and displaces acidic drugs from plasma protein binding sites. Furthermore, it inhibits the metabolism of ethanol while ethanol promotes formation of trichloroethanol, the active metabolite of chloral hydrate ("Mickey Finn" or "knockout drops"). Typical initial oral doses in alcoholic withdrawal are 1.0–2.0 g. It is too irritating to administer parenterally. The half-life is 6–8 hours.

Alpha-adrenergic agonists. Clonidine is a centrally active imidazoline derivative effective in treating alcohol or opiate withdrawal. An open trial compared clonidine with a carbamazepine-neuroleptic combination and found both regimens effective (Walinder et al. 1981), although this study lacked placebo controls. Two placebo-controlled studies indicated that clonidine (0.15 mg bid or tid orally or 5 μg/kg) was effective in reducing tremor, sweating, heart rate, blood pressure, tension, anxiety, and depression (Bjorkvist 1975; Wilkins et al. 1983). In a double-blind comparison, clonidine was not as effective as chlormethiazole for patients with major alcohol withdrawal symptoms (Robinson et al. 1989). Clonidine was not effective in preventing seizures or hallucinations and was associated with orthostatic hypotension and drowsiness. For milder withdrawal, clonidine may be as effective as chlordiazepoxide (Baumgartner and Rown 1987). Clonidine also blocks alcohol withdrawal symptoms in laboratory animals (Kostowski and Trazaskowska 1980). The mechanism of action is inhibition of brain noradrenergic activity via alpha-receptor agonist activity. Its side effects are hypotension, dry mouth, and light-headedness and, like propranolol, it may mask sedative-hypnotic symptoms of withdrawal.

The alpha-adrenergic agonist lofexidine has less hypotensive and sedative effects than clonidine, and studies suggest it is also effective in withdrawal (Cushman et al. 1985). In one trial, 0.4–2.4 mg/day in four divided oral doses were used for the first 3 days of withdrawal (Brunning et al. 1986). From day 4 on, dosage was decreased by 50% daily. The mean daily dose by the end of the second day was 1.36 mg and by the fifth day was 0.34 mg. All alpha-adrenergic agonists cause hypotension, a serious side effect, and, with the exception of low-abuse potential, offer no advantages over the benzodiazepines. One study suggests a relative subsensitivity of alpha-adrenoceptors in alcoholics in withdrawal, leading to noradrenergic overactivity, which could explain some symptoms of withdrawal and the efficacy of clonidine and lofexidine (Nutt et al. 1988).

Barbiturates. Pentobarbital, phenobarbital, and secobarbital are effective in the treatment of withdrawal and provide excellent anticonvulsant activity. Their greater tendency to induce respiratory depression and abuse, as well as to interact with a number of other drugs, make the benzodiazepines a better first line of treatment. The barbiturates are still widely used in Europe and are believed by some clinicians to be useful in the rare patient refractory to benzodiazepines. Some authorities still recommend phenobarbital as a first-line agent (Smith 1989). When phenobarbital is used, a 15-mg/day dose is considered approximately equivalent to 30 ml of 80–100 proof alcohol. Using this formula, a typical patient who is consuming a quart per day of distilled spirits would require a 500-mg/day dose of phenobarbital.

Neuroleptics. Delirium may occur in severe cases of withdrawal. Psychotic symptoms are best treated with haloperidol, 0.5–2.0 mg intramuscularly every 2 hours until symptoms abate, although no more than five doses should be given in 24 hours (Jaffe and Ciraulo 1985). Neuroleptics produce hypotension and lower seizure threshold and are not indicated in the absence of psychotic symptoms. Chlorpromazine should not be used because intramuscular administration to patients with delirium tremens may lead to cardiovascular collapse and death.

Paraldehyde. Once an important treatment for alcohol withdrawal, paraldehyde is obsolete (Gessner 1979). Its only formulation is as a noxious-smelling liquid. Oral administration causes gastric irritation. Intramuscular administration causes pain and sterile abscesses. Intravenous administration risks fat embolization. Rectal administration causes proctitis, and absorption is slow and erratic. Furthermore, paraldehyde is hepatotoxic and may lead to respiratory depression, apnea, and death.

Anticonvulsants. One or more grand mal seizures may occur during withdrawal, seizures that in animal studies are not blocked by phenytoin (Sellers and Kalant 1975). The anticonvulsant effects of benzodiazepines are sufficient for patients without histories of seizure disorder. Mephenytoin, phenacemide, paramethadione, and valproic acid are effective in prophylaxis of alcohol withdrawal seizures in animals (Gessner 1979; Shaw 1982). For those patients with preexisting seizure disorders and currently taking phenytoin, a dose of 300 mg/day with up to 400 mg/day of chlordiazepoxide has proven effective (Sampliner and Iber 1974). If the patient has not been taking phenytoin for five days, then an intravenous loading dose should be administered. Phenytoin, 10 mg/kg, is given in 250–500 ml of 5% dextrose in water over 1–4 hours.

Carbamazepine. Repeated seizures during withdrawal may be due to kindling of neuronal excitability in cortical and subcortical tissues. Carbamazepine seems to inhibit limbic activity. Studies indicate carbamazepine is as effective as chlormethiazole and tiapride in treating dysphoric symptoms of withdrawal (Agricola 1982; Bjorkqvist et al. 1976; Brune and Busch 1971; Chu 1979; Post et al. 1983; Poutanen 1979; Ritola and Malinen 1981) and delirium tremens. It is administered in a divided daily dose of 600–800 mg during the first 48 hours of abstinence, and then reduced by 200 mg/day.

Ethanol. Ethanol is not recommended for treatment of alcohol withdrawal symptoms. It is toxic to organs; prolongs metabolic disturbances; interacts with other medications; and, in moderate to severe withdrawal, requires administration of excessive amounts of fluid. It is of questionable efficacy in severe withdrawal, although a clinical trial in a small number of burn patients prevented withdrawal symptoms (Hansbrough et al. 1984).

The Late Withdrawal Syndrome

Wellman (1954) described a characteristic set of symptoms found in abstinent alcoholics with a history of "repeated blackouts and at least occasional evidence of intolerance [i.e., loss of tolerance] of alcohol" (p. 526). These symptoms include irritability, depression, insomnia, fatigue, restlessness, a sense of aloneness, and distractibility. They develop within days to weeks of withdrawal and persist with decreasing intensity up to 18 months, after which they may occur in waves of lesser intensity as late as 5–10 years. Severe symptoms usually occur within the first 6 months, and depression "frequently becomes paranoidal [sic] and the distractibility becomes confusion" (p. 526). The physical signs described by Wellman resemble a hyperadrenergic state: bright red flushed facies, diaphoresis, tachycardia, muscle twitching, anxiety, confusion, and, somewhat paradoxically, hypotension. These anxiety symptoms appear as "attacks" lasting from 30 minutes to a few hours and are most common during the first 6 months of abstinence.

Although the late withdrawal syndrome has not been carefully studied, clinicians and researchers alike have observed long-lasting mood and somatic disturbances in abstinent alcoholics. Abnormalities in the cold pressor response (Kissin et al. 1959), sleep architecture (Lester et al. 1973), electroencephalogram (Pfefferbaum et al. 1979), and mood (Wellman 1954) have all been reported. Persistence of abnormalities, however, is not in itself evidence of withdrawal. A withdrawal syndrome occurs on abrupt discontinuation of a drug after prolonged intake, is time-limited, and is reversed by administration of that drug or by drugs with cross-tolerance. Many long-lasting effects are no doubt the consequences of alcohol-induced damage and not a true withdrawal syndrome. Furthermore, many of the symptoms are the psychological sequelae of interpersonal and intrapsychic disruption caused by alcoholism.

POSTWITHDRAWAL TREATMENT

For many years, myths about the untreatability of alcoholism, its inevitable fatal outcome, and psychiatrists' lack of interest in alcoholic patients dominated public thinking about this problem. Stories of inadequate or poor care, missed diagnosis, or inappropriate prescription of tranquilizers led many alcoholic patients to mistrust physicians in general and psychiatrists in particular. It was not uncommon to hear angry attacks on psychiatry, coupled with claims that the AA approach was the only realistic option for all alcoholics. Many psychiatrists recounted histories of ungrateful, often unpleasant patients who seemed unable to sustain sobriety despite the therapist's apparently heroic efforts. Such treatment failures were often attributed to the patients' lack of motivation and led many psychiatrists to assume that working with alcoholic patients was a waste of their time.

More recently a growing body of scientific research and clinical experience has demonstrated the fallacy of these assumptions. Rather than blaming the patients for their alleged lack of motivation and resistance to treatment, it is becoming clear that the successful management of alcoholism requires the application of specific treatment techniques. Of particular importance is the recognition that alcoholism is a chronic, relapsing condition that requires a long-term commitment to treatment. Successful therapists must be comfortable with both occasional relapses and their personal inability to control either the patient or the course of the alcoholism. With more difficult patients, particularly those with other major psychiatric disorders, treatment must often be geared to the amelioration and control of symptoms, rather than to cure. This is no different from the expectations physicians have regarding many other chronic conditions. Therapists skilled in the management of alcoholism can expect to see a significant and positive response in most of their patients. Given the prevalence of alcoholism among psychiatric patients, it is vital that psychiatrists be familiar with the basic management techniques that are spelled out in this chapter.

Early Psychiatric Interventions With Alcoholism

During the early 1900s, most psychiatrists had remarkably little interest or experience working with alcoholic patients. Because of assumptions about the "primitive" nature of the "character pathology" thought to underly all of the addictions, early psychoanalysts believed that alcoholics were untreatable. One notable alcoholic patient, Roland H, underwent an apparently successful analysis by Carl Jung. When the patient later relapsed, he returned to Zurich seeking further treatment. Jung advised him that his case was hopeless and that further psychiatric treatment would be of no benefit. In what has come to be seen as a prophetic observation in the history of the AA movement, Jung then stated that the only thing that could save the patient was a "conversion experience," a major personality reorganization that was fueled by a powerful emotional experience. The patient eventually did undergo such a conversion experience and joined the Oxford Movement, a prominent religious reform organization of the 1920s and 1930s. He remained sober and attributed this to the "spiritual steps" practiced by members of the Oxford Movement. Bill Wilson heard of Roland H and followed a similar course in his own successful effort to achieve sobriety. He then went on to found AA, basing AA's Twelve Steps on the spiritual steps of the Oxford Movement (AA World Services 1957).

In one of the few early optimistic reports in the literature, Robert Knight (1938) of the Menninger Clinic described the long-term psychoanalytic treatment of alcoholics in an inpatient setting. Other analysts were less successful in their work with such patients, and eventually such approaches were disparaged as being impractical and unsuccessful, if not actually harmful. Such techniques often precipitate drinking bouts in patients who have no other effective way to cope with anxiety (Vaillant 1981). Until a patient has achieved stable sobriety, traditional forms of uncovering or anxiety-provoking psychotherapy should be avoided. Despite the recognized value of insight-oriented psychotherapy for a wide variety of other psychiatric complaints, such unmodified approaches to psychotherapy cannot be recommended as a basic treatment for alcoholism.

Psychopharmacologic approaches were also seen to be limited, if not clearly dangerous. Although the benzodiazepines became the standard medication for detoxification, it also became apparent that this class of drugs had abuse potential among alcoholic patients.

Given the problems with these standard psychiatric treatments, are there any effective alternatives for the alcoholic? Fortunately, research studies have identified a variety of innovative approaches that give psychiatry a major role to play in the treatment of alcoholism.

Treatment Outcome Studies

With the establishment of the National Institute on Alcohol Abuse and Alcoholism (NIAAA) in 1970, a major commitment was made to fund a broad spectrum of treatment approaches. As Chafetz (1962) had shown in his study of emergency room intervention with skid row alcoholics, even notoriously "unmotivated" patients would respond given appropriate attention. In 1976 NIAAA published an 18-month follow-up on patients treated in these federally funded programs (Chafetz 1976). Despite the variety of treatment approaches employed, the results were remarkably consistent and positive. More than 70% of all patients treated showed improvement, and this was usually apparent within 6 months of entering treatment. In many cases only minimal intervention was necessary; recovery appeared to be related more to the intensity than to the duration of treatment. Of particular controversy was the finding that abstinence was not always necessary as a condition for improvement (Chafetz 1976). It was not possible to document the superiority of any one treatment approach. As a result, the findings of this study were difficult to explain and raised doubts about the need for more expensive, professionally staffed programs.

These doubts about the value of psychiatric intervention were amplified by Edwards' study (1977), which suggested that a simple warning and the advice not to drink again, were as effective as more comprehensive treatment. Although described as a "no treatment" approach, the patients in this study were tracked on a monthly basis, and there was ongoing contact with family members. Rather than being an example of the value of "no treatment", this study may well have documented the power of an intervention similar to probationary supervision.

One of Vaillant's most provocative research findings (1983) was the observation that the presence of any other nonalcohol-related psychiatric diagnosis was related to a poorer outcome. Among those alcoholics able to return to social drinking, only 23% had a history of some other psychiatric diagnosis. This increased to 33% in the group who achieved stable sobriety and to 45% in the group who continued to drink in a progressive alcoholic pattern (Vaillant 1983). This observation is paralleled by the work of McLellan et al. (1983, 1986) who did a series of 6-month follow-up studies on more than 1,000 alcoholics and drug addicts in a variety of treatment programs. In these studies, the clearest predictor of treatment outcome was the presence of a second psychiatric diagnosis and a high rating on a scale of overall severity of psychiatric symptomatology. Patients with no other diagnosis did well in all types of treatment settings; those with severe psychiatric problems did poorly in all programs. In general, patients did better if they received specific treatment for their psychiatric problems and if they had a longer treatment period.

Rounsaville et al. (1987) found similar results in their 1-year follow-up of 266 alcoholic patients. Men with no other diagnosis had the best outcome; those with a major depression, antisocial personality disorder, or other drug abuse did poorly. In women, a better outcome was associated with a history of preexisting major depression. It was suggested that this subgroup was more likely experiencing a form of secondary alcoholism and apparently was more amenable to treatment. Another study of 100 male alcoholic Veterans Administration patients demonstrated a positive relationship between the severity of alcohol dependence and the prevalence of additional psychiatric symptoms (Schaefer et al. 1987).

These more recent treatment evaluation studies provide a clearer picture of the interplay between alcoholism and other psychiatric conditions and also help to delineate an alcoholic population in which psychiatric treatment is a necessary part of any effective intervention program.

Contemporary Psychiatry and the Treatment of Alcoholism

Despite the current limitations of pharmacotherapy and some forms of psychotherapy, psychiatrists have several key roles to play in the treatment of alcoholism. One major function is that of being "gate-keepers." We are well placed to identify, evaluate, and recommend treatment for many of the individuals most at risk for developing severe alcoholism. Skills in early intervention and the effective management of pathological denial should be routine among all practitioners. All alcoholics require careful psychiatric diagnosis to identify symptoms secondary to the alcoholism and to rule out the presence of other primary psychiatric diseases. Patients with no other psychopathology can ordinarily be referred to AA, those with more complicated problems will clearly do better if referred to alcoholism programs that can also provide a comprehensive range of psychiatric treatment or to psychiatrists skilled in working with alcoholic patients. Failure to properly identify this subgroup of alcoholics will inevitably lead to poor treatment outcomes.

All psychiatrists need to become comfortable with the techniques most effective in the treatment of alcoholism, including the use of confrontation and the specialized psychotherapy techniques described by Dodes and Khantzian (Chapter 11). Anxiety-provoking therapies should be avoided or used with great restraint. AA should be the central core of most treatment plans (Chapter 12); psychiatrists need to be skilled in referral to AA and should be prepared to work comfortably with patients involved in such self-help programs. It is equally important to know which patients cannot tolerate participation in such a program and how to work out an alternative treatment plan. Family therapy and couples treatment may also play a major part in work with this population; this type of professional intervention can be a natural compliment to the Alanon and Alateen programs.

Work with patients with more severe alcoholism, especially those with other major psychiatric disorders, requires a high level of sophistication in psychopharmacology and psychotherapy. Although the prognosis is guarded with such "dual diagnosis" patients, it is clearly an area in which the skills of a well-trained psychiatrist are most in demand. Using the approaches described in this chapter, we can expect a more than adequate response from our patients—clear evidence that contemporary psychiatry has an essential part to play in the treatment of alcoholism.

Psychopharmacologic Treatment in the Postwithdrawal Phase

Coexistent psychiatric symptoms are commonplace in hospitalized alcoholics (V Hesselbrock et al. 1985), especially those admitted to general psychiatric wards (see Table 1-8) (Ciraulo and Ciraulo 1988). When detoxification, psychotherapy, and behavorial techniques fail or are not indicated, the physician may prescribe psychotropic medications.

There are five general precepts of prescribing psychoactive drugs to alcoholics. First, determine the diagnosis. Oftentimes intoxication and withdrawal mimic psychopathology. Anxiety and depression can be symptoms of withdrawal alone, and the clinician must take a careful history to make a differential diagnosis. For example, depression or anxiety that antedates the onset of problem drinking, worsens during chronic alcohol consumption, and is improved but not entirely eliminated during abstinence suggests an autonomous or primary psychiatric disorder.

Second, prescribe drugs that have low abuse potential. Drugs with low abuse potential are characterized by little or no mood change after a single dose and a long elimination half-life, which prevents withdrawal symptoms. Buspirone, for example, has virtually no euphoric effects after a single dose. Differences exist even among the benzodiazepines. Alprazolam produces a rapid euphoric effect in alcoholics (Ciraulo et al. 1988a), whereas halazepam, a precursor of desmethyldiazepam, does not (Jaffe et al. 1983). Any benzodiazepine that has a slow onset of mood effects (e.g., chlordiazepoxide, halazepam, prazepam, and clorazepate) would be expected to have lower potential for abuse than diazepam or alprazolam.

Table 1-8. DSM-III Axis I diagnoses of 88 alcoholics requiring psychiatric admission

Diagnosis	*n*	%
Bipolar disorder	20	23
Posttraumatic stress disorder	12	14
Major depression	10	11
Schizophrenia (all types)	8	9
Dysthymic disorder	5	6
Agoraphobia and/or panic	4	5
Paranoid disorder	2	2
Dementia associated with alcoholism	2	2
Alcohol hallucinosis	2	2

Source. Adapted from Ciraulo and Ciraulo (1988).

Third, prescribe drugs that have low lethality in overdose. Between 15% and 25% of suicides are alcoholics (Barraclough et al. 1974; Robins 1981). Coexistent psychopathology may increase the risk for suicide among alcoholics (Berglund 1984; Holloway et al. 1984; Murphy et al. 1979; Thorarinsson 1979). Fourth, dispense limited amounts of medication and maintain frequent patient contact. Finally, perform random urine or plasma toxicology screens in cases where they may be helpful to determine if other drugs are being misused.

Anxiolytics

Beta-blockers. The prototype drug for this class is propranolol. It appears to be especially effective in performance anxiety and in anxiety associated with hyperadrenergic states. Dosage range is 40–320 mg/day in divided doses. Pulse reductions to 60–65 may be a useful guide in individualizing doses. Although doses of up to 1 g/day have been reported in the literature (Carlsson and Fasth 1976), we are unaware of such high doses being used clinically. Propranolol is contraindicated in bronchial asthma, congestive heart failure, serious bradycardia and greater than first-degree heart block, and cardiogenic shock.

Buspirone. Buspirone is an anxiolytic with a high affinity for serotonin (5-HT$_{1A}$) receptors and moderate affinity for brain D_2-dopamine receptors. It differs from the benzodiazepines in that it has no sedative, muscle relaxant, or anticonvulsant activity. It has no potential for abuse and does not interact with ethanol. It neither binds to the benzodiazepine receptor nor affects GABA binding. Buspirone is not cross-tolerant with ethanol, benzodiazepines, or barbiturates and cannot, therefore, be used to treat withdrawal. Common initial doses of 15 mg/day (5 mg three times a day) are used, with the maximum daily dose being 60 mg. Because buspirone is oxidatively metabolized, the clinician should anticipate that recently abstinent alcoholics without liver disease may require higher doses than nonalcoholic anxious patients. In our clinical experience, a small but significant subgroup of anxious alcoholics respond favorably to buspirone. Those that do also seem to maintain abstinence. Bruno and Casten (1987) have reported a decrease in alcohol consumption in anxious alcoholics on buspirone compared with placebo.

Benzodiazepines.   Although most studies indicate that benzodiazepines have potential for abuse in alcoholic patients, they can be useful adjuncts in some anxious alcoholics (Ciraulo et al. 1988c). We believe that there is a spectrum of abuse potential among members of this class and prefer clordiazepoxide, clorazepate, halazepam, and prazepam for anxious alcoholics. Although several studies have also shown oxazepam to have less abuse potential, its shorter elimination half-life makes it less than ideal for this purpose. We advise that clinicians avoid the use of diazepam or alprazolam when possible. In cases of panic disorder, clonazepam appears to be a better choice for alcoholics than alprazolam. For some individuals, the benzodiazepines can trigger feelings of intoxication similar to alcohol, but this is not true for all alcoholics or for all benzodiazepines. Animal studies show that diazepam may increase ethanol consumption, whereas chlordiazepoxide and phenazepam may actually decrease consumption.

MAO inhibitors.   MAO inhibitors may be particularly useful in alcoholics with "atypical depressions" characterized by anxiety, dysphoria, hypersomnia, phobias, increased appetite, and weight gain. Drawbacks of the MAO inhibitors are dietary and drug restrictions and the potential for hepatic toxicity with the hydrazine derivative phenelzine.

Other agents.   Sedative antidepressants such as doxepin, trazodone, and amitriptyline, and the antihistamine hydroxyzine are occasionally used to treat anxious alcoholics. Antidepressants are particularly useful in phobic and panic anxiety. The tricyclic antidepressants present a risk for lethal overdose in this population.

Antidepressants

The role of antidepressants in alcoholism remains controversial (Ciraulo and Jaffe 1981). Although their efficacy has not been established, adequately designed studies are lacking. Most fail to differentiate subtypes of depression or to use acceptable diagnostic criteria, measure both changes in depression and alcohol consumption, use adequate doses of antidepressant, or monitor plasma levels. Despite the generally equivocal findings in the literature, antidepressants do improve both affective and somatic symptoms occurring during withdrawal. However, after 3 weeks of abstinence, no drug-placebo differences are usually evident.

Clinical experience suggests that in the absence of coexistent depression, there is little to gain by using a tricyclic antidepressant in alcoholism. The use of heterocyclic serotonergic agents is still under investigation, although preliminary data indicate that they reduce ethanol consumption in animals and problem drinkers (Naranjo 1985). In our clinical practice, fluoxetine (a serotonin reuptake inhibitor) has been useful in treating alcoholic patients with persistent depression, improving mood and decreasing the desire to drink.

From a practical standpoint, most alcoholics who appear depressed while drinking or during detoxification will not need antidepressant therapy. If significant improvement is not seen within 2 weeks of discontinuing drinking, however, it is likely that antidepressant therapy is indicated. For example, it is not uncommon to see alcoholics in withdrawal with Beck Depression Inventory (Beck 1978) scores in the severely depressed range immediately on admission for detoxification. Within 2 weeks, the mean scores are generally in the mildly depressed range. Approximately 5% of alcoholic patients admitted will have major depression. Invariably, these patients will continue to have severely depressed scores by 2 weeks, and antidepressant medication should be started. Some experts suggest that antidepressant treatment begin no sooner than 4 weeks after detoxification (Brown and Schuckit 1988), but in our experience if some improvement has not occurred by week 2, it is unlikely that it will. For most patients, of course, the physician has more to work with than merely symptom profile and severity. Past history of drug-responsive depression may lead clinicians to prescribe antidepressants sooner than 2 weeks.

When prescribing antidepressants to recently abstinent alcoholics, dosage adjustments must be made. Several studies now indicate that, in the absense of cirrhosis, metabolism of imipramine, desipramine, amitriptyline, and 2-OH imipramine are enhanced (Ciraulo et al. 1982, 1988b, 1990; Sandoz et al. 1983). In the case of imipramine, doses may require twofold increases; with desipramine, slightly lower increases are necessary. It is prudent to monitor plasma levels of antidepressants in recovering alcoholics, because the enzyme induction is probably reversible.

Disulfiram

Disulfiram (Antabuse) is a widely used alcohol deterrent (Jaffe and Ciraulo 1985; McNichol et al. 1987). Its therapeutic application is straightforward: persons taking disulfiram become mildly to violently ill if they ingest ethyl alcohol. Fear of this reaction is presumed to act as a deterrent to alcohol consumption.

Following oral administration, disulfiram is rapidly metabolized to diethyldithiocarbamate (DDC). DDC inhibits enzyme systems by chelating trace metals, and itself degrades into diethylamine and several other compounds, including carbon disulfide. Its effective half-life is about 24 hours, but inhibition of aldehyde dehydrogenase is irreversible.

The onset of action of disulfiram is slow (approximately 12 hours) with a maximum effect at 24–48 hours. It has a long duration of action because new enzyme must be synthesized, which may take 6–14 days. The duration of the disulfiram-ethanol reaction (DER) varies from 30 minutes to several hours.

Disulfiram inhibits a variety of enzymes such as dopamine beta-hydroxylase (DBH), xanthene oxidase, hexokinase, 3-phosphoglyceraldehyde dehydrogenase, beta-hydroxybutyrate dehydrogenase, and d-amino acid oxidase. Of most importance, however, is the inhibition of acetaldehyde oxidoreductase (acetaldehyde dehydrogenase), leading to the accumulation of acetaldehyde and the onset of the DER. In addition to the DER, clinicians should be aware of the possibility of multiple drug interactions, altered levels of neurotransmitters, and toxic symptoms from disulfiram or its metabolites.

DER symptoms vary in nature and severity. A mild DER begins with increasing heart rate and blood pressure; leads to breathlessness, chills, nausea, vomiting, and hypotension; and terminates with a period of sedation and sleep (McNichol et al. 1987). A mild DER may occur at therapeutic doses of disulfiram (250 mg) with doses of ethanol as low as 0.125–0.15 g/kg of body weight, the equivalent of 36 ml of 80 proof spirit (Peachey 1981a, 1981b, 1984). In its more severe form, the DER involves intense tachycardia, electrocardiographic changes, myocardial infarction, cerebrovascular hemorrhage, and cerebral infarction. The hypotensive phase may lead to bradycardia or cardiac arrest secondary to vagal stimulation associated with vomiting and retching. Convulsions, congestive heart failure, and cardiovascular collapse may also occur in severe cases. These severe reactions are generally limited to disulfiram doses over 500 mg/day interacting with more than 2 ounces of alcohol. Peachey (1984) stated that severe acetaldehyde-mediated reactions can occur at 250 mg of disulfiram if 0.5 g/kg of ethanol is ingested. Mild reactions may occur at blood alcohol concentrations as low as 5–10 mg/100 mL, with a moderate reaction at 50–100 mg/100 mL, and unconsciousness developing at 125–150 mg/100 mL.

Increased acetaldehyde levels are responsible for many aspects of the DER, and there is a good correlation between the cardiovascular symptoms and acetaldehyde levels; 4-methylpyrazol, which blocks acetaldehyde production, has been used to treat the DER. Hypotension, on the other hand, cannot be explained by increased acetaldehyde, because when administered alone it causes a pressor response (Egle et al. 1973; Tottmar and Hellstrom 1979). This was previously explained as the result of inhibition of DBH activity, which, by impairing norepinephrine synthesis, permits acetaldehyde to depress the myocardium directly and causes a vasodilatory effect in coronary and peripheral vessels (Gailis 1975; Goldstein and Nakajima 1967; Goldstein et al. 1964; Musacchio et al. 1966; Nakano et al. 1974; Nguyen and Gailis 1974; Truitt and Walsh 1971). Inhibition of DBH may not entirely explain the adverse effect because hypotension is also seen in the ethanol reaction induced by cyanamide and the inky cap mushroom, *Coprinus atramentarius,* even though they do not inhibit DBH (Carlsson et al. 1978; Cornsbruch and Derwort 1968; Fischer 1945).

Other drugs that inhibit aldehyde dehydrogenase result in similar reactions when ethanol is administered. Some MAO inhibitors increase blood acetaldehyde levels in mice given ethanol. Pargyline causes 20-fold increases and deprenyl and clorgyline 2-fold increases; nialamide and tranylcypromine are only weakly active (Dembiec et al. 1976). Twenty hours after pargyline administration, 30% of aldehyde dehydrogenase activity returns.

Tolbutamide and chlorpropamide may also cause an alcohol flushing reaction, probably through the effect of a metabolite, which inhibits aldehyde dehydrogenase (Barnett et al. 1981; Fitzgerald et al. 1962; Perez 1974). Metronidazole also causes a reaction to ethanol, but does not appear to act via elevation of acetaldehyde levels (Goodwin and Reinhard 1972; Kalant et al. 1971; Madalena and De Mattos 1967; Rothstein and Clancy 1970). A number of other chemicals also cause altered sensitivity and adverse responses to ethanol. Included here are antibiotics (the beta lactam cephalosporins, moxalactam, cefamandole, and cefoperazone), hydrogen sulfide, tetraethyllead, pyrogallol, 4-bromopyrazole, and coprine (1-aminocyclopropanol), the active ingredient in the inky cap mushroom (Fried 1980; Sellers et al. 1981).

Conservative measures are the best course of treatment for DER. Modified Trendelenburg position for hypotension and cholinergic blockers for vagal-induced bradycardia are advised. One study found that 4-methylpyrazol inhibited the metabolism of alcohol to acetaldehyde and caused a prompt fall in blood acetaldehyde levels, which decreased DER symptoms (Lindros et al. 1981).

There is also some evidence that ascorbic acid (vitamin C) reduces the effects of DER. An intravenous dose of 1 g of ascorbic acid given during severe DER has relieved symptoms. Symptoms recur within 1–2 hours, however, necessitating further doses of ascorbic acid (McNichol et al. 1987).

Distinct from DER, disulfiram may produce its own side effects. These include drowsiness, lethargy, peripheral neuropathy, hepatoxicity, seizures, elevated serum acetone and cholesterol, optic neuritis, and hypertension. Because hepatotoxic effects may be fatal if the drug is not discontinued, it is important to monitor liver enzymes periodically. Limb anomalies may occur in babies born to women taking disulfiram, but a causative relationship is not established (Nora et al. 1977). Disulfiram and DDC increase brain dopamine and decrease norepinephrine levels by inhibiting dopamine beta-hydroxylase. This may explain depression and psychosis, which can occur during disulfiram treatment. Alcoholics with low CSF DBH, platelet MAO, plasma amine oxidase, or high red cell catechol-o-methyltransferase activity may be predisposed to psychotic symptoms secondary to disulfiram. Psychotic reactions are more common in patients with preexisting psychiatric disorders (e.g., depression, schizophrenia, or borderline disorders) or who have other side effects such as fatigue and lethargy. Higher doses (500 mg) are more likely to induce psychotic symptoms than lower ones (250 mg) (Major et al. 1979a, 1979b; Sellers et al. 1981).

In addition to its intrinsic side effects, patients on disulfiram run the risk of DER caused by consumption of substances containing latent alcohol, such as sauces, cough syrups, or vinegars containing wine. After-shaves or other facial lotions containing alcohol are not contraindicated because alcohol is not normally absorbed through the skin, although some people do develop erythema.

According to one authority (Peachey 1984), the contraindications for disulfiram are cardiovascular disease (angina, coronary artery disease, cardiac arrhythmias, cardiomyopathy, and untreated or uncontrolled hypertension), hepatic dysfunction (hepatitis, cirrhosis, hepatic encephalopathy, esophageal varices, and hepatorenal syndrome), organic brain disorders, pulmonary insufficiency, pregnancy, psychiatric disorders (suicidal ideation and poor impulse control), renal failure, and previous adverse reaction.

Relative contraindications are the need for treatment with vasodilators, beta-adrenergic antagonists, MAO inhibitors, tricyclic antidepressants, or antipsychotic agents, because they may increase morbidity of the DER. Sellers et al. (1981) recommended an initial complete mental and physical examination, including a laboratory screen and electrocardiogram as well as psychosocial assessment. This is followed by a monthly repeat of mental and physical examinations, a quarterly repeat of selected laboratory work, and a semiannual repeat of all initial exams. Some clinicians believe that such stringent criteria and routine examinations may largely preclude the use of disulfiram in most alcoholics or raise the cost of its use to prohibitive levels (Gragg 1982). Liver function tests, especially early in treatment, are essential to detect chemical hepatitis, which may be fatal. We find no contraindication to combining disulfiram with tricyclic antidepressants, provided that allowances are made for alterations in metabolism of the latter (Ciraulo et al. 1985). Disulfiram interacts with drugs that are oxidatively metabolized and may inhibit the metabolism of phenytoin, warfarin, isoniazid, rifampin, diazepam, antipyrine, imipramine, and desipramine. In general, a potential disulfiram patient should be lucid regarding the commitment he or she is undertaking and the consequences that will arise from attempted drinking.

Disulfiram should be given orally in doses of 250 mg/day.

Higher doses are not recommended because they increase side effects and toxic hazards without increasing therapeutic benefit. For the occasional patient who is able to drink without consequence while taking 250 mg, it may be necessary to increase the dose to 500 mg. Subcutaneous implantation in the abdominal wall has been tried as an alternative route of administration, but blood levels of disulfiram and metabolites are too low by this method and the 100-mg implants used are rapidly depleted (Bergstrom et al. 1982; Sellers et al. 1981; Wilson et al. 1980).

The therapeutic effect of disulfiram is primarily psychological. The pharmacologic effects of the DER loom in the background, coercing abstinent alcoholics to stay that way. The most comprehensive study of disulfiram efficacy (Fuller et al. 1986) studied three groups: 202 men taking disulfiram at a therapeutic dose of 250 mg, 204 men taking 1 mg of disulfiram, and 199 taking placebo. All received counseling and bimonthly treatment analysis for a year, including blood and urine ethanol analyses. The researchers found no significant differences among the groups in terms of total abstinence, time to first drink (breaking abstinence), employment, or social stability. On the other hand, among those who did drink, those on 250 mg of disulfiram reported fewer drinking days (49.0 $\pm$ 8.4 versus 75.4 $\pm$ 11.9) than those on 1 mg or no disulfiram (86.5 $\pm$ 13.6). The researchers concluded that "disulfiram may help reduce drinking frequency after relapse, but does not enhance counseling in aiding alcoholic patients to sustain continuous abstinence or delay the resumption of drinking" (p. 1449).

Despite a number of studies and clinical reports, questions remain concerning the efficacy and risks of disulfiram. On the one hand, experienced clinicians find it useful in a subpopulation of well-motivated alcoholics. On the other hand, research studies indicate that neither abstinence rates nor social functioning is improved with disulfiram, although total days drinking is reduced. In light of its limited efficacy, its adverse effects, and the danger of DER, some clinicians question its value. The ideal disulfiram patient is one who seeks abstinence, wants to use disulfiram, and has no medical or psychological contraindications.

Calcium Carbimide

Calcium carbimide (Temposil or Abstem) is an alcohol deterrent drug that is not available in the United States, but is widely used in

Canada and Europe. It is hydrolyzed in the gut to carbimide (cyanimide). It differs from disulfiram in several important ways. It is a reversible inhibitor of aldehyde dehydrogenase, with a rapid onset of action (within 1 hour) and a short duration of action (24 hours). Because of this, it is often given in two daily doses of 50 mg each. It does not inhibit DBH or the hepatic mixed function oxidase system and is less likely to have behavioral toxicity or to interfere with the metabolism of other drugs.

As with disulfiram, the intensity of the reaction depends on the amount of ethanol ingested and the dose of calcium carbimide (Peachey 1980). One important difference, however, is that if alcohol ingestion occurs within 2–4 hours of taking calcium carbimide, the reaction is more severe than if alcohol were taken later (e.g., 12 hours postdose). At ethanol doses of 0.25 g/kg, changes occur up to 12 hours after a 50-mg dose, and with 0.5 g/kg up to 24 hours.

Calcium carbimide is relatively free of adverse effects. It has antithyroid activity in animals (Benitz et al. 1965), but may not pose a serious clinical problem (Brunner-Orne 1962). Authorities recommend periodic thyroid function tests for patients on calcium carbimide. Although peripheral neuropathy (Reilly 1976) and hepatocyte inclusion bodies (Vazquez and Cervera 1980) have been reported, a causative link to calcium carbimide has not been established.

Conditioned Aversion to Alcohol

Pairing alcohol consumption with an unpleasant stimulus, such as electric shock, succinylcholine, or drugs that induce nausea and vomiting, has been used to produce conditioned aversion to alcohol. Emetine and apomorphine are commonly used in chemical aversion programs, and 3-year abstinence rates of 50% have been reported (Neubuerger et al. 1981).

MEDICAL CONSEQUENCES OF ALCOHOLISM

Wernicke-Korsakoff's Syndrome

Greenberg and Diamond (1985) discussed Wernicke-Korsakoff's syndrome as a result of alcoholism. Wernicke's encephalopathy is an acute neurologic illness seen in alcoholics and others with nutritional deficiency states. It is characterized by the triad of ophthalmoplegia, ataxia, and confusion. The ocular abnormalities include nystagmus (horizontal, vertical, and rarely rotatory), lateral rectus palsies, conjugate gaze palsies (horizontal alone, both horizontal and vertical, and rarely internuclear, ophthalmoplegia), and pupillary abnormalities (anisocoria and slowly reactive pupils). These symptoms reflect lesions in the sixth and third nerve nucleii, pretectal region, periaqueductal gray, vestibular complex, and cerebellum.

Of patients with Wernicke's syndrome, 90% have ataxia that is cerebellar in type affecting the legs and gait, but less commonly involving arms or speech. The confusional state appears as inattention, drowsiness, disorientation, and, in severe cases, coma. Hypothermia, vestibular paresis, peripheral neuropathy, and findings associated with chronic alcoholism also may be present in the patient.

The neuropathologic findings indicate selective involvement of the paraventricular gray matter of the diencephalon and brain stem. Microscopically, areas of demyelination and glial proliferation are seen. Myelinated fibers are affected to a greater extent than cell bodies. Lesions vary with time, with microglia predominant in the acute phase and fibrous astrocytes in older lesions.

The treatment of Wernicke's encephalopathy is administration of parenteral thiamine, 50–100 mg/day. Oral thiamine is poorly absorbed in alcoholic patients. Some improvement may be seen within hours of treatment, but maximum improvement may take weeks. Complete recovery of gaze palsies and confusion usually occurs, but gait ataxia and nystagmus persist in 40% of cases. There is a 17% mortality rate during the acute phase.

Approximately 80% of patients who survive develop Korsakoff's syndrome (alcohol amnestic disorder), which is a memory disorder characterized by amnesia (anterograde and retrograde) in an otherwise alert patient. Such patients may be impaired in orientation to time and place and unable to recall names or lists, but may adequately repeat digits (immediate recall). Impairment of remote memory is variable, but there is a general tendency for recent memory to be more severely impaired. Patients appear indifferent to the memory loss, and confabulation may be prominent.

Lesions of the mammillary body, medial dorsal nucleus of the thalamus, and medial pulvinar are the characteristic neuropathologic findings. Many authorities believe that vitamin deficiency alone is not responsible for Korsakoff's syndrome, but that the direct neurotoxic effects of ethanol are also of importance.

In contrast to Wernicke's syndrome, the amnestic syndrome does not significantly improve in more than half of patients. Clinical reports have suggested that arginine vasopressin may be of value in improving the memory disturbance, but the evidence does not support routine use.

Alcoholic Dementia

DSM-III-R defines this syndrome as dementia—an impairment in short- and long-term memory, associated with impairment of abstract thinking, impaired judgment, other disturbances of higher cortical function, or personality change—following prolonged and heavy ingestion of alcohol, for which all other causes of dementia have been ruled out. It is distinguished from Korsakoff's syndrome because the latter spares the intellectual functions other than memory.

Alcoholic dementia is characterized by impairment on visuospatial tasks, such as block design or maze tests. Clinicians should be aware that performance in copying tasks, a common office screening procedure, may show no impairment. While neuropsychological tests clearly establish memory deficits, the amnesia is usually not as severe as Korsakoff's syndrome or Alzheimer's disease. Impairment of abstracting abilities and psychomotor function has also been observed.

Chronic alcoholism leads to a number of neuropathologic changes that may lead to dementia. Although some aspects focus on frontal lobe atrophy as primary in alcoholic dementia, others suggest that ventricular dilation, atrophy in the area surrounding the third ventricle, or even diffuse cortical atrophy may underlie the dementia.

Other Neurologic Consequences

Cerebellar degeneration occurs in a substantial number of alcoholics (Allsop and Turner 1966). In one study, 30% of alcoholics referred for treatment had atrophy of the cerebellar vermis; of these, 67% had atrophy involving both cerebellar hemispheres (Freund 1985).

Corpus callosum degeneration (Marchiafava-Bignami disease) is a rare neurologic condition occurring in alcoholics; it may also be seen in nonalcoholics. It was initially thought to be etiologically related to drinking Italian wines; however, it has also been reported in other countries. Clinical symptoms include dementia, psychosis, seizures, aphasia, apraxia, and paresis. It is usually fatal within 6 months after onset.

Central pontine myelinolysis has been reported in alcoholics, but is also seen after exposure to organic solvents and after overly vigorous treatment of hyponatremia. It clinically presents as acute onset of pseudobulbar palsy, quadraplegia, impaired ocular movements, slurred speech, dysphasia, and hypoactive gag and cough reflexes.

Gastrointestinal Consequences of Alcoholism

The various gastrointestinal consequences of alcoholism have been discussed by Korsten and Lieber (1985) and Lieber (1982).

Effects on the liver.   Alcoholic steatosis or fatty liver presents clinically as an enlarged, nontender, smooth liver on physical examination. Histologic features include fat within intracytoplasmic vacuoles, displacement of the nucleus, distorted mitochondrial structure, and dilation of the endoplasmic reticulum. Perivenular fibrosis may be a precirrhotic lesion. Liver enzymes correlate poorly with histologic changes. The etiology of steatosis appears to be the increased NADH/NAD ratio that occurs during oxidation of ethanol. Abstinence, improved nutrition, dietary restriction of fat, and administration of anabolic steroids have been advocated as treatment for fatty liver.

Alcoholic hepatitis.   Alcoholic hepatitis presents with fever, anorexia, right upper quadrant pain, and jaundice and may mimic the signs and symptoms of extrahepatic biliary obstruction. Elevated serum glutamate dehydrogenase and the aspartate transaminase–alanine transaminase ratio (greater than 1 in 55% of patients with alcoholic hepatitis) may serve as an index of inflammation and necrosis. Corticosteroids and propylthiouracil may be used in the treatment of alcoholic hepatitis, but their efficacy is not established. Long-term survival is improved with abstinence or decreased consumption.

Alcoholic cirrhosis.   The onset of cirrhosis is heralded by anorexia, weight loss, and weakness. Physical findings include hepatomegaly, jaundice, and secondary signs such as ascites, asterixis, edema, testicular atrophy, gynecomastia, spider angiomata, splenomegaly, gastrointestinal hemorrhage, peritonitis, palmar erythema, and Dupuytren's contracture. Laboratory studies show hypoalbuminemia, hyperglobulinemia, elevation of beta and gamma globulins (beta-gamma bridging), and low or absent alpha- and prebeta-lipoprotein bands. Liver enzyme studies may show only mild abnormalities.

Early in the illness, a uniformly nodular liver is found, which as the disease progresses becomes irregular. Cholestasis, iron deposits, fatty infiltration, inflammation, and fibrosis are seen microscopically. These changes result in reduced hepatic blood flow and formation of extrahepatic portosystemic shunts.

Ascites is a complication of cirrhosis. Treatment consists of restriction of dietary sodium and/or administration of diuretics. Spironolactone is the preferred agent because even though the thiazide diuretics enhance sodium excretion, they may induce hypokalemia and azotemia. Weight loss of 2 lb/day is optimal.

Renal failure may occur in the presence of severe hepatic disease and is occasionally triggered by gastrointestinal hemorrhage, rapid diuresis, or paracentesis.

Hepatic encephalopathy may begin with mild changes in personality and then progress to drowsiness, confusion, and lack of responsiveness. Asterixis may be prominent. Elevated serum and CSF ammonia levels and increased CSF glutamine and alpha-keto-glutaramate are characteristic. Electroencephalogram may be helpful in making the diagnosis. Typical precipitants of hepatic encephalopathy include azotemia, gastrointestinal blood loss, infection, dietary protein, hypokalemia, and constipation. Lactulose, neomycin, protein restriction (or a substitution of vegetable protein for animal protein), potassium supplementation, and bowel cleansing have been used to reduce ammonia production in the gastrointestinal tract.

Esophageal and gastric varices may also occur in cirrhotics, and hepatic coma and renal failure may follow a bleed. Vasopressin is typically used to treat the variceal hemorrhage, but the options include balloon tamponade, injection sclerosis, portal systemic anastomosis, and other operative procedures. Propranolol has been used in long-term management to reduce portal flow.

Effects on the pancreas. Alcoholic pancreatitis typically develops after 10–15 years of heavy drinking and presents with severe upper abdominal pain, which radiates to the back and is relieved by leaning forward. Ileus and fever may also be present. If a pseudocyst develops, an abdominal mass may be palpated. Pancreatic ascites may be detected by shifting dullness. In addition to these physical findings, a plain film of the abdomen ("KUB") may reveal pancreatic calcification or ileus. Ultrasound can be used to determine pancreatic ascites, presence of pseudocysts, and status of the common bile duct.

Endoscopic retrograde cholangiography may also be useful in assessing duct status. Serum amylase is usually elevated, but may be normal in chronic cases. Complications of pancreatitis include pancreatic insufficiency, pseudocyst formation, glucose intolerance, and pancreatic ascites.

Other gastrointestinal effects. Alcoholics have an increased incidence of esophageal cancer and have altered esophageal peristalsis. They may have gastrointestinal blood loss secondary to esophagitis, gastritis, duodenitis, varices, peptic ulceration, or Mallory-Weiss syndrome; glossitis, stomatitis, enlargement of the parotid glands, and altered salivary secretion may also occur.

Hematologic Effects

Folate deficiency secondary to alcoholism results in megaloblastic anemia. The mean corpuscular volume is usually increased, but may be within normal limits in the presence of iron deficiency. In severe cases, thrombocytopenia and granulocytopenia may also occur. Red cell folate is a better measure of tissue levels than serum folate concentrations. Pernicious anemia should be considered in these patients, and serum B_{12} levels should be measured. Sideroblastic anemia, secondary to pyridoxine deficiency, may also occur in alcoholics (Hines and Cowan 1970). In alcoholics with liver disease, target cells, acanthocytosis, stomatocytes, and hemolytic anemia may occur.

Abnormalities of white cells have also been reported. In addition to granulocytopenia, functional abnormalities that impair immunological activity occur and may be the mechanism by which alcoholics show decreased resistance to infection.

Ethanol directly reduces platelet production and decreases platelet survival time, frequently resulting in thrombocytopenia in chronic alcoholics. Clinical consequences of this reduction are rare, and normal platelet counts typically return during abstinence.

Cardiovascular Consequences

Van Theil and Gavaler (1985b) discussed the cardiovascular consequences of alcoholism.

Hypertension. Studies of the work force indicate that employees identified as problem drinkers have higher mean systolic and diastolic blood pressures and rates of hypertension greater than twice that of controls. Although studies of inpatient alcoholics have not shown a high rate of hypertension, elevated blood pressure is seen in a substantial number of alcoholics on admission. In most cases, however, it normalizes 1 or 2 weeks postdetoxification. Cross-sectional studies of the general population have yielded conflicting data; however, there is evidence to suggest that a linear relationship exists between blood pressure and alcohol consumption (1–5 drinks/day). The effect is small, with a 1–2 mm Hg increase in blood pressure per drink.

Alcoholic cardiomyopathy. Alcoholic cardiomyopathy presents with fatigue, dyspnea on exertion, hepatomegaly, paroxysmal nocturnal dyspnea, orthopnea, palpitations, atrial fibrillation, conduction defects, edema, cough, abnormal P waves, and decreased QRS voltage on electrocardiogram. On auscultation, a third and fourth heart sound, rales, and holosystolic and systolic ejection murmurs are heard. Cardiomegaly is seen by X ray and detected by lateral displacement of the apical pulse on physical examination. Cardiac catheterization reveals high diastolic pressures, reduced cardiac output, and pulmonary hypertension. Heart tissue of patients with alcoholic cardiomyopathy shows muscle fiber hypertrophy and degeneration, fibrosis, areas of endocardial fibroelastosis, mural thrombosis, and chronic inflammatory cells. Mitochondrial damage and endoplasmic reticulum distension are seen on electron micrographs (Urbano-Marquez et al. 1989).

In a study of 310 patients with primary myocardial disease followed from 1962 to 1970, 93% were judged to be secondary to alcoholism (Demakis et al. 1974).

Cardiac arrhythmias. Arrhythmias may be the consequence of cardiac disease and/or a direct effect of ethanol or acetaldehyde. The so-called holiday heart syndrome is atrial fibrillation that develops in patients without heart disease after periods of excessive alcohol consumption. Ventricular fibrillation may occur during intoxication, and cardiac arrest has also been reported.

High-density lipoproteins (HDLs). Lipoproteins serve to transport lipids in the bloodstream. HDLs are the smallest lipoproteins and are divided into at least two subfractions HDL_2 and HDL_3, which have differing lipid-to-protein ratios. The amount of cholesterol carried by the HDL may be a predictor of coronary heart disease, with higher levels associated with lower risk. HDL_2-cholesterol levels may be a better predictor than total HDL cholesterol. The protein components of HDL may vary, but apoprotein A is the most common and is divided into types A-I and A-II, which may also predict cardiac risk.

Alcoholics without severe liver disease have higher levels of HDL cholesterol than controls. Levels return to normal within 2 weeks of abstinence. In cross-sectional studies of the general population, alcohol consumption and HDL cholesterol are positively correlated, especially in older subjects. No consistent findings have been reported concerning the effect of alcohol on HDL subfractions or apoproteins.

The clinical implications of these findings are unclear, although moderate ethanol consumption (up to 60 ml/day) is associated with a lower risk of nonfatal myocardial infarction. Large amounts of ethanol do not have this protective effect. Furthermore, alcohol may primarily increase HDL_3, whereas HDL_2 is believed to have the cardioprotective effect (Korsten and Lieber 1985).

Endocrine Consequences

Plasma cortisol is increased in alcoholics, and symptoms resembling Cushing's syndrome may be present (Mendelson et al. 1971).

Alcohol alone, in the absence of liver disease, affects gonadal function, but cirrhosis will also alter it. Acute doses of ethanol lower serum testosterone (Van Thiel and Gavaler 1985a). In chronic alcoholics, testosterone clearance is enhanced, and testosterone synthesis is depressed. Decreased luteinizing hormone levels and altered binding at the Leydig cell receptor may also occur. Irreversible damage to the testes ultimately results, a direct effect of ethanol and/or acetaldehyde. At the same time, estrogen levels rise. The resulting clinical picture is testicular atrophy, loss of facial hair, breast enlargement, decreased libido, and impotence.

Endocrine effects in alcoholic women are less well studied than in men. Chronic alcoholism, however, is known to be associated with amenorrhea, luteal phase dysfunction, anovulation, early menopause, and hyperprolactinemia (Mello 1988). Amenorrhea may persist for months or years, even with abstinence. The mechanism of these alterations remains uncertain. Studies of the general population indicate that women who had one or more alcoholic drinks per day were more likely than those who drank less to have spontaneous abortions in the second trimester but not the first trimester.

Thyroid function. Although clinical hypothyroidism is not common in alcoholics, a persistent blunted thyroid-stimulating hormone response to protirelin is seen in abstinent alcoholics. Liver disease may also affect thyroid function.

Metabolic effects. Hypoglycemia, ketosis, and hyperuricemia may also be seen in alcoholics.

Respiratory Consequences

Alcoholics have a high incidence of respiratory tract infections, particularly pneumococcal pneumonia and gram-negative infections. Aspiration pneumonia and lung abscesses are also common.

Alcoholic Myopathy

Alcoholic myopathy may present as muscle weakness, atrophy, tenderness, and pain. Creatine phosphokinase (CPK-MM) is elevated, and myoglobin may be present in the urine. Weakness is usually proximal, and the distribution may be confined to one limb or symmetrical. Occasionally it is evident only by decreased muscle strength or elevated serum CPK-MM, aspartate aminotransferase, and lactate dehydrogenase. In its severe form, there may be rapidly progressing rhabdomyolysis with myoglobinuria, hyperkalemia, renal failure, and even death.

Fetal Alcohol Syndrome

The harmful effects of ethanol on the fetus have been known since antiquity, as evidenced by biblical references and the writings of the Greek philosophers. The English language literature on the subject dates to at least the early 1700s, when the lifting of restrictions on distilling gin created a major social problem in England (Warner and Rosett 1975). Over the next 200 years, the problem of fetal effects of ethanol received a great deal of study; however, during the period of Prohibition in the United States (1920–1933), very little appeared on the subject. When the topic was taken up again by medical investigators, the tone was less ominous. In fact, the idea of harmful effects of ethanol on the fetus was generally dismissed as biased and moralistic, no doubt a reaction to the temperance movement. There was a rediscovery of the fetal toxicity of ethanol in the late 1960s and early 1970s. Lemoine et al. (1968) studied 127 children of alcoholic mothers in France and found low birth weight, retarded growth and development, craniofacial abnormalities, cardiovascular defects, low intelligence, and impaired school performance. In the United States, Jones et al. (1973, 1974) reported children of alcoholic mothers with similar developmental problems and anomalies. Clarren and Smith (1978) identified three principal features of the fetal alcohol syndrome: central nervous system effects, growth deficiency, and facial abnormalities.

Central nervous system effects include mild to moderate mental retardation, microcephaly, poor coordination, hypotonia, irritability in infancy, and hyperactivity in childhood. Although slight improvement in intellectual function with growth may be seen in some cases, persistence of the deficit is the rule.

At birth, infants with the fetal alcohol syndrome have lower lengths and weights, and as children remain 2 standard deviations below the mean. These children generally show normal levels of growth hormone, cortisol, and gonadotropins. They may have diminished adipose tissue.

There is a distinctive facial appearance associated with fetal alcohol syndrome. These children show short palpebral fissures, a hypoplastic upper lip with thin vermilion, absent or diminished philtrum, and midfacial hypoplasia. The ear may show posterior rotation of the helix and altered conchal shape. Retrognathia in infancy and micrognathia or relative prognathia in adolescence may also be present.

Various other features are less commonly reported and include other eye findings such as ptosis, strabismus, epicanthal folds, myopia, and blepharophimosis. Approximately half of the children with fetal alcohol syndrome have hypoplasia of the optic nerve head and increased tortuosity of the retinal vessels, especially the arteries (Stromland 1987). Cardiac murmurs, atrial septal defect, or other anomalies may be seen. Musculoskeletal defects such as aberrant palmar creases, pectus excavatum, and others have also been reported. Prominent lateral palatine ridges, cleft lip or palate, and small teeth with faulty enamel have been observed. Hemangiomas and labial hypoplasia are frequent associated features.

The amount of maternal alcohol ingestion required to induce congenital defects is unknown. Animal studies have typically used high doses. A study in humans found that 11% of women who drank 1–2 ounces of absolute alcohol per day gave birth to children with symptoms of fetal alcohol syndrome (Hanson et al. 1978). Others suggest that even one daily drink may be associated with lower-than-average birth weight (Little et al. 1986). Smith (1979) suggested that as little as two drinks per day have a mild effect on total growth and development. Many experts recommend total abstinence as the safest policy for pregnant women and for those planning pregnancy (Blume 1985-86).

The cause of fetal alcohol syndrome is most likely the direct toxic effect of ethanol or acetaldehyde on the fetus. Ethanol is also toxic to the placenta and impairs transport of amino acids, zinc, or other nutrients to the fetus. Other possible placental effects include decreased placental folate receptor activity, decreased protein synthesis, collapsed umbilical vessels, and villitis (Fisher 1985).

CONCLUSIONS

The origins of alcoholism are complex. Biological and psychological factors are of etiologic and therapeutic importance. Genetic findings have fueled a research effort into physiological etiologies of alcoholism. Identification of biological risk factors, such as abnormal electroencephalograms, altered enzyme activity, or disturbed receptor-effector coupling, provides hope for understanding the biological and physiologic basis of alcoholism.

Yet the answer to an individual's alcohol problem will not likely be found only at the biochemical level. In fact, the separation of psychological and biological factors is really an artificial one. Every thought or feeling we have is based in our neurochemistry, which is, in turn, influenced by cognition. Investigators are beginning to examine the relationship, and intriguing hypotheses have been generated linking certain personality traits with neurotransmitter dysfunction. We eagerly await the testing of these hypotheses.

Alcoholism is the major drug problem confronting our society. More than 10 million Americans experience problems because of drinking. Alcoholism is the most common psychiatric diagnosis in adult males in the United States. Emergency room visits and hospital stays are common for alcoholics; alcohol-related health expenditures account for about 12% of the nation's total health care costs.

Although we have made significant advances in understanding the nature of alcoholism, much remains to be done. Understanding the role of serotonin and serotonergic drugs in alcoholism is one exciting area that has reached our treatment programs. AA continues to be the mainstay of treatment, but research on cognitive-behavior therapy and individual psychotherapy indicates an important role for these modalities as well. The synthesis of biological and psychosocial research and its subsequent clinical applications present a challenge for the next decade. We hope that our nation continues to make alcohol research and treatment an important national priority.

References

AA World Services: Alcoholics Anonymous Comes of Age. New York, AA World Services, 1957

Abraham K: The psychological relations between sexuality and alcoholism (1908), in Selected Papers on Psychoanalysis, 3rd Edition. Translated by Bryan D, Strachey A. New York, Basic Books, 1957, pp 80–89

Agarwal DP, Harada S, Goedde H: Racial differences in biological sensitivity to ethanol: the role of alcohol dehydrogenase and aldehyde dehydrogenase isoenzymes. Alcoholism: Clinical and Experimental Research 5:12–16, 1981

Agricola R: Treatment of acute alcohol withdrawal syndrome with carbamazepine: a double-blind comparison with tiapride. J Int Med Res 10:160–165, 1982

Alexopoulos GS, Lieberman KW, Frances R, et al: Platelet MAO during the alcohol withdrawal syndrome. Am J Psychiatry 138:1254–1255, 1981

Alkana RL, Parker ES, Malcolm RD, et al: Interaction of apomorphine and amantadine with ethanol in men. Alcoholism: Clinical and Experimental Research 6:403–411, 1982

Allsop J, Turner B: Cerebellar degeneration associated with chronic alcoholism. J Neurol Sci 3:238–258, 1966

Altshuler HL, Shippenberg TS: Tetrahydroisoquinoline and opioid substrates of alcohol action. Prog Clin Biol Res 90:329–344, 1982

Altshuler HL, Phillips PE, Feinhandler DA: Alteration of ethanol self-administration by naloxone. Life Sci 26:679–688, 1980

American Psychiatric Association: Diagnostic and Statistical Manual of Mental Disorders, 3rd Edition, Washington, DC, American Psychiatric Association, 1980

American Psychiatric Association: Diagnostic and Statistical Manual of Mental Disorders, 3rd Edition, Revised. Washington, DC, American Psychiatric Association, 1987

Arvola A, Forsander O: Comparison between water and alcohol consumption in six animal species in free-choice experiments. Nature 191: 819–820, 1961

Bales RF: Cultural differences in rates of alcoholism. Quarterly Journal of Studies on Alcohol 6:480–499, 1946

Bales RF: Attitudes toward drinking in the Irish culture, in Society, Culture and Drinking Patterns. Edited by Pittman DJ, Snyder CR. New York, John Wiley, 1962, pp 157–187

Banerjee SP, Sharma VK, Khanna JM: Alteration in beta adrenergic receptor binding during ethanol withdrawal. Nature 276:407–409, 1978

Bannister P, Losowsky M: Cell receptors and ethanol. Alcoholism: Clinical and Experimental Research 10:50S–54S, 1986

Barboriak JJ, Jacobson GR, Cushman P, et al: Chronic alcohol abuse and high density lipoprotein cholesterol. Alcoholism: Clinical and Experimental Research 4:346–349, 1980

Barnett AH, Gonzalez-Auvert C, Pyke DA, et al: Blood concentrations of acetaldehyde during chloropropamide-alcohol flush. Br Med J 283: 939–941, 1981

Barraclough B, Bunch J, Nelson B, et al: A hundred cases of suicide: clinical aspects. Br J Psychiatry 125:355–373, 1974

Baumgartner GR, Rown RC: Clonidine versus chlordiazepoxide in the management of acute alcohol withdrawal syndrome. Arch Intern Med 107:880–884, 1987

Bean MH: Denial and the psychological complications of alcoholism, in Dynamic Approaches to the Understanding and Treatment of Alcoholism. Edited by Bean MH, Zinberg NE. New York, Free Press, 1981, pp 55–96

Beck AT: Depression Inventory. Philadelphia, PA, Philadelphia Center for Cognitive Therapy, 1978

Begleiter H, Porjesz B, Bihari B, et al: Event-related brain potentials in boys at risk for alcoholism. Science 225:1493–1496, 1984

Belfrage P, Berg B, Hagerstrand I, et al: Alteration of lipid metabolism in healthy volunteers during long-term ethanol intake. Eur J Clin Invest 7:127–131, 1977

Benitz KF, Kramer AW, Dambach G: Comparative studies on the morphologic effects of calcium carbimide, propylthiouracil and disulfiram in male rats. Toxicol Appl Pharmacol 7:128–162, 1965

Berglund M: Suicide in alcoholism: a prospective study of 88 suicides, I: the multidimensional diagnosis at first admission. Arch Gen Psychiatry 41:888–891, 1984

Bergstrom B, Ohlin H, Lindblom PE, et al: Is disulfiram implantation effective? Lancet 1:49–50, 1982

Bjorkvist SE: Clonidine in alcohol withdrawal. Acta Psychiatr Scand 52: 256–263, 1975

Bjorkqvist SE, Isohanni M, Makela R, et al: Ambulant treatment of alcohol withdrawal symptoms with carbamazepine: a formal multicentre double-blind comparison with placebo. Acta Psychiatr Scand 53:333–342, 1976

Blum K, Noble EP, Sheridan PJ, et al: Allelic association of human dopamine D$_2$ receptor gene in alcoholism. JAMA 263:2055–2060, 1990

Blume SB: Is social drinking during pregnancy harmless? there is reason to think not. Adv Alcohol Subst Abuse 5:202–219, 1985-86

Boggan WO, Meyer JS, Middaugh LD, et al: Ethanol, calcium, naloxone in mice. Alcoholism: Clinical and Experimental Research 3:158–161, 1979

Bohman M: Genetic aspects of alcoholism and criminality. Arch Gen Psychiatry 35:269–276, 1978

Bohman M, Sigvardsson S, Cloninger R: Maternal inheritance of alcohol abuse. Arch Gen Psychiatry 38:965–969, 1981

Bolos AM, Dean M, Lucas-Derse S, et al: Population and pedigree studies reveal a lack of association between the dopamine D2 receptor gene and alcoholism. JAMA 264:3156–3160, 1990

Brick J, Horowitz GP: Tolerance and cross-tolerance to morphine and ethanol in mice selectively bred for differential sensitivity to ethanol. J Stud Alcohol 44:770–779, 1983

Brown SA, Schuckit MA: Changes in depression among abstinent alcoholics. J Stud Alcohol 49:412, 1988

Brune F, Busch H: Anticonvulsive-sedative treatment of delirium alcoholism. Quarterly Journal of Studies on Alcohol 32:334–342, 1971

Brunner-Orne M: Evaluation of calcium carbimide in the treatment of alcoholism. Journal of Neuropsychiatry 3:163–167, 1962

Brunning J, Mumford JP, Keaney FP: Lofexidine in alcohol withdrawal states. Alcohol Alcohol 21:167, 1986

Bruno F, Casten G: Buspirone treatment of alcoholic patients. Data presented at the Hospital and Community Psychiatry meeting, Boston, MA, 1987

Carlsson A, Henning P, Lindberg P, et al: On the disulfiram-like effect of coprine, the pharmacologically active principle of Coprinus atramentarius. Acta Pharmacologica et Toxicologica 42:292–297, 1978

Carlsson C, Fasth BG: A comparison of the effects of propranolol and diazepam in alcoholics. Br J Addict 71:321–326, 1976

Castelli WP, Doyle JT, Gordon T, et al: Alcohol and blood lipids. Lancet 2:153–155, 1977

Cerderlof R, Friberg L, Lundman T: The interactions of smoking, environment and heredity and their implications for disease aetiology. Acta Med Scand 302(suppl 612):1261–1268, 1977

Chafetz ME: Alcoholism and alcoholic psychoses, in Comprehensive Textbook of Psychiatry, 2nd Edition, Vol 2. Edited by Freedman AM, Kaplan HE, Sadock BJ. Baltimore, Williams & Wilkins, 1975, pp 1331–1348

Chafetz ME: Alcoholism, the response of the National Institute of Alcohol Abuse and Alcoholism. Psychiatric Annals 6:69–96, 1976

Chafetz ME, Blane HT, Abram HS, et al: Establishing treatment relations with alcoholics. J Nerv Ment Dis 134:395–409, 1962

Chalmers DM, Rinsler MG, MacDermott S, et al: Biochemical and haematological indicators of excessive alcohol consumption. Gut 22:992–996, 1981

Chan AW: Racial differences in alcohol sensitivity. Alcohol Alcohol 21:93–104, 1986

Chick J, Longstaff M, Kreitman MP, et al: Plasma [alpha]-amino-n-butyric acid leucine ratio and alcohol consumption in working men and in alcoholics. J Stud Alcohol 43:583–587, 1982

Chu NS: Carbamazepine: prevention of alcohol withdrawal seizures. Neurology 29:1397–1401, 1979

Church AC, Feller D: The influence of mouse genotype on the changes in brain cyclic nucleotide levels induced by acute alcohol administration. Pharmacol Biochem Behav 10:335–338, 1979

Ciraulo DA, Ciraulo AM: Substance abuse, in Handbook of Clinical Psychopharmacology, 2nd Edition. Edited by Tupin JP, Shader RI. Northvale, NJ, Jason Aronson, 1988, p 131

Ciraulo DA, Jaffe JH: Tricyclic antidepressants in the treatment of depression associated with alcoholism. J Clin Psychopharmacol 1:146–150, 1981

Ciraulo DA, Kramer P, Alderson L, et al: Imipramine disposition in alcoholics. J Clin Psychopharmacol 2:2–7, 1982

Ciraulo DA, Barnhill JG, Boxenbaum HG: Pharmacokinetic interaction of disulfiram and antidepressants. Am J Psychiatry 142:1373–1374, 1985

Ciraulo DA, Barnhill JG, Greenblatt DJ, et al: Abuse liability and clinical pharmacokinetics of alprazolam in alcoholic men. J Clin Psychiatry 49:333–337, 1988a

Ciraulo DA, Barnhill JG, Jaffe JH: Clinical pharmacokinetics of imipramine and desipramine in alcoholics and normal volunteers. Clin Pharmacol Ther 43:509–518, 1988b

Ciraulo DA, Sands BF, Shader RI: Critical review of liability for benzodiazepine abuse among alcoholics. Am J Psychiatry 145:1501–1506, 1988c

Ciraulo DA, Barnhill J, Jaffe JH, et al: Clinical pharmacokinetics of 2-hydroxyimipramine in alcoholics and normal volunteers. J Stud Alcohol 51:366–372, 1990

Clarren SK, Smith DW: The fetal alcohol syndrome. N Engl J Med 298:1063–1067, 1978

Cloninger CR: Neurogenetic adaptive mechanisms in alcoholism. Science 236:410–416, 1987

Cloninger CR, Reich T, Wetzel R: Alcoholism and the affective disorders: familial associations and genetic models, in Alcoholism and the Affective Disorders. Edited by Goodwin D, Ericson C. New York, Spectrum, 1979, pp 57–86

Cloninger CR, Sigvardsson S, Bohman M: Childhood personality predicts alcohol abuse in young adults. Alcoholism: Clinical and Experimental Research 12:494, 1988

Coffman JA, Petty F: Plasma GABA levels in chronic alcoholics. Am J Psychiatry 142:1204–1205, 1985

Cornsbruch U, Derwort A: Klinishe Erfahrugen und biochemische Aspekte bei der Behandlung des Alkoholismus mit Calcium carbimid (DIPSAN). International Pharmacopsychiatry 1:143–157, 1968

Cox WM: The alcoholic personality: a review of the evidence. Progress in Experimental Personality Research 9:89–148, 1979

Cruz-Coke R: Color blindness and cirrhosis of the liver. Lancet 2:1064–1065, 1964

Cruz-Coke R, Varela A: Inheritance of alcoholism: its association with color blindness. Lancet 2:1282–1284, 1966

Cushman P, Forbes R, Lerner W, et al: Alcohol withdrawal syndromes: clinical management with lofexidine. Alcoholism: Clinical and Experimental Research 9:103–108, 1985

Danielsson B, Ekman R, Fex G, et al: Changes in plasma high density lipoproteins in chronic male alcoholics during and after abuse. Scand J Clin Lab Invest 38:113–119, 1978

Demakis JG, Proskey A, Rahimtoola SH, et al: The natural course of alcoholic cardiomyopathy. Ann Intern Med 80:293–297, 1974

Dembiec D, McNamee D, Cohen G: The effect of pargyline and other monoamine oxidase inhibitors on blood acetaldehyde levels in ethanol intoxicated mice. J Pharmacol Exp Ther 197:332–339, 1976

Devenji P, Robinson GM, Kapur BM, et al: High density lipoprotein cholesterol in male alcoholics with and without severe liver disease. Am J Med 71:589–594, 1981

Diamond I, Wrubel B, Estrin W, et al: Basal and adenosine receptor-stimulated levels of cAMP are reduced in lymphocytes from alcoholic patients. Proc Natl Acad Sci USA 84:1413–1416, 1987

Diehl AM, Potter J, Boitnott J, et al: Relationship between pyridoxal 5'-phosphate deficiency and aminotransferase levels in alcoholic hepatitis. Gastroenterology 86:632–636, 1984

Dienstag JL, Carter EA, Wands JR, et al: Plasma [alpha]-amino-n-butyric acid to leucine ratio: nonspecificity as a marker for alcoholism. Gastroenterology 75:561–565, 1978

Dodson RA, Johnson WE: Effects of ethanol, arecoline, atropine and nicotine, alone and in various combinations, on rat cerebellar cyclic guanosine 3', 5'-monophosphate. Neuropharmacology 18:871–876, 1979

Dolinsky ZS, Schnitt JM: Discriminant function analysis of clinical laboratory data: use in alcohol research, in Recent Advances in Alcoholism, Vol 6. Edited by Galanter M. New York, Plenum, 1988, pp 367–385

Donovan JM: An etiologic model of alcoholism. Am J Psychiatry 143:1–11, 1986

Drejer K, Theilgaard A, Teasdale TW, et al: A prospective study of young men at high risk for alcoholism: neuropsychological assessment. Alcoholism: Clinical and Experimental Research 9:498–502, 1985

Edwards G: Alcohol dependence: provisional description of a clinical syndrome. Br Med J 1:1058–1061, 1976

Edwards G, Oxford J, Egert S, et al: Alcoholism: a controlled trial of "treatment" and "advice." J Stud Alcohol 38(5):1004–1031, 1977

Egle JL Jr, Hudgins PM, Lai FM: Cardiovascular effects of intravenous acetaldehyde and propionaldehyde in the anaesthetised rat. Toxicol Appl Pharmacol 24:636–664, 1973

Elmasian R, Neville H, Woods D, et al: Event-related brain potentials are different in individuals at high and low risk for developing alcoholism. Proc Natl Acad Sci USA 79:7900–7903, 1982

Engel J, Liljequist S: The effect of long-term ethanol treatment on the sensitivity of the dopamine receptors in the nucleus accumbens. Psychopharmacology 49:253, 1976

Eriksson CJP: Ethanol and acetaldehyde metabolism in rat strains genetically selected for their ethanol preference. Biochem Pharmacol 22:2283–2292, 1973

Ewing JA, Rouse BA: Identifying the hidden alcoholic. Paper presented at the 29th International Conference on Alcoholism and Drug Dependence, Sidney, Australia, February 2–6, 1970

Ewing JA, Rouse BA, Pellizzari ED: Alcohol sensitivity and ethnic background. Am J Psychiatry 131:206–210, 1974

Feldman DJ, Pattison EM, Sobell LC, et al: Outpatient alcohol detoxification: initial findings on 564 patients. Am J Psychiatry 132:407–412, 1975

Fenna D, Mix L, Schaefer O, et al: Ethanol metabolism in various racial groups. Can Med Assoc J 105:472–475, 1971

Ferko AP, Bobyock E, Chernick WS: Regional rat brain content of adenosine 3′, 5′-cyclic monophosphate and guanosine 3′, 5′-cyclic monophosphate after acute and subacute treatment with ethanol. Toxicol Appl Pharmacol 4:447–455, 1982

Fischer I: Saregen svampforgiftning (translation: Peculiar mushroom poisoning). Svenska Lakartidningen 42:2513–2515, 1945

Fisher SE: Ethanol: effect on fetal brain growth and development, in Alcohol and the Brain: Chronic Effects. Edited by Tarter RE, Van Thiel DH. New York, Plenum, 1985, p 265

Fitzgerald MG, Gaddie R, Malins JM, et al: Alcohol sensitivity in diabetics receiving chlorpropamide. Diabetes 2:40–43, 1962

Forsander O, Eriksson K: Forekommer det etnolgiska skillnader i alkoholens amnesomattningen (in Swedish). Alkoholpolitik 37:315, 1974

Fox JE: Outpatient alcoholism coverage to be tried. U.S. Medicine 19:24–25, 1983

Freud S: The Complete Letters of Sigmund Freud to Wilhelm Fleiss. Edited and translated by Masson JM. Cambridge, MA, Harvard University Press, 1985

Freund G: Neuropathology of alcohol abuse, in Alcohol and the Brain: Chronic Effects. Edited by Tarter RE, Van Thiel DH. New York, Plenum, 1985, pp 3–17

Freund G, Ballinger WE: Loss of cholinergic muscarinic receptors in the frontal cortex of alcohol abusers. Alcoholism: Clinical and Experimental Research 12:630, 1988

Frezza M, DiPadova C, Pozzato G, et al: High blood alcohol levels in women: the role of decreased gastric alcohol dehydrogenase activity and first-pass metabolism. N Engl J Med 322:95–99, 1990

Fried R: Biochemical actions of anti-alcoholic agents. Substance and Alcohol Actions/Misuse 1:5, 1980

Frosch WA, Milkman H: Ego functions in drug users. Natl Inst Drug Abuse Res Monogr Ser 12:142–156, 1977

Fuller R, Branchey L, Brightwell DR, et al: Disulfiram treatment of alcoholism: a Veterans Administration cooperative study. JAMA 256: 1449–1455, 1986

Gabrielli WF, Mednick SA, Volavka J, et al: Electroencephalograms in children of alcoholic fathers. Psychophysiology 19:404–407, 1982

Gailis L: Cardiovascular effects of acetaldehyde: evidence for the involvement of tissue SH-groups. Finnish Foundation for Alcohol Studies 23:47–66, 1975

Gerrein JR, Rosenberg CM, Manohar V: Disulfiram maintenance in outpatient treatment of alcoholics. Arch Gen Psychiatry 28:798–802, 1973

Gessner PK: Drug therapy of the alcohol withdrawal syndrome, in The Biochemistry and Pharmacology of Ethanol. Edited by Majchrowicz E, Noble E. New York, Plenum, 1979, pp 375–434

Giller E, Hall H: Platelet MAO activity in recovered alcoholics after long-term abstinence. Am J Psychiatry 140:114–115, 1983

Giller EM, Nocks J, Hall H, et al: Platelet and fibroblast monoamine oxidase in alcoholism. Psychiatry Res 12:339–347, 1984

Goldman GD, Volicer L, Gold BF, et al: Cerebrospinal fluid GABA and cyclic nucleotides in alcoholics with and without seizures. Alcoholism 5:431–434, 1981

Goldstein D: Pharmacology of Alcohol. New York, Oxford University Press, 1983

Goldstein D: Alcohol and biological membranes, in Alcoholism: Biomedical and Genetic Aspects. Edited by Goedde JW, Agarwal DP. New York, Pergamon, 1989, pp 87–98

Goldstein M, Nakajima K: The effect of disulfiram on catecholamine levels in the brain. J Pharmacol Exp Ther 157:96–102, 1967

Goldstein M, Anagnoste B, Lauber E, et al: Inhibition of dopamine-[beta]-hydroxylase by disulfiram. Life Sci 3:763–767, 1964

Goodwin DW: Is Alcoholism Hereditary? New York, Oxford University Press, 1976

Goodwin DW: Alcoholism and heredity. Arch Gen Psychiatry 36:57–61, 1979

Goodwin DW: Genetic determinants of alcoholism, in The Diagnosis and Treatment of Alcoholism. Edited by Mendelson JH, Mello NK. New York, McGraw-Hill, 1985, pp 72–79

Goodwin DW, Reinhard J: Disulfiram-like effect of trichomonoacidal drugs: a review and double-blind study. Quarterly Journal of Studies on Alcohol 33:734–740, 1972

Goodwin DW, Schulsinger F, Hermansen L, et al: Alcohol problems in adoptees raised apart from alcoholic biological parents. Arch Gen Psychiatry 28:238–243, 1973

Goodwin DW, Schulsinger F, Guze SB, et al: Alcoholism and the hyperactive child syndrome. J Nerv Ment Dis 160:349–353, 1975

Gragg DM: Drugs to decrease alcohol consumption. N Engl J Med 306:747, 1982

Greenberg DA, Diamond I: Wernicke-Korsakoff syndrome, in Alcohol and the Brain: Chronic Effects. Edited by Tarter RE, Van Thiel DH. New York, Plenum, 1985, pp 295–314

Greenblatt DJ, Shader RI: Treatment of the alcohol withdrawal syndrome, in Manual of Psychiatric Therapeutics: Practical Psychopharmacology and Psychiatry. Edited by Shader RI. Boston, MA, Little, Brown, 1975, p 211

Gross GA: The use of propranolol as a method to manage acute alcohol detoxification. J Am Osteopath Assoc 82:206–207, 1982

Haertzen AC, Martin WR, Ross FE, et al: Psychopathic State Inventory (PSI): development of a short test for measuring psychopathic states. Int J Addict 15:137–146, 1980

Hanna EZ: Toward determining the importance of context in drinking behavior. Alcoholism (NY) 3:178, 1979

Hansbrough JF, Zapata-Sirvent RL, Carroll WJ, et al: Administration of intravenous alcohol for prevention of withdrawal in alcohol burn patients. Am J Surg 148:266–269, 1984

Hanson JW, Streissguth AP, Smith DW: The effects of moderate alcohol consumption during pregnancy on fetal growth and morphogenesis. J Pediatr 92:457–460, 1978

Harada S, Agarwal DP, Goedde HW: Aldehyde dehydrogenase polymorphism and alcohol metabolism in alcoholics. Alcohol 2:391–392, 1985

Harris RA: Alteration of alcohol effects by calcium and other inorganic cations. Pharmacol Biochem Behav 10:527–534, 1979

Hartung GH, Foreyt JP, Mitchell RE, et al: Effect of alcohol intake on high-density cholesterol levels in runners and in inactive men. JAMA 249:747–750, 1983

Hathaway SR, McKinley JC: Minnesota Multiphasic Personality Inventory. Minneapolis, MN, University of Minnesota, 1943

Herrington RE, Jacobsen GR, Daley ME, et al: Use of the plasma [alpha]-amino-n-butyric acid: leucine ratio to identify alcoholics. J Stud Alcohol 42:492–499, 1981

Hesselbrock MN, Meyer RE, Keener JJ: Psychopathology in hospitalized alcoholics. Arch Gen Psychiatry 42:1050–1055, 1985

Hesselbrock VM, Stabenau JR, Hesselbrock MN: Minimal brain dysfunction and neuropsychological test performance in offspring of alcoholics, in Recent Advances in Alcoholism, Vol 3. Edited by Galanter M. New York, Plenum, 1985, p 65

Hill SY, Aston C, Rabin B: Suggestive evidence of genetic linkage between alcoholism and the MNS blood group. Alcoholism (NY) 12:811–814, 1988

Hines JD, Cowan DH: Studies on the pathogenesis of alcohol-induced sideroblastic bone-marrow abnormalities. N Engl J Med 283:441–446, 1970

Ho AKS, Tsai CS: Effects of lithium on alcohol preference and withdrawal. Ann NY Acad Sci 273:371–377, 1976

Hoberman HD, Chiodo SM: Elevation of the hemoglobin A1 fraction in alcoholism. Alcoholism: Clinical and Experimental Research 6:260–266, 1982

Hoffman H, Loper RG, Kammeier MLP: Identifying future alcoholics with MMPI scales. Quarterly Journal of Studies on Alcohol 35:490–498, 1974

Hoffman P, Tabakoff B: Alterations in dopamine receptor sensitivity by chronic ethanol treatment. Nature 268:551, 1977

Hoffman PL, Tabakoff B: Effects of ethanol on Arrhenius parameters and activity of mouse striatal adenylate cyclase. Biochem Pharmacol 31:3101–3106, 1982

Hoffman PL, Tabakoff B: Ethanol's action on brain biochemistry, in Alcohol and the Brain: Chronic Effects. Edited by Tarter RE, Van Thiel DH. New York, Plenum, 1985, pp 19–68

Holloway HC, Hales RE, Watanabe HK: Recognition and treatment of acute alcohol withdrawal syndromes. Psychiatr Clin North Am 7:729–743, 1984

Hruska RE, Silbergeld EK: Inhibition of ^{3}H-spiroperidol binding by in vitro addition of ethanol. J Neurochem 35:750–752, 1980

Hultber B, Isaksson A, Tiderstrom G: [beta]-hexoaminidase, leucine aminopeptidase, cystidylaminopeptidase, hepatic enzymes and bilirubin in serum of chronic alcoholics with acute ethanol intoxication. Clin Chim Acta 105:317–323, 1980

Hunt WA, Majchronwicz E: Alterations in the turnover of brain norepinephrine and dopamine in alcohol-dependent rats. J Neurochem 23:549–552, 1974

Hunt WA, Redos JD, Dalton TK, et al: Alterations in brain cyclic guanosine 3', 5'-monophosphate levels after acute and chronic treatment with ethanol. J Pharmacol Exp Ther 201:103–109, 1977

Hunt WA, Majchronwicz E, Dalton TK: Alterations in neurotransmitter activity after acute and chronic ethanol treatment studies of transmitter interactions. Alcoholism 3:359, 1979

Isaksson A, Blance C, Hultber B, et al: Influence of ethanol on the human serum level of [beta]-hexosaminidase. Enzyme 33:162–166, 1985

Ishii H, Okuno F, Shigeta Y, et al: Enhanced serum glutamic oxaloacetic transaminase activity of mitochondrial origin in chronic alcoholics, in Currents in Alcoholism, Vol 5. Edited by Galanter M. New York, Grune & Stratton, 1979, pp 101–108

Israel MA, Kimura H, Kuriyama K: Changes in activity and hormonal sensitivity of brain adenylate cyclase. Biochem Pharmacol 31:3101–3106, 1982

Iturriaga H, Pereda T, Estevez A, et al: Serum immunoglobulin A changes in alcoholic patients. Ann Clin Res 9:39, 1977

Jacob MS, Zilm DH, Macleod SM, et al: Propranolol-associated confused states during alcohol withdrawal. J Clin Psychopharmacol 3:185, 1983

Jaffe JH, Ciraulo DA: Drugs used in the treatment of alcoholism, in Diagnosis and Treatment of Alcoholism. Edited by Mendelson JH, Mello NK. New York, McGraw-Hill, 1985, pp 355–389

Jaffe JH, Ciraulo DA: Alcoholism and depression, in Psychopathology and Addictive Disorders. Edited by Meyer RE. New York, Guilford, 1986, pp 293–320

Jaffe JH, Ciraulo DA, Nies A, et al: Abuse potential of halazepam and of diazepam in patients recently treated for acute alcohol withdrawal. Clin Pharmacol Ther 34:623–630, 1983

Jellinek EM: Phases of alcohol addiction. Quarterly Journal of Studies on Alcohol 13:673–684, 1952

Jellinek EM: The Disease Concept of Alcoholism. New Haven, CT, College & University Press, 1960

Jessor R: Perceived opportunity, alienation, and drinking behavior. J Pers Soc Psychol 15:215–222, 1970

Jones JD, Morse RM, Hurt RD: Plasma alpha-amino-n-butyric acid/leucine ration in alcoholics. Alcoholism: Clinical and Experimental Research 5:363–365, 1981

Jones K, Smith DW, Ulleland CN, et al: Pattern of malformation in offspring of chronic alcoholic women. Lancet 1:1267–1271, 1973

Jones K, Smith DW, Streissguth AP, et al: Outcome in offspring of chronic alcoholic women. Lancet 1:1076–1078, 1974

Jonsson E, Nilsson T: Alkoholkonsumption ho s monozygota och dizogota tvillingar (in Swedish). Nord Hyg Tidsk 49:21, 1968

Kaij L: Alcoholism in twins. Studies on the Etiology and Sequels of Abuse of Alcohol. Stockholm, Almqvist and Wiksell, 1960

Kaij L, Dock J: Grandsons of alcoholics. Arch Gen Psychiatry 32:1379–1381, 1975

Kalant H: Interactions of ethanol and neuropeptides, in Research Advances in New Psychopharmacological Treatments for Alcoholism. Edited by Naranjo CA, Sellers EM. New York, Excerpta Medica, 1985, pp 69–86

Kalant H, LeBlanc E, Guttman M, et al: Metabolic and pharmacologic interaction of ethanol and metronidazole in the rat. Can J Physiol Pharmacol 50:476–484, 1971

Kaprio J, Koskenvuo M, Langinvainio H, et al: Genetic influences on use and abuse of alcohol: a study of 5638 adult Finnish twin brothers. Alcoholism: Clinical and Experimental Research 11:349–356, 1987

Kernberg OF: Borderline Conditions and Pathological Narcissism. Northvale, NJ, Jason Aronson, 1975

Kessel N, Grossman G: Suicide in alcoholics. Br Med J 2:1671–1672, 1961

Khantzian EJ: Opiate addiction: a critique of theory and some implications for treatment. Am J Psychother 28:59–70, 1974

Khantzian EJ: Psychopathology, psychodynamics, and alcoholism, in Encyclopedic Handbook of Alcoholism. Edited by Pattison EM, Kaufman E. New York, Gardner, 1982, pp 581–597

Kissin B, Schenker V, Schenker A: The acute effects of ethyl alcohol and chlorpromazine on certain physiological functions in alcoholics. Quarterly Journal of Studies on Alcohol 20:480–492, 1959

Knight R: The psychodynamics of chronic alcoholism. J Nerv Ment Dis 86:538–548, 1937

Knight RP: The psychoanalytic treatment in a sanatorium of chronic addiction to alcohol. JAMA 111:1443–1448, 1938

Knop J: Premorbid assessment of young men at high risk for alcoholism, in

Recent Advances in Alcoholism, Vol 3. Edited by Galanter M. New York, Plenum, 1985, p 53

Knop J, Goodwin D, Teasdale TW, et al: A Danish prospective study of young males at high risk for alcoholism, in Longitudinal Research in Alcoholism. Edited by Goodwin DW, Van Dusen DT, Mednick SA. Boston, MA, Kluwer-Nijhoff, 1984, pp 107–122

Kohut H: The Analysis of the Self. New York, International Universities Press, 1971

Kopun M, Propping P: The kinetics of ethanol absorption and elimination in twins and supplementary repetitive experiments in single subjects. Eur J Clin Pharmacol 11:337–344, 1977

Korri UM, Nuutinen H, Salaspuro M: Increased blood acetate: a new laboratory marker of alcoholism and heavy drinking. Alcoholism: Clinical and Experimental Research 9:468–471, 1985

Korsten MA, Lieber CS: Medical complications of alcoholism, in The Diagnosis and Treatment of Alcoholism. Edited by Mendelson JH, Mello NK. New York, McGraw-Hill, 1985, p 21

Kostowski W, Trazaskowska E: Effects of lesion of the locus coeruleus and clonidine treatment on ethanol withdrawal syndrome in rats. Pol J Pharmacol Pharm 32:617, 1980

Kraus ML, Gottlieb LD, Horwitz RI, et al: Randomized clinical trial of atenolol in patients with alcohol withdrawal. N Engl J Med 313:905–909, 1985

Krystal H: Alexithymia and psychotherapy. Am J Psychother 33:17–31, 1979

Lemoine P, Harroussea H, Borteyru JP, et al.: Les enfants de parents alcooliques: anomalies observees a proposa de 127 cas. Quest Medical 25:477–482, 1968

Lester BK, Rundell OH, Cowden LC, et al: Chronic alcoholism, alcohol, and sleep. Advances in Experimental and Biological Medicine 35:261–279, 1973

Lieber CS: Medical Disorders of Alcoholism: Pathogenesis and Treatment. Philadelphia, PA, WB Saunders, 1982

Liljequist S: Effects of dependence-producing drugs on neurotransmitters and neuronal excitability, in Proceedings European Society on Neurochemistry. Edited by Neuhoff V. New York, Verlag Chemie, 1978, pp 359–373

Lindros KO, Stowell A, Pikkarainen P, et al: The disulfiram (Antabuse)-alcohol reaction in male alcoholics: its efficient management by 4-methylpyrazole. Alcoholism: Clinical and Experimental Research 5:528–530, 1981

Lister RG, Nutt DJ: Alcohol antagonists: the continuing quest. Alcoholism: Clinical and Experimental Research 12:566, 1988

Little RE, Asker RL, Sampson PD, et al: Fetal growth and moderate drinking in early pregnancy. Am J Epidemiol 123:270–278, 1986

Luthin GR, Tabakoff B: Effects of ethanol on calmodulin levels in mouse striatum and cerebral cortex. Alcoholism: Clinical and Experimental Research 8:68–72, 1984

Alcoholism   85

MacAndrew C: The differentiation of male alcoholic outpatients from non-alcoholic psychiatric outpatients by means of the MMPI. Quarterly Journal of Studies on Alcohol 26:238–246, 1965

Mack JC: Alcoholism, A.A., and the governance of the self, in Dynamic Approaches to the Understanding and Treatment of Alcoholism, Edited by Bean MN, Zinberg NE. New York, Free Press, 1981, pp 128–162

Madalena JC, De Mattos HG: Use of metronidazole in alcoholism. Hospital (Rio de Janeiro) 71:481–488, 1967

Major LF, Murphy DL: Platelet and plasma amine oxidase activity in alcoholic individuals. Br J Psychiatry 132:548–554, 1978

Major LF, Ballenger JC, Goodwin FK, et al: Cerebrospinal fluid homovanillic acid in male alcoholics: effects of disulfiram. Biol Psychiatry 12:635–642, 1977

Major LF, Lerner P, Ballenger JC, et al: Dopamine beta-hydroxylase in the cerebrospinal fluid: relationship to disulfiram induced psychosis. Biol Psychiatry 14:337, 1979a

Major LF, Murphy DL, Gershon ES, et al: The role of plasma amine oxidase, platelet monoamine oxidase, and red cell catechol-O-methyltransferase in severe behavioral reactions to disulfiram. Am J Psychiatry 136:679–684, 1979b

Markley HG, Mezey E: Induction of alcohol withdrawal by nalorphine in chronic alcoholic patients. Int J Addict 13:395–402, 1978

Matloff DS, Seligran MJ, Kaplan MM: Hepatic transaminase activity in alcoholic liver disease. Gastroenterology 78:1389–1392, 1980

Mayfield D, McLeod G, Hall P: The CAGE questionnaire: validation of a new alcoholism screening instrument. Am J Psychiatry 131:1121–1123, 1974

McCarty D, Ewing JA: Are the endorphins involved in mediating the mood effects of ethanol? Alcoholism: Clinical and Experimental Research 7:271–275, 1983

McLellan AT, Luborsky L, Woody GE, et al: Predicting response to alcohol and drug abuse treatments. Arch Gen Psychiatry 40:620–625, 1983

McLellan AT, Luborsky L, O'Brien CP: Alcohol and drug abuse treatment in three different populations: is there improvement and is it predictable? Am J Drug Alcohol Abuse 12:101–120, 1986

McNichol RN, Ewing JA, Faiman M: Disulfiram (Antabuse®): A Unique Medical Aid to Sobriety: History, Pharmacology, Research, Clinical Use. Springfield, IL, Charles C Thomas, 1987

Mello NK: Alcohol Abuse and Reproductive Function in Women, in Recent Developments in Alcoholism, Vol 6. Edited by Galanter M. New York, Plenum, 1988, pp 253–276

Mendelson JH, Ogata M, Mello NK: Adrenal function and alcoholism, I: serum cortisol. Psychosom Med 33:145–157, 1971

Meyers RD, Melchior CM: Differential actions on voluntary alcohol intake of tetrahydroisoquinolines or a beta-carboline infused chronically in the ventricle of the rat. Pharmacol Biochem Behav 7:381–392, 1977

Michaelis EK, Mulvaney, MJ, Freed WJ: Effects of acute and chronic ethanol intake on synaptosomal glutamate binding activity. Biochem Pharmacol 27:1685–1691, 1978

Michaelis EK, Change HH, Roy S, et al: Ethanol effects on synaptic glutaanol intake on synaptosomal glutamate binding activity. Biochem Pharmacol 27:1685–1691, 1978

Michaelis EK, Change HH, Roy S, et al: Ethanol effects on synaptic gluta-mate receptor functions and on membrane lipid organization. Pharmacol Biochem Behav 18 (suppl 1):1–6, 1983

Miller LG, Greenblatt DJ, Barnhill JG, et al: Differential modulation of benzodiazepine receptor binding by ethanol in LS and SS mice. Pharmacol Biochem Behav 29:471–477, 1988

Miller NS, Goodwin DW, Jones FC, et al: Antihistamine blockade of alcohol-induced flushing in orientals. J Stud Alcohol 49:16–20, 1988

Morgan Y, Milsom JP, Sherlock S: Ratio of plasma [alpha]-amino-n-butyric acid to leucine as an empirical marker of alcoholism: diagnostic value. Science 197:1183–1185, 1977

Moser J: Prevention of Alcohol-Related Problems. Toronto, Alcoholism and Drug Addiction Research Foundation, 1980

Moss HB, Gutherie S, Linnoila M: Enhanced thyrotropin response to thyrotropin releasing hormone in boys at risk for development of alcoholism. Arch Gen Psychiatry 43:1137–1142, 1987

Mueller GC: Synthesis of phosphatidylethanol: a potential marker for adult males at risk for alcoholism. Proc Natl Acad Sci USA 85:9778–9782, 1988

Murphy GE, Armstrong JW Jr, Hermele SL, et al: Suicide and alcoholism: interpersonal loss confirmed as a predictor. Arch Gen Psychiatry 36:65–69, 1979

Musacchio JM, Goldstein M, Anagnoste B, et al: Inhibition of dopamine-beta-hydroxylase by disulfiram in vivo. J Pharmacol Exp Ther 152: 56–61, 1966

Musto DF: The American Disease. New Haven, CT, Yale University Press, 1973

Myers JK, Weissman MW, Tischler GL, et al: Six-month prevalence of psychiatric disorders in three communities. Arch Gen Psychiatry 41:959–967, 1984

Myers RD, Critcher EC: Naloxone alters alcohol drinking induced in the rat by tetrahydropapaveroline (THP) infused ICV. Pharmacol Biochem Behav 16:827–836, 1982

Nakano J, Gin AC, Nakano SK: Effects of disulfiram on cardiovascular responses to acetaldehyde and ethanol in dogs. Quarterly Journal of Studies on Alcohol 35:620–634, 1974

Nalpas B, Vassault A, Le Guillou A, et al: Serum activity of mitochondrial aspartate aminotransferase: a sensitive marker of alcoholism with or without alcoholic hepatitis. Hepatology 5:893–896, 1984

Naranjo CA: Moderation of ethanol drinking: role of enhanced serotenergic neurotransmission, in Research Advances in New Psychopharmacological Treatments for Alcoholism. Edited by Naranjo CA, Sellers EM. New York, Excerpta Medica, 1985, p 171

National Council on Alcoholism Criteria Committee: Criteria for the diagnosis of alcoholism. Ann Intern Med 77:249–258, 1972

National Institute on Drug Abuse: National Household Survey on Drug

Abuse: Main Findings 1985 (DHHS Publ No ADM-88-1586). Rockville, MD, US Department of Health and Human Services, 1988

Neubuerger OW, Matarazzo JD, Schmitz RE, et al: Behavioral-chemical treatment of alcoholism: an outcome replication. J Stud Alcohol 42:806–810, 1981

Nguyen MH, Gailis L: Effect of acetaldehyde on the isolated, non-working guinea pig heart: independence of the coronary flow increase from changes in heart rate and oxygen consumption. Can J Physiol Pharmacol 52:602–612, 1974

Nora AH, Nora JJ, Blu J: Limb reduction anomalies in infants born to disulfiram-treated alcoholic mothers (letter). Lancet 2:664, 1977

Nordberg A, Larsson C, Perdahl E, et al: Changes in cholinergic activity in human hippocampus following chronic alcohol abuse. Pharmacol Biochem Behav 18 (suppl 1):397–400, 1983

Nutt D, Molyneux S, Clark E: Alpha-2-adrenoceptor function in alcohol withdrawal: a pilot study of the effects of IV clonidine in alcoholics and normals. Alcoholism: Clinical and Experimental Research 12:14–18, 1988

Orenberg EK, Renson J, Barchas JD: The effects of alcohol on cyclic AMP in mouse brain. Neurochem Res 1:659–667, 1976a

Orenberg EK, Zarcone VP, Renson JF et al: The effects of ethanol ingestion on cyclic AMP, homovanillic acid and 5-hydroxyindoleacetic acid in human cerebrospinal fluid. Life Sci 19:1669–1672, 1976b

Panteghini M, Falsetti F, Chiari E, et al: Determination of aspartate aminotransferase isoenzymes in hepatic diseases: preliminary findings. Clin Chim Acta 128:133–140, 1983

Partanen J, Bruun K, Markkanen T: Inheritance of Drinking Behavior. New Brunswick, NJ, Rutgers University Center of Alcohol Studies, 1966

Pattison EM: Types of alcoholism reflective of character disorders, in Character Pathology Theory and Treatment. Edited by Zales MR. New York, Brunner/Mazel, 1984, pp 84–116

Peachey JE: A comparative review of the pharmacological and toxicological properties of disulfiram and calcium carbimide. J Clin Psychopharmacol 1:21–26, 1981a

Peachey JE: The disulfiram and calcium carbimide acetaldehyde-mediated ethanol reactions. Pharmacol Ther 15:89–97, 1981b

Peachey JE: Clinical uses of the alcohol-sensitizing drugs, in Pharmacological Treatments for Alcoholism. Edited by Edwards G, Little J. New York, Croom Helm, 1984, p 531

Peachey JE, Brien JF, Loomis CW: A study of the calcium carbimide-ethanol interaction in man: symptom response. Alcoholism: Clinical and Experimental Research 4:322–329, 1980

Peeples EE: Taste sensitivity to phenylthiocarbamide in alcoholics. Masters thesis, Stetson University, Deland, Florida, as cited in Goodwin DW: Genetic determinants of alcoholism, in The Diagnosis and Treatment of Alcoholism. Edited by Mendelson JH, Mello NK. New York, McGraw-Hill, 1985, p 73

Perez A: Modification of ethanol metabolism in the rat by disulfiram and metronidazole. Thesis, Purdue University, West Lafayette, IN, 1974

Pfefferbaum A, Horvath TB, Roth WT, et al: Event-related potential changes in chronic alcoholics. Electroencephalogr Clin Neurophysiol 47:637–647, 1979

Pollock VE, Volavka J, Goodwin DW, et al: The EEG after alcohol administration in men at risk for alcoholism. Arch Gen Psychiatry 40: 857–861, 1983

Porteus SD: The Porteus Maze Test. San Antonio, TX, Psychological Corporation, 1933

Post RM, Ballenger JC, Putnam F, et al: Carbamazepine in alcohol withdrawal syndromes: relationship to the kindling model. J Clin Psychopharmacol 3:205–207, 1983

Poutanen P: Experience with carbamazepine in the treatment of withdrawal symptoms in alcohol abusers. Br J Addict 74:201–204, 1979

Puchois P, Fontan M, Gentilini JL, et al: Serum apolipoprotein A-II, a biochemical indicator of alcohol abuse. Clin Chim Acta 185:185–189, 1984

Rabin RA, Molinoff PB: Activation of adenylate cyclase by ethanol in mouse striatal tissue. J Pharmacol Exp Ther 216:129–134, 1981

Rabin RA, Wolfe BB, Dibner MD, et al: Effects of ethanol administration and withdrawal in neurotransmitter receptor systems in mice. J Pharmacol Exp Ther 213:491–496, 1980

Rado S: The psychoanalysis of pharmacothymia. Psychoanal Q 2:1–23, 1933

Reed TE, Kalant H, Gibbins RJ, et al: Alcohol and acetaldehyde metabolism in Caucasians, Chinese and Amerinds. Can Med Assoc J 115: 851–855, 1976

Reilly TM: Peripheral neuropathy associated with citrated calcium carbimide. Lancet 1:911–912, 1976

Reitan RM: Halstead-Reitan Neuropsychological Test Battery. Tucson, AZ, Neuropsychology Laboratory, University of Arizona, 1979

Rej R: Aspartate aminotransferase activity and isoenzyme proportions in human liver tissues. Clin Chem 24:1971–1979, 1978

Riley EP, Freed EX, Lester D: Selective breeding of rats for differences in reactivity to alcohol: an approach to an animal model of alcoholism, I: general procedures. J Stud Alcohol 37:1535–1547, 1976

Ritola E, Malinen L: A double-blind comparison of a carbamazepine and clomethiazole in the treatment of alcohol withdrawal syndrome. Acta Psychiatr Scand 64:254–259, 1981

Robins E: The Final Months: A Study of the Lives of 134 Persons Who Committed Suicide. New York, Oxford University Press, 1981

Robinson BJ, Robinson GM, Maling TJB, et al: Is clonidine useful in the treatment of alcohol withdrawal? Alcoholism: Clinical and Experimental Research 13:95–98, 1989

Roe A: The adult adjustment of children of alcoholic parents raised in foster homes. Quarterly Journal of Studies on Alcohol 5:378–393, 1944

Rothstein E, Clancy DD: Combined use of disulfiram and metronidazole in treatment of alcoholism. Quarterly Journal of Studies on Alcohol 31:446–47, 1970

Rounsaville BJ, Dolinsky ZS, Babor TF, et al: Psychopathology as a predictor of treatment outcome in alcoholics. Arch Gen Psychiatry 44:505–513, 1987

Rush B: Inquiry into the effects of ardent spirits upon the human body and mind (1785). Quarterly Journal of Studies on Alcohol 4:321–341, 1943

Ryback RS, Eckhardt MJ, Pautler CP: Biochemical and hematological correlates of alcoholism. Res Commun Chem Pathol Pharmacol 27:533–550, 1980

Salaspuro M: Conventional and coming laboratory markers of alcoholism and heavy drinking. Alcoholism: Clinical and Experimental Research 10 (suppl):55–125, 1986

Sampliner R, Iber FL: Diphenylhydantoin control of alcohol withdrawal seizures: results of a controlled study. JAMA 230:1430–1432, 1974

Sandoz M, Vandel S, Vandel B, et al: Biotransformation of amitriptyline in alcoholic depressive patients. Eur J Clin Pharmacol 24:615–621, 1983

Schaefer MR, Sobieraj K, Hollyfield RL: Severity of alcohol dependence and its relationship to additional psychiatric symptoms in male alcoholic inpatients. Am J Drug Alcohol Abuse 13:435–447, 1987

Schuckit MA: Differences in plasma cortisol after ethanol in relatives of alcoholics and controls. J Clin Psychiatry 45:374-379, 1984a

Schuckit MA: Subjective responses to alcohol in sons of alcoholics and controls. Arch Gen Psychiatry 41:879–884, 1984b

Schuckit MA: Ethanol-induced body sway in men at high alcoholism risk. Arch Gen Psychiatry 42:375–379, 1985

Schuckit MA: Goodwin DW, Winokur G: A half-sibling study of alcoholism. Am J Psychiatry 128:1132–1136, 1972

Schuckit MA, Sweeney S, Huey L: Hyperactivity and the risk for alcoholism. J Clin Psychiatry 48:275–277, 1987

Schuckit MA, Risch SC, Gold EO: Alcohol consumption, ACTH level, and family history of alcoholism. Am J Psychiatry 145:1391–1395, 1988

Sellers EM, Kalant H: Alcohol intoxication and withdrawal. N Engl J Med 294:757–762, 1975

Sellers EM, Naranjo CA, Peachey JE: Drugs to decrease alcohol consumption. N Engl J Med 305:1255–1262, 1981

Selzer ML: The Michigan Alcoholism Screening Test: the quest for a new diagnostic instrument. Am J Psychiatry 27:89–94, 1971

Seto A, Tricomi S, Goodwin DW, et al: Biochemical correlates of ethanol-induced flushing in orientals. J Stud Alcohol 39:1–11, 1978

Shaw GK: Alcohol dependence and withdrawal. Br Med Bull 38:99–102, 1982

Shaw S, Lieber CS: Increased plasma amino-n-butyric acid (AANB) due to excess hepatic production: a biochemical marker of alcoholism. Clin Res 25:449A, 1977

Shaw S, Lieber CS: Plasma amino acid abnormalities in the alcoholic: respective role of alcohol, nutrition, and liver injury. Gastroenterology 74:677–682, 1978

Shaw S, Stimmel B, Lieber CS: Plasma [alpha]-amino-n-butyric acid to leucine ratio: an empirical biochemical marker of alcoholism. Science 194:1057–1058, 1976

Shaw S, Worner TM, Borysow MF, et al: Detection of alcoholism relapse: comparative diagnostic value of MCV, GGTP, and AANB. Alcoholism: Clinical and Experimental Research 3:297–301, 1979

Shen A, Jacobyansky A, Smith T, et al: Cyclic adenosine 3',5'-monophosphate, adenylate cyclase and physical dependence on ethanol: studies with tranylcypromine. Drug Alcohol Depend 2:431–440, 1977

Sheppard JR, Albersheim P, McClearn G: Aldehyde dehydrogenase and ethanol preference in mice. J Biol Chem 245:2876–2882, 1970

Shippenberg TS, Altshuler HL: A drug discrimination analysis of ethanol-induced behavioral excitation and sedation: the role of endogenous opiate pathways. Alcohol 2:197–201, 1985

Sinclair JD, Rusi M, Airaksinen MM, et al: Relating TIQ's, opiates, and ethanol. Prog Clin Biol Res 90:365–376, 1982

Smith BR, Amit Z, Aragon CMG, et al: Neurobiological correlates of ethanol self-administration: the role of acetaldehyde, in Research Advances in New Psychopharmacological Treatments for Alcoholism. Edited by Naranjo CA, Sellers EM. New York, Excepta Medica, 1985, pp 45–67

Smith DE: Use of psychotropic drugs in alcoholism treatment: a summary. Addictions Alert 2:48, 1989

Smith DW: The fetal alcohol syndrome. Hosp Prac [Off] 14:121–128, 1979

Stamatoyanopoulos G, Chen S-H, Kukio M: Liver alcohol dehydrogenase in Japanese: high population frequency of atypical form and its possible role in alcohol sensitivity. Am J Hum Genet 27:789–796, 1975

Stevens VJ, Fantl WJ, Newman CB, et al: Acetaldehyde adducts with hemoglobin. J Clin Invest 67:361–369, 1981

Stone AR, Neustadt JO, Imber SD, et al: An interview method for assessing alcoholism. Am J Orthopsychiatry 35:564–572, 1965

Strauss GD, Sack DA, Lesser I: Which veterans go to VA psychiatric hospitals for care: a pilot study. Hosp Community Psychiatry 36:962–965, 1985

Stromland K: Ocular involvement in the fetal alcohol syndrome. Surv Ophthalmol 31:277–284, 1987

Sullivan JL, Stanfield CN: Platelet monoamine oxidase and serum dopamine-b-hydroxylase activity in chronic alcoholics. Arch Gen Psychiatry 35:1209–1212, 1978

Sullivan JL, Cavenar JO, Maltbie AA, et al: Familial biochemical and clinical correlates of alcoholics with low platelet monoamine oxidase activity. Biol Psychiatry 14:385, 1979

Sutherland FH, Schroeder HG, Tordella CL: Personality traits and the alcoholic. Quarterly Journal of Studies on Alcohol 11:547–561, 1950

Swinson RP: Genetic markers and alcoholism, in Recent Developments in Alcoholism. Edited by Galanter M. New York, Plenum, 1983, pp 9–24

Swinson RP, Madden JS: ABO blood groups and ABH substance secretion in alcoholics. Quarterly Journal of Studies on Alcohol 34:64–70, 1973

Syme L: Personality characteristics and the alcoholic. Quarterly Journal of Studies on Alcohol 18:288–302, 1957

Sytinsky IA, Guzikov BM, Gomanko MV, et al: The gamma-aminobutyric acid (GABA) system in brain during acute and chronic ethanol intoxication. J Neurochem 25:43–48, 1975

Tabakoff B, Hoffman PL: Biochemical pharmacology of alcohol, in Psychopharmacology: The Third Generation of Progress. Edited by Meltzer HY. New York, Raven, 1987, pp 1521–1533

Tabakoff B, Munoz-Marcus M, Fields JZ: Chronic ethanol feeding produces an increase in muscarinic cholinergic receptors in mouse brain. Life Sci 25:2173–3180, 1979

Tabakoff B, Luthin GR, Saito T, et al: Effects of ethanol on receptor-adenylate cyclase coupling. Federal Process 42:902, 1983

Tabakoff B, Hoffman PL, Lee JM, et al: Differences in platelet enzyme activity between alcoholics and nonalcoholics. N Engl J Med 318:134–139, 1988

Tanna VL, Wilson AF, Winokur G, et al: Possible linkage between alcoholism and esterase-D. J Stud Alcohol 49:472–476, 1988

Tarter RE, Hegedus AM, Gavaler JS: Hyperactivity in sons of alcoholics. J Stud Alcohol 46:259–261, 1985a

Tarter RE, Alterman AI, Edwards KL: Vulnerability to alcoholism in men: a behavior-genetic perspective. J Stud Alcohol 46:329–356, 1985b

Thorarinsson AA: Mortality among men alcoholics in Iceland, 1951–74. J Stud Alcohol 40:704–718, 1979

Tottmar O, Hellstrom E: Blood pressure response to ethanol in relation to acetaldehyde levels and dopamine-beta-hydroxylase activity in rats pretreated with disulfiram, cyanamide and coprine. Acta Pharmacologica et Toxicologica 45:2272–2281, 1979

Towle AC, Sze PY: Chronic ethanol reduces brain calmodulin levels. Transactions of the American Society of Neurochemistry 12:88, 1981

Triana E, Frances RJ, Stokes PE: The relationship between endorphins and alcohol induced subcortical activity. Am J Psychiatry 137:491–493, 1980

Truitt EB Jr, Walsh MJ: The role of acetaldehyde in the actions of ethanol, in The Biology of Alcoholism, Vol 1. Edited by Kissin B, Begleiter H. New York, Plenum, 1971, 161–195

Urbano-Marquez A, Estruch R, Navarro-Lopez F: The effects of alcoholism on skeletal and cardiac muscle. N Engl J Med 320:409–415, 1989

Vaillant GE: Dangers of psychotherapy in the treatment of alcoholism, in Dynamic Approaches to the Understanding and Treatment of Alcoholism. Edited by Bean MH, Zinberg NE. New York, Free Press, 1981, pp 36–54

Vaillant GE: The Natural History of Alcoholism: Causes, Patterns and Paths to Recovery. Cambridge, MA, Harvard University Press, 1983

Van Thiel DH, Gavaler JS: Endocrine effects of chronic alcohol abuse: hypothalamic-pituitary-gonadal axis, in Alcohol and the Brain: Chronic Effects. Edited by Tarter RE, Van Thiel DH. New York, Plenum, 1985a, pp 69–77

Van Thiel DH, Gavaler JS: Myocardial effects of alcohol abuse: clinical and physiologic consequences, in Recent Advances in Alcoholism, Vol

3. Edited by Galanter M. New York, Plenum, 1985b, pp 181–187

Varela A, Rivera L, Mardones J, et al: Color vision defects in non-alcoholic relatives of alcoholic parents. Br J Addict 64:67, 1969

Vazquez JJ, Cervera S: Cyanamide-induced liver in alcoholics. Lancet 1:361–362, 1980

Vesell ES, Page JG, Passananti GT: Genetic and environmental factors affecting ethanol metabolism in man. Clin Pharmacol Ther 12:192, 1971

Volavka J, Pollock V, Gabrielli WF, et al: The EEG in persons at risk for alcoholism, in Recent Advances in Alcoholism, Vol 3. Edited by Galanter M. New York, Plenum, 1985, p 21

Volicer L, Hurter BP: Effects of acute and chronic ethanol administration and withdrawal on adenosine 3′,5′-monophosphate and guanosine 3′,5′-monophosphate levels in the rat brain. J Pharmacol Exp Ther 200:298–305, 1977

von Hungen K, Baxter CF: Sensitivity of rat brain adenylate cyclase to activation by calcium and ethanol after chronic exposure to ethanol. Biochem Biophys Res Commun 106:1078–1082, 1982

Walinder J, Balldin J, Bokstrom K, et al: Clinidine suppression of the alcohol withdrawal syndrome. Drug Alcohol Depend 8:345–348, 1981

Warner RH, Rosett HL: The effects of drinking on offspring: an historical survey of the American and British literature. J Stud Alcohol 36:1395–1420, 1975

Wechsler D: Wechsler Adult Intelligence Scale-Revised. San Antonio, TX, Psychological Corporation, 1981

Wellman M: The late withdrawal symptoms of alcoholic addiction. Can Med Assoc J 70:526, 1954

Whitfield EL, Thompson G, Lamb A, et al: Detoxification of 1,024 alcoholic patients without psychoactive drugs. JAMA 293:1409–1410, 1978

Wiberg A, Gottfies CG, Oreland L: Low platelet monoamine oxidase activity in human alcoholics. Med Biol 55:181–186, 1977

Wilkins AJ, Jenkins WJ, Steiner JA; Efficacy of clonidine in treatment of alcohol withdrawal state. Psychopharmacology 81:78–80, 1983

Wilson A, Davidson WJ, Blanchard R: Disulfiram implantation: trial using placebo implants and two types of controls. J Stud Alcohol 41:4299–4436, 1980

Witkin HA, Karp SA, Goodenough DR: Dependence in alcoholics. Quarterly Journal of Studies on Alcohol 20:493–504, 1959

Wolff PH: Ethnic differences in alcohol sensitivity. Science 175:449–450, 1972

Wolff PH: Vasomotor sensitivity to alcohol in diverse Mongoloid populations. Am J Hum Genet 25:193–199, 1973

Yamamoto HA, Harris RA: Calcium-dependent ^{86}Rb efflux and ethanol intoxication: studies of human red blood cells and rodent brain synaptosomes. Eur J Pharmacol 88:357–363, 1983

Yoshida K, Engle J, Liljequist S: The effect of chronic ethanol administration on high affinity ^{3}H-nicotinic binding in rat brain. Archives of Pharmacology 321:74–76, 1982

Zilm DH, Sellers EH, MacLeod SM, et al: Propranolol effect on tremor in alcohol withdrawal. Ann Intern Med 83:234–236, 1975

Zimmer R, Cramer J, Athen D, et al: Changes in cerebrospinal fluid cyclic nucleotides in alcohol-dependent patients suffering from delerium tremens. Biol Psychiatry 17:837–843, 1982

Zinberg NE: Alcohol addiction: toward a more comprehensive definition, in Dynamic Approaches to the Understanding and Treatment of Alcoholism. Edited by Bean MH, Zinberg NE. New York, Free Press, 1981, pp 97–127

Zung WWK: Self-Rating Depression Scale. Cincinnati, OH, Merrell-National Laboratories, 1974

Chapter 2

Opioids

Jerome H. Jaffe, M.D.
Steven Epstein, M.D.
Domenic A. Ciraulo, M.D.

A BRIEF HISTORY

In the mid-19th century, it was the custom for doctors to frequently prescribe morphine (first isolated from opium by Seturner in 1806) and other opium preparations. The public also had ready access to opium and purified drugs in grocery stores and pharmacies. Medicinal mixtures and nostrums, usually unlabelled as to contents, often contained opium or morphine. By the end of the century, many physicians had come to recognize that chronic use of morphine was a disorder (morphinism), although others in society viewed it as a vice. After the passage of the Harrison Act in 1914, legal use of opioids was restricted and opioids were no longer available except by prescription. Within a few years, increasing numbers of people were using opioids obtained illicitly. Some U.S. Supreme Court decisions at this time appeared to support the position that the prescription of an opioid to an addict was not the proper practice of medicine and was, therefore, illegal. Physicians who prescribed opioids to addicts were tried and censored, and a few were imprisoned. By the early 1920s, people addicted to opioids often were denied hospital treatment for medical problems.

Between the 1930s and the late 1950s, it was recognized that addiction itself needed to be treated, but prolonged hospitalization was essentially the only treatment recommended and available. In the late 1950s, the first therapeutic community for drug addicts was established. In the early 1960s, California and New York initiated compulsory commitment for treatment. At about the same time, Dole and Nyswander (1965) showed that maintenance on daily doses of methadone led to reduction in heroin use and in associated criminal activity. The use of narcotic antagonists for treatment of opiate addiction was also tried at this time. By the 1970s, concern about the increasing number of heroin addicts, along with the recognition that many opioid addicts could return to active, law-abiding participation in society during and after treatment, led to expansion of community-based treatment programs and of resources for research (Jaffe 1989). Currently, there is extensive research under way in areas related to opioid dependence, from the characterization of opioid receptors and second messengers to the psychosocial and pharmacological treatment of opioid-dependent people.

PREVALENCE AND NATURAL HISTORY

The National Institute on Drug Abuse National Household Survey on Drug Abuse (National Institute on Drug Abuse 1988) found that 1.2% of persons aged 18–25 reported using heroin at some time in their lives. However, less than 0.5% reported use during the preceding month. (Household surveys may underestimate use since they do not sample individuals in jail or hospitals or those without fixed residences.) In urban areas, heroin use among men is approximately three times that among women.

Misuse of other opioids is far more common than heroin use. As is true for heroin, nonmedical use of opioids other than heroin is predominantly a problem of young adults. Lifetime use varies by race and socioeconomic class. College graduates are less likely to use opioids than high school dropouts. Health professionals have a much higher incidence than others with comparable education.

Opioid dependence rarely results from the prescribing of opioids temporarily for treatment of acute pain or pain of terminal illness. Even use in chronic pain does not inevitably lead to opioid abuse and dependence. In a study of chronic opioid use to treat nonmalignant pain, problems developed in only 2 of 38 patients, both of whom had a prior history of drug abuse (Portenoy and Foley 1986). If patients are properly screened and treatment is monitored, opioids can be vital drugs for analgesia of chronic pain not responsive to nonopioid treatment.

Pentazocine (Talwin) and the antihistamine tripelennamine (a blue tablet), known as "Ts and blues," produce an effect that is both opioid-like and reinforcing when they are injected intravenously in combination. In the late 1970s, this combination became a significant problem in certain urban areas of the United States. In 1983, the oral preparation of Talwin was replaced with Talwin Nx, a Talwin-naloxone combination that includes 0.5 mg of the opioid antagonist. At this dose, naloxone is inactive orally but, if injected intravenously, it blocks some of the effects of pentazocine. Although there continue to be some reports of abuse of Talwin Nx (Reed and Schnoll 1986), the reformulation has significantly reduced pentazocine abuse (Baum et al. 1987).

Although many who experiment with opioids experience euphoria or symptom relief with the first use, some experimenters use these drugs only a few times and then avoid further use because of a cognitive appreciation of the risks or because of unpleasant side effects such as nausea or vomiting. Even for those who become dependent, the most common pattern in Western cultures where the drug is illegal is one of alternating periods of use and abstinence, whether voluntary or brought about by external pressure. Typically, without supervision, within 6 months after detoxification as many as two-thirds will relapse, most of these within the first few months.

Addicts who voluntarily abstain often state they do so simply because they are tired of their life-styles of constant drug seeking and frequent encounters with the law. The average time from addiction to first treatment is now approximately 2–3 years. Opioid addicts who do not seek treatment have less psychopathology, fewer legal problems, more adequate social functioning, but not less drug dependence (Rounsaville and Kleber 1985b). Many opioid users recover without ever having formal treatment. For those arrested, time from first use to first arrest ranges from 6 months to 5 years. In the 1970s, some experts estimated the average length of active addiction from the first use to be about 9 years. "Maturing out" (or stopping opioid use as an overall result of the passage of time) is less likely for addicts involved in crime and drug dealing (Anglin et al. 1986).

The life-styles of opioid addicts in Great Britain and the United

States who are involved in treatment are far from uniform. Some, like health professionals, may hold jobs; others, "Loners," live mainly on legitimate earnings supplemented by some criminal activities or live on welfare. The stereotypical "junkies" socialize within an addict subculture and earn their income primarily from illegal activities, including drug dealing (Stimson and Oppenheimer 1982).

There have been several long-term follow-up studies of addicts who sought treatment from publicly supported programs. In one study, selected daily opioid users who entered treatment in 1969–1974 were followed up 12 years after initial treatment; 24% of the males had used opioids daily during the previous year, and 25% reported they had never returned to daily opioid use (Simpson and Marsh 1986; Simpson et al. 1982, 1986). Of the sample, 35% never relapsed after they had quit. During the previous year, 13% had been arrested, and 29% had spent time in jail or prison.

Another study interviewed more than 10,000 drug addicts who entered treatment during 1979–1981 and reinterviewed a sample of these individuals 3–5 years later (Hubbard et al. 1989). Heroin use declined during and following treatment. For those who stayed in treatment, regular use of heroin declined from 63.5% before treatment to 17.5% 3–5 years later. In general, physicians and other health professionals have a remarkably good prognosis when their license to practice is made contingent on continued abstinence and their drug use is monitored by random urine tests. Most studies report abstinence rates of 65–75% 1–2 years after initial treatment (Herrington et al. 1982). Somewhat lower success has been reported for anesthesia residents. One study reported that only 34% of parenteral opioid abusers in residency training for anesthesia successfully reentered training, compared with 70% of anesthesiology residents who abused other substances (Menk et al. 1990).

Currently, there are no reliable means to predict an individual's long-term prognosis as measured by drug use, work, crime, and psychological adjustment. Although the achievement of even temporary abstinence is associated with improvement in a number of factors (legal problems in particular), simply attaining abstinence does not ensure complete psychosocial adjustment. Therefore, other problem areas must be addressed as well. In general, outcome in a particular area (e.g., work or crime) is best predicted by past behavior with respect to that area (Kosten et al. 1987a; Rounsaville et al. 1987).

PHARMACOLOGY

The term *opioid* currently refers to any exogenous substance that acts as an agonist at any of several receptors. Opioid antagonists are drugs that bind to a receptor but produce no actions. The poppy plant, *Papaver somniferum*, from which opium is obtained, is grown in many areas of the world. Morphine constitutes 10% of opium, and codeine can be obtained directly from opium. Semisynthetic opioids such as heroin and oxycodone are obtained directly or indirectly from morphine. There are other distinct chemical classes of drugs with opioid actions, including the methadones.

Central nervous system effects of opioids include analgesia, sedation, "mental clouding" (apathy and difficulty concentrating), mood changes, nausea, and vomiting. In abstinent addicts, euphoria is greater and mental clouding is less pronounced than in normal subjects. Tolerance develops to these effects with chronic use. Opioids acutely inhibit gonadotropin-releasing hormone and corticotropin-releasing hormone secretion but tolerance develops with chronic use. Therefore, male methadone patients who have been maintained for more than a year on stable doses generally have been found to have normal levels of cortisol, luteinizing hormone, and testosterone (for general references, see Jaffe 1990; Jaffe and Martin 1990).

Major gastrointestinal effects include decreased gut motility and changes in secretion of gastric and intestinal fluids. Morphine and most mu agonists cause pupillary constriction. Some tolerance to this effect may develop, but addicts with high opioid levels will still have miosis. Respiratory depression is the usual cause of death from opioid overdose.

After rapid intravenous injection of an opioid, the user experiences warm skin flushing and a "rush" that lasts about 45 seconds. In one retrospective study, the most common feelings associated with the rush were pleasure, relaxation, and satisfaction. Although at one time the rush was classically reported to be similar to a sexual orgasm, in a study of the phenomenon such a feeling was reported in only 18% of men and 10% of women (Seecof and Tennant 1987).

Opioids are easily absorbed subcutaneously and intramuscularly, as well as from the gastrointestinal tract, nasal mucosa (e.g., when heroin is used as snuff), and lung (e.g., when opium is smoked). About 90% of the excretion of morphine occurs during the first 24 hours, but traces are detectable in urine for over 48 hours. Heroin (diacetylmorphine) is hydrolyzed to monoacetylmorphine, which is then hydrolyzed to morphine. Morphine and monoacetylmorphine are responsible for the pharmacologic effects of heroin. Heroin produces effects more rapidly than morphine because it is more lipid soluble and therefore crosses the blood-brain barrier faster. In the urine, heroin is detected as free morphine and morphine glucuronide (for general references, see Jaffe and Martin 1990).

Endogenous Opioids

More than a dozen endogenous opioid peptides have been characterized. These are grouped into three families: endorphins, enkephalins, and dynorphins. Each family has separate pathways, genetic bases, and precursors, and each probably binds preferentially to certain opioid receptor types. Active opioid peptides produced from breakdown of the polypeptide precursors may be present in neurons that contain other peptide and nonpeptide neurotransmitters. In addition, enzyme differences lead to variations in ratios of the peptides formed from precursor breakdown (Akil et al. 1984; Goldstein 1984). For these and other reasons, the process of delineating clearly the normal physiologic roles of the various endogenous opioids has been difficult. Furthermore, there is as yet no clear association between endogenous opioid activity and opioid depdendence (O'Brien et al. 1982).

Receptors

In addition to the three major types of opioid receptors (mu, kappa, and delta), there is also evidence for other receptor types (e.g., epsilon and lambda), which may be the preferential binding sites for certain endogenous peptides (for references, see Jaffe and Martin 1990). There is also evidence that subtypes of mu receptors exist (Callahan and Pasternak 1987). Another receptor type, sigma, unlike the others, is not antagonized by naloxone and may not be a true opioid receptor. None of the clinically available opioid agonists or antagonists are entirely selective for any one type of receptor, although there are now compounds under investigation that are highly selective in their actions. Therefore, available opioid drugs have clinical effects that are caused by the net pattern of activation and/or antagonism at more than one receptor site at a given dose level. Furthermore, degree of activation at a given receptor type may vary a great deal from one species to another. Further, since the affinity of a drug for the various receptors differs, the effect of the drug may shift with dose changes. For example, a drug that has primarily mu actions and relatively low affinity for the kappa receptor may nevertheless begin to exert kappa actions if the dose is raised to high levels. The drug nalorphine, once used widely as an antagonist, has antagonistic actions at the mu receptor, but also has some partial agonist actions at kappa. As the dose was raised, nontolerant individuals experienced dysphoria as a result of these kappa actions. (For references for the following discussion on the three major types of opioid receptors, see Jaffe [1990] and Jaffe and Martin [1990].)

Mu.   Mu-receptor activation leads to euphoria, analgesia, indifference to pain, respiratory depression, and miosis. These receptors are located in the thalamus, periaqueductal gray, substantia gelatinosa of the spinal cord, and other areas. Morphine and methadone bind preferentially to mu receptors. Activation of mu receptors is associated with increases in prolactin and growth hormone and decreases in luteinizing hormone, follicle-stimulating hormone, and beta-endorphin (Jaffe and Martin 1990). Euphorigenic effects may be linked in part to release of dopamine from dopaminergic neurons originating in the ventral tegmental area and connecting to the nucleus accumbens and frontal cortex.

Kappa.   Kappa receptors also produce analgesia, but often have dysphoric effects. On the other hand, kappa agonists such as pentazocine may induce euphoria in some people, although the reason for this effect is not well understood. Kappa agonists appear to decrease dopamine release from ventral tegmental dopaminergic neurons. They have effects in spinal cord and on the gastrointestinal and genitourinary tracts that are distinct from and sometimes antagonistic to those of mu and delta agonists. Kappa agonists do not suppress mu agonist withdrawal and do not exhibit cross-tolerance with mu agonists. Dynorphins may be endogenous kappa agonists, but their action is quite complex.

Delta.   Delta-receptor activation produces analgesia. Other effects are not as well understood. These receptors are most concentrated in the limbic system. Enkephalins such as Met-enkephalin appear to be endogenous delta agonists.

ETIOLOGY

Multiple factors interact in complex ways to result in opioid dependence. It is difficult to delineate, even for a specific individual, the precise etiology of dependence. In addition, each of the etiologic factors discussed below may play variable roles in initiation of use, maintenance of use, relapse, and recovery. Keeping in mind all of these potential factors is essential when formulating a treatment plan for each individual.

Learning Factors

Opioids can be reinforcing by directly inducing pleasurable effects or by reducing aversive affects or the experience of noxious stimuli. They may reduce pain or anxiety and for some users decrease boredom, relieve the experience of intense aggression, and increase self-esteem. Social approval among peers may be a factor in initial opioid use. The rituals of injecting opioids often become associated with a "high," so that even an occasional placebo injection may still elicit pleasurable effects. Even after tolerance has developed to some of the effects of opioids, the rush may still be experienced briefly after an iv injection. Animal studies indicate that low doses of opioids lower the threshold for producing reinforcing (pleasurable) effects by means of self-administration of electrical currents to certain brain regions. Tolerance to this effect does not seem to occur. The experience of withdrawal relief also contributes to the repeated opioid use. Because of heroin's brief duration of action, withdrawal occurs several times a day, and its repeated relief leads to a strongly reinforced behavior pattern.

The paraphernalia and setting associated with drug use can become cues indicating that a high or relief of distress is possible. Craving or desire to use the drug is increased in the presence of such stimuli. Withdrawal symptoms may also become conditioned to such stimuli. The addict may experience conditioned withdrawal as an increase in craving or desire to use opioids (McLellan et al. 1986; Meyer and Mirin 1979; Wikler 1980). However, the most intense craving appears to be elicited by conditions associated with opioid use rather than those associated with withdrawal. The role that conditioned phenomena play in relapse and perpetuation of use is presently unknown; however, the work in research settings suggests that these phenomena may be clinically important and that their extinction may be helpful in treatment (Childress et al. 1988).

Social and Environmental Factors

In general, the use of such drugs as marijuana and alcohol precedes the use of opioids (Clayton and Voss 1981; Kandel and Faust 1975). Although one cannot predict definitively which users will proceed to opioid use, those who do generally have low self-esteem, disrupted families, and/or difficult relationships with their parents. The increased availability of opioids in inner cities of major urban centers contributes to initiation of use and relapse. It is particularly difficult to avoid use and relapse in areas with high unemployment, poor school systems, and high crime, since living in such an area may contribute to the very affects opioid use temporarily relieves.

Brief experimentation with illicit opioids rarely leads to dependence, but persons who use opioids commonly escalate to daily use, at least once per month for at least a brief period. In Vietnam, experimentation with opioids was widespread; 73% of the soldiers who used opioids at least five times became dependent; however, 88% of enlisted men who became addicted to heroin did not become readdicted at any time in the 3 years after return, and 56% did not use opioids at all during that time (Robins et al. 1975).

Psychodynamic Factors

Psychodynamic theory of opioid addiction is predicated on the belief that underlying psychopathology is the key element in the etiology of opioid use and relapse. Some analysts view defects in the self as primary etiologic factors in opioid abusers. Ego defenses against intolerable affects, particularly rage, are also felt to be deficient (Khantzian and Schneider 1986; Wurmser 1979). Evidence that psychopathology precedes opioid use includes the fact that many users show evidence of conduct disorder prior to first use of opioids. Epidemiological studies find a higher prevalence of anxiety, affective disorders, bipolar disorder, and alcoholism, as well as antisocial personality among individuals who meet lifetime criteria for drug dependence (Regier et al. 1990).

Family

The commonly held belief that disruptions in the family cause opioid abuse has not been proven. However, there is a strong association between disturbed family relationships and opioid use. Most urban heroin addicts come from single-parent families. Family systems in two-parent families are often disturbed as well. For example, the opposite-sex parent is often overly involved with the drug abuser while the same-sex parent is distant or punitive. A stable maladaptive pattern may develop, the maintenance of which could be threatened by the recovery of the identified patient, the addict. Thus family therapy is often essential in helping the user to break the addictive cycle (Kaufman 1986; Stanton 1982). It is also important to remember that alcoholism and drug abuse, as well as depression and antisocial personality, are common in the families of opioid users (Rounsaville et al. 1991).

Biology

There is little evidence of a genetic vulnerability that is specific for opioid dependence. Dole and Nyswander (1967) postulated that a preexisting metabolic deficiency could lead to dependence or that changes induced by opioid use could perpetuate dependence. Dole (1988) more recently hypothesized that opioid receptor dysfunction is a primary etiologic factor. However, there is no clear support for these theories at the present time. Antisocial personality and alcoholism are more common in opioid users. Since both of these disorders appear to be influenced by genetic factors, it is possible that a link with genetic factors in opioid use may some day be discovered.

TOLERANCE AND WITHDRAWAL

Tolerance

Although tolerance develops with extended use of all opioids, it does not develop uniformly to all of their actions. With mu-receptor opioids, some euphoric, miotic, endocrine, and constipating effects may persist after tolerance has developed to the analgesic, respiratory depressant, and sedative effects. That changes in noradrenergic sensitivity may occur with chronic opioid use is suggested by the following: 1) opioids inhibit the activity of adrenergic neurons in the locus coeruleus; 2) naloxone causes increased locus coeruleus activity in opioid-dependent animals; 3) chronic opioid treatment results in supersensitivity of other neurotransmitter systems, such as those involving dopamine, acetylcholine, and serotonin; and 4) alpha$_2$ agonists (which inhibit adrenergic activity), such as clonidine, diminish the severity of adrenergic signs of opioid withdrawal (Redmond and Krystal 1984). One would expect that central opioid receptor changes would be present in dependent animals, but consistent evidence has not yet been found. Changes in linkage between G proteins and other intracellular mechanisms may also play a role in tolerance.

Some degree of tolerance to the euphorigenic effects of heroin in addicts may develop in 1–2 weeks (Meyer and Mirin 1979). Therefore, the addict who desires a rush or a high progressively increases the dose. Although some build up to extraordinarily high doses, there is always a dose capable of causing death from respiratory depression. Physical dependence and tolerance occur more rapidly in former addicts; morphine addicts can reach a dose of 500 mg/day within 10 days of resumption of use. Tolerance largely disappears after withdrawal; addicts have unwittingly taken fatal doses by returning to their previous doses after detoxification. Receptor upregulation may occur with chronic administration of opioid antagonists and may render addicts treated with these agents more sensitive to opioids when the antagonists are discontinued.

Withdrawal

Administration of sufficient doses of an opioid antagonist after only a single therapeutic dose of morphine results in withdrawal phenomena (Bickel et al. 1987; Heishman et al. 1989; Jones 1979). Some degree of physical dependence develops in people who are given opioids regularly for more than a few days. However, very few become chronic users. Physical dependence and the presence of tolerance and withdrawal symptoms thus cannot be viewed as the only causes of continued use and relapse. However, the presence of physical dependence clearly contributes to difficulty with or fear of withdrawing and tendency to relapse.

Intensity of withdrawal depends on the following factors: 1) dose of the opioid used (however, increasing beyond the equivalent of 500 mg/day of morphine does not significantly increase severity), 2) duration of use, 3) rate of removal of opiods from receptors, and 4) extent of continuous use. Generally, the character of the signs and symptoms is opposite to that of the acute agonist effects. For example, constipation occurs during acute treatment, and bowel hypermotility occurs with withdrawal. Individual sensitivity may affect the nature of the withdrawal syndrome. For example, stomach cramps predominate in some, muscle aches in others. The character of withdrawal is generally similar among agents that have similar profiles of receptor activity. Also, generally, the shorter the duration of action of the drug, the more severe is the withdrawal syndrome, and the more rapid is the onset of symptoms and shorter the total duration of the symptoms. With short-acting drugs such as heroin and morphine, early symptoms may occur between 8 and 12 hours after the last dose. Severe syndromes peak from 48 to 72 hours. In some individuals, subjective symptoms predominate over objective signs. Untreated, the acute phase of morphine or heroin withdrawal lasts 7–10 days. Withdrawal from kappa agonists (e.g., nalorphine) is generally mild and of a qualitatively distinct character. The onset of withdrawal with longer-acting drugs such as methadone or *l*-alpha-acetylmethadol (LAAM) can be delayed until 1–3 days after the last dose. Peak symptoms often may not occur until days 3–5. Withdrawal from methadone includes complaints of pain, which patients state originates from muscle or bone. Meperidine withdrawal develops within 3 hours after the last dose, peaks in from 8 to 12 hours, and generally ends in 4–5 days. With meperidine, subjective symptoms such as craving and restlessness may be much more severe than autonomic changes. Codeine withdrawal is comparatively less severe.

A protracted abstinence syndrome may follow the acute opioid withdrawal syndrome and last for many weeks (Martin et al. 1973). In one study of heroin addicts detoxified with methadone, withdrawal distress peaked at day 20, the final day of methadone, and it was not until day 40 that addicts' symptom scores reached normal levels (Gossop et al. 1987). During this phase, there may be excessive somatic concerns, decreased stress tolerance, poor self-image, and disturbed sleep. Opioid effects are especially reinforcing at this time, perhaps providing one explanation for early relapse (Cushman and Dole 1973; Martin et al. 1973).

Formerly, ratings of withdrawal severity from drugs such as heroin, morphine, and methadone made use of the Himmelsbach Scale (Himmelsbach 1941), which emphasized "objective" or measurable signs over subjective reports. Using such a system, the sequence of signs observed were as shown in Table 2-1.

However, more recent work giving greater weight to subjective aspects of withdrawal distress has shown that drug users experience mood changes, fatigue, dysphoria, and vague discomforts many hours before such signs as lacrimation or yawning can be detected. When buprenorphine, a partial mu agonist, is withdrawn, no changes are observed using the Himmelsbach Scale, but a withdrawal syndrome is readily measured using an opioid withdrawal symptom checklist (Fudala et al. 1990a).

Personality variables, state of mind at time of withdrawal, and expectations of severity of symptoms all may affect withdrawal severity (Kleber 1981). One study found that merely providing addicts information about the withdrawal syndrome resulted in lower levels of withdrawal symptomatology (Green and Gossop 1988). Naloxone will rapidly induce a severe withdrawal syndrome, which peaks within 30 minutes and then declines rapidly. Until the antagonist is eliminated, only partial suppression of the withdrawal syndrome is possible, and then only by using very high opioid doses, which may cause respiratory depression when naloxone is metabolized.

Table 2-1. Signs and symptoms of opiate withdrawal

Early	Middle	Late
Lacrimation	Restless sleep	Increased severity of earlier symptoms
Yawning	Dilated pupils	Tachycardia
Rhinorrhea	Anorexia	Nausea
Sweating	Gooseflesh	Vomiting
	Restlessness	Diarrhea
	Irritability	Abdominal cramps
	Tremor	Tachycardia
		Increased blood pressure
		Mood lability
		Depression
		Muscle spasms
		Weakness
		Bone pain

Source. Adapted from Ciraulo and Ciraulo 1988.

OPIOID DETOXIFICATION

At present in the United States, methadone is the most commonly used drug to treat withdrawal symptoms. It is the only opioid federally approved for this purpose. Detoxification can be accomplished over a period as long as 6 months in an ambulatory methadone maintenance program or as brief as several days in a hospital setting. The goal in brief detoxification is to make the experience less distressing, but the suppression of all withdrawal symptoms should not be expected. If the daily opioid dose is known, one can administer the pharmacologically equivalent methadone dose. The following doses, given im, are approximately equivalent as analgesics to 7–10 mg of methadone im: morphine 10 mg, hydromorphone (Dilaudid) 1.5 mg, codeine 120 mg, oxycodone (Percodan) 10–15 mg, meperidine (Demerol) 80–100 mg, heroin 3 mg, levorphanol (Levo-Dromoran) 2–3 mg, fentanyl (Sublimaze) 0.1 mg, and sufentanil (Sufenta) 0.01 mg. Because of methadone's longer duration of action and oral efficacy, it is possible to suppress withdrawal with lower doses of oral methadone than would be predicted from these analgesic equivalents.

For patients taking street heroin, initial dosage of methadone is usually 15–20 mg orally. If withdrawal symptoms or signs persist, one may repeat the dose in a few hours. Although some addicts with access to pure drugs may require higher doses, generally 40 mg/day of methadone is adequate. Once a stabilizing dosage has been found, methadone can be reduced about 10–20% per day to achieve full detoxification within 10 days. The rate of decrease can be more rapid if clonidine is used (see below). To facilitate compliance in outpatient detoxification, the period may need to be prolonged. Reasonable tapering schedules are 10% per week from high doses and 3% per week from doses less than 20 mg (Senay et al. 1977).

Relapse rates after detoxification are very high. Although extension of withdrawal period for up to 6–8 weeks does not appear to improve outcome, patients who have been maintained on methadone and who have a good therapeutic relationship are more successful.

Clonidine

Clonidine, an alpha$_2$ agonist used primarily as an antihypertensive, is another agent now commonly used for detoxification (Table 2-2). Since the late 1970s, clonidine repeatedly has been shown to suppress

Table 2-2. Protocol for administration of clonidine (dose mg/day)

	Detoxification	
Day	From short-acting opioid (heroin, oxycodone)	From methadone (25 mg or less)
1	0.3–0.6 (includes 0.1 test dose)	0.3–0.6 (includes 0.1 test dose)
2	0.4–0.8	0.4–0.6
3–6	0.6–1.2 Then reduce daily dose by 50% each subsequent day. Daily reductions should not exceed 0.4.	0.5–0.8
6–10		0.6–1.2 Then reduce daily dose by 50% each subsequent day. Daily reductions should not exceed 0.4.

Note. Clonidine alone may not adequately treat insomnia, diarrhea, muscle aches, restlessness, irritability, or other withdrawal symptoms, which may require other medications. For this reason many programs use lower doses of clonidine than outlined above, in combination with oral opioids.
Source. Adapted from Kleber and Kosten 1984.

many of the autonomic symptoms of the withdrawal syndrome (Gold et al. 1978; Kleber et al. 1985). Patients taking opioids can be switched to oral clonidine in doses starting at 0.1–0.3 mg three to four times per day (up to 2.5 mg/day). Doses greater than 1.0 mg/day are not recommended for outpatient settings. Also limiting use of clonidine on an outpatient basis are two major side effects: hypotension, which may be marked, and sedation.

Detoxification is more successful when the patient is switching from a stable methadone dose with the support of ongoing therapy than when coming directly from the street for detoxification from heroin. Some believe that detoxification with clonidine can be more rapid than with methadone, at least on an outpatient basis. One important limitation of clonidine is that, while autonomic signs of withdrawal are suppressed, subject-reported symptoms such as lethargy, restlessness, insomnia, and craving are not well relieved (Charney et al. 1981; Jasinski et al. 1985). Anxiety may be alleviated with benzodiazepines, and preliminary data suggest that low-dose propranolol may reduce restlessness (Roehrich and Gold 1987).

Clonidine has been used in combination with naltrexone to facilitate rapid withdrawal as well as to ease rapid transition to treatment with the antagonist. Patients are usually begun on both clonidine and very low doses of naltrexone on day 1. Clonidine is given in divided doses adjusted for severity of withdrawal up to 2–2.5 mg/day. Naltrexone doses are gradually increased to 50–150 mg/day by approximately day 5 or 6; 80–90% of patients are able to complete transition to naltrexone in less than 1 week (Charney et al. 1986; Kleber et al. 1987; Vining et al. 1988).

Buprenorphine

At this writing, buprenorphine (Buprenex) is available in the United States only as an injectable analgesic. Buprenorphine is a partial mu-receptor agonist, with most of the properties of morphine, but with a longer duration of analgesic actions. Given chronically in high doses (4–8 mg/day sublingually or subcutaneously), it attenuates or blocks opioid-induced euphoria. It is not clear whether this is a result of cross-tolerance or some other action at the receptor. It is now under investigation as an agent for detoxification and maintenance. Hospitalized heroin addicts reduced self-administration of heroin when given 8 mg of buprenorphine subcutaneously (Mello and Mendelson 1980). In a 17-week maintenance study, buprenorphine (8 mg sublingually) appeared to suppress heroin use as well or better than 60 mg of oral methadone and significantly better than 20 mg of oral methadone (Johnson et al. 1990).

One virtue of buprenorphine as a detoxification agent is that, properly managed, it can be used immediately after methadone or illicit opioid use without precipitating withdrawal symptoms (Fudala et al. 1990a; Kosten and Kleber 1988). In one study, sublingual buprenorphine appeared to be as effective as methadone in a 7-week detoxification (Bickel et al. 1987). Furthermore, although direct comparisons to low-dose methadone have not been carried out, the buprenorphine withdrawal syndrome appears to be quite mild, with few subjects requesting drugs for relief (Fudala et al. 1990a; Jasinski et al. 1978; Kosten and Kleber 1988; Mello and Mendelson 1980). After 6 weeks of 8 mg buprenorphine sublingually daily, withdrawal was measurable by a symptom checklist and appeared to peak at about 72 hours after the last dose. No increase in withdrawal symptoms was observed with the Himmelsbach Scale, which emphasizes physiological signs and symptoms (Fudala et al. 1990a). The low severity of buprenorphine withdrawal seems to facilitate rapid induction of naltrexone after buprenorphine discontinuation (Kosten and Kleber 1988). An additional benefit of buprenorphine is that risk of overdose may be low. As a partial agonist, there appears to be a ceiling effect as dose is increased so that respiratory depression greater than that caused by 30–60 mg of morphine is not produced (Jasinski et al. 1978). Buprenorphine suppresses cocaine self-administration in non-human primates (Mello et al. 1990). In uncontrolled trials, buprenorphine was reported to reduce cocaine use among patients formerly maintained on methadone (Kosten and Kleber 1988) and to have some antidepressant properties (Kosten et al. 1990). However, no reduction of cocaine use was observed in a double-blind controlled study (Fudala et al. 1990b).

Other Drugs

Lofexidine and guanabenz are other alpha$_2$ agonists that suppress some elements of the withdrawal syndrome. Lofexidine may be less sedating and hypotensive than clonidine (Washton and Resnick 1981).

ASSOCIATED PROBLEMS

Medical Complications and Life Expectancy

Before 1980, the mortality rate among younger addicts was up to 20 times higher than that among controls; it was 2–3 times higher for older addicts. The higher mortality rate was due to factors such as overdose, suicide, homicide, and infection. About 1–1.5% of addicts who sought treatment died each year (Joe and Simpson 1987; Stimson and Oppenheimer 1982). With the spread of human immunodeficiency virus (HIV) infection, which is transmitted among opioid users by needle sharing and sexual contact, these figures will undoubtedly rise.

Infections are common with use of intravenous opioids. Recent estimates are that more than 50% of those in clinics in the northeastern region of the United States are HIV positive. The lethality and prevalence of HIV are the bases for the controversial argument for clean needle distribution to addicts. A study by Ball et al. (1988) indicated that standard methadone maintenance significantly reduces needle sharing. Other transmittable infections include hepatitis and malaria. Two of three heroin addicts have abnormal liver function tests (which may be contributed to by alcoholism), and up to 50% may have hepatitis B antibody levels. Tuberculosis is more common in heroin addicts than in the general population. Other infectious complications include endocarditis, meningitis, brain abscess, and septicemia.

Embolic phenomena may occur from particulate matter such as talc or starch when pills are used for injections, or if drugs are filtered through cigarette filters or cotton. Pulmonary emboli may result in pulmonary hypertension and right ventricular failure. Septic emboli may be a cause of staphylococcal pneumonitis.

Approximately 75% of all addicts have lymphadenopathy (which may be due to particulate contaminants). Vein sclerosis and contaminant-related lymphatic obstruction may cause extremity edema. Ulceration and other dermatologic changes are often present in those who "skin pop."

Women and Pregnant Patients

Treatment programs must be attuned to the special problems of female addicts. Women who are opioid addicts have fewer vocational skills than men and show more depression and lower self-esteem. Women's opioid use appears to be particularly influenced by having an ongoing relationship with an addicted partner. Therefore, including the male partner in therapy or helping the female addict to separate from him may be an integral part of treatment (Anglin et al. 1987). Opioid-dependent women are more likely than men to seek treatment because of medical problems.

Opioid withdrawal is much more dangerous for the fetus than for the adult. Withdrawal in the pregnant addict can cause fetal death or miscarriage. Since continued heroin use or high-dose methadone maintenance can result in a severe withdrawal syndrome after delivery, many believe methadone maintenance at 10–40 mg/day is best. However, these lower doses are clearly less effective than doses above 60 mg in suppressing illicit iv opioid use. In light of the risk of HIV infection associated with continued iv drug use, clinicians must consider several factors and individualize treatment for each patient. There appear to be no uniform long-term effects of maternal methadone maintenance on children followed up to 7 years of age (Rosen and Johnson 1985). When mothers are maintained on low methadone doses, neonatal withdrawal is usually mild and readily manageable with low-dose paregoric (Finnegan et al. 1984). If pregnancy has begun when the woman is on high-dose methadone, there could be a slow taper of 1 mg every 3 days. If complete withdrawal is desired, it should occur during the second trimester.

Psychiatric Disorders

High levels of global severity of psychopathology adversely influence the course of opioid dependence as well as response to all forms of treatment. It is unclear whether specific diagnoses selectively influence outcome (Kosten et al. 1986a; McLellan 1986; McLellan et al. 1983; Rounsaville et al. 1986b; Woody et al. 1984), although in the case of alcoholism, researchers have shown an effect of diagnosis even after accounting for variance due to overall severity. There have been a number of studies assessing prevalence of psychiatric disorders among opioid-dependent persons. In one study of 533 treated opioid addicts, lifetime prevalence rates using Research Diagnostic Criteria (RDC) (Spitzer et al. 1978) were assessed (Rounsaville et al. 1982). The most common diagnoses, with percentages for men and women, respectively, were: affective disorder (70.7%, 85.4%), with major depression the most prevalent (48.4%, 69.2%); alcoholism (37%, 26.9%); antisocial personality (29.5%, 16.9%); and anxiety disorders (13.2%, 25.4%), with phobic disorder the most prevalent (8.2%, 13.9%). RDC require that the diagnosis of antisocial personality be independent of the need for drugs; using DSM-III criteria (American Psychiatric Association 1980), 54% of the population studied would have met criteria for antisocial personality disorder. In this study, 70.3% met criteria for a current episode of psychiatric disorder, the most common of which were: major depression (23.8%), alcoholism (13.7%), and phobic disorder (9.2%).

Comparable lifetime prevalence of psychiatric disorders were obtained in another study of 133 persons, which also found that 47% received a concurrent DSM-III diagnosis of substance abuse or dependence (Khantzian and Treece 1985). The most frequently abused substances were sedative-hypnotics (23%), alcohol (14%), and cannabis (13%). Similar rates of psychiatric disorders are found in other studies of drug abusers (Mirin et al. 1986; Woody et al. 1983).

Although such diagnoses do not imply causality, and in many cases, opioid dependence causes or exacerbates psychiatric problems, some causal link seems likely (Regier et al. 1990).

Alcoholism.   Opioid-dependent people who abuse alcohol appear to have greater psychological difficulties and to lead more unstable lives than opioid addicts without alcohol problems (Barr and Cohen 1987). Affective disorders and alcoholism often coexist in this population (Mirin et al. 1986; Rounsaville et al. 1982). Alcoholism apparently mitigates against successful treatment of opioid addiction (Green and Jaffe 1977; Joseph and Appel 1985). Psychological treatment for alcoholism may be provided, and disulfiram (Antabuse) can be used safely with methadone, but it is difficult to determine if such measures are beneficial (Ling et al. 1983).

Polydrug use.   Many opioid users are also dependent on nonopioids. As is true when the secondary substance is alcohol, those with combined addictions have greater psychiatric problems (Hartog and Tusel 1987; Kosten et al. 1987c). Those who abuse nonopioids also appear to have greater difficulties in treatment programs and have poorer treatment outcomes. In one retrospective self-report study, abuse of nonopioids and particularly of cocaine was higher during periods of active opioid addiction than during periods of nonaddiction (Nurco et al. 1988).

A 2.5-year follow-up study of opioid addicts in methadone maintenance treatment found that prevalence of cocaine use only slightly declined and that severity of cocaine use in users actually increased, particularly in those with depressive disorders (Kosten et al. 1987c). These data obtained during the rising phase of the current cocaine epidemic indicate that methadone and counseling alone are insufficient to prevent or ameliorate cocaine use. Pilot data from one program suggested that desipramine can decrease cocaine craving in methadone-maintained patients (Kosten et al. 1987d), but other programs have not observed similar beneficial results (Arndt et al. 1990).

Affective disorders.   Affective disorders are the most common psychiatric problems in opioid addicts. Many others will have subsyndromal depressive symptoms. However, even without specific treatment for depression, many will report less depression within the first few months after beginning opioid treatment (Mirin et al. 1988).

In one study, current depression was seen in 25.9% of a sample but in only 12.7% at 2.5-year follow-up (Rounsaville et al. 1986a). Depressed patients improve about equally in outpatient drug-free therapy, therapeutic communities, and methadone maintenance when there is no correction for severity of depression (Ginzburg et al. 1984). However, some patients who had no symptoms initially may develop them during the course of treatment.

Lithium can be combined safely with methadone and naltrexone and thus should be considered for patients with bipolar disorders. Controlled studies of antidepressants have yielded mixed results. Some have not shown that such treatment results in significant improvement (Kleber et al. 1983) beyond that seen with placebo, but plasma samples were not obtained to ensure therapeutic levels. In other studies, depressed patients maintained on methadone responded better to doxepin than to placebo (Woody et al. 1975). For those with major depression that persists for several weeks after detoxification, antidepressant treatment should nonetheless be strongly considered. Methadone reduces the metabolism of desipramine so that clinical responses or side effects may be seen with relatively low doses (Manny et al. 1989).

Anxiety and schizophrenia. Anxiety disorders and schizophrenia have not been well studied in this population. For those with an anxiety disorder and an affective disorder, an antidepressant such as doxepin could be used. Schizophrenia is seen in fewer than 1% of those treated for opioid dependence. Opioids appear to have antidopaminergic effects and thus may have some antipsychotic effects. Antipsychotic medications can be used along with methadone or naltrexone.

Crime. Crime increases 150–300% for opioid-dependent persons when they are actively addicted (Anglin and McGlothlin 1984; Nurco et al. 1984). Conversely, decreases in crime are seen when opioid use is reduced. More than 50% of heroin addicts have been arrested before they ever started using opioids; for them, criminal activity during addiction may be seen as an exacerbation of previous behavior. For those without a history of crime, criminal behavior does not generally occur when opioids are supplied through legal channels or at low cost.

Treatment of opioid dependence reduces criminal behavior and costs to society (Hubbard et al. 1989). Civil commitment to treat opioid addiction is beneficial as determined by social measures as well as by reduced opioid use (Anglin 1988). Long-term treatment in a therapeutic community may be particularly helpful in reducing criminal behavior. It is, of course, unreasonable to expect that treatment of opioid dependence will entirely eliminate criminal behavior, especially in those who were involved with crime prior to opioid use.

TREATMENT

There is no consensus about the most effective treatment for opioid dependence. Each individual needs to be evaluated extensively, with attention paid to a number of factors: 1) motivation for a particular type of treatment; 2) presence of psychopathology; 3) presence of other substance abuse; 4) availability and feasibility of various types of treatment; and 5) success or failure of previously tried treatments. More often than not, a combination of treatment methods is practiced. Therefore, even for programs focused on the use of a medication, counseling and/or psychotherapy may play a critical role. In addition, the necessity for acute detoxification must always be assessed prior to determining appropriate long-term treatment. Detoxification alone is usually unsuccessful in preventing relapse, so strong efforts must be made to interest the detoxifying addict in further treatment.

Major treatment categories are: 1) short-term detoxification, usually with methadone or clonidine; 2) maintenance treatment with methadone or naltrexone; 3) outpatient drug-free treatment, which may include formal relapse prevention programs; and 4) the therapeutic community. Some private residential chemical dependency programs emphasizing a twelve-step approach to recovery also offer treatment to opioid-dependent individuals. Therapists in each of these settings may have experience ranging from prior addiction and experiential training to advanced degrees in the health professions. An addict often has experience with more than one treatment modality in his or her career. For example, the user may first be detoxified, then relapse, enter methadone maintenance, eventually be detoxified from methadone, and finally continue successfully with outpatient drug-free treatment. It is often difficult to ascertain for such individuals what was the key ingredient for recovery.

Polysubstance users often supplement one of these programs with self-help groups such as Narcotics Anonymous, Alcoholics

Anonymous, and Cocaine Anonymous. Narcotics Anonymous has, since its inception in 1947, approached opioid addiction from a perspective similar to that of Alcoholics Anonymous (for an overview, see Peyrot 1985). Mental health practitioners may use individual, group, or family therapy to treat opioid-dependent individuals who have significant psychopathology. Both opioid dependence and concomitant psychopathology should be addressed, regardless of the treatments chosen.

Methadone Maintenance

Methadone maintenance was first introduced in 1964 by Dole and Nyswander (1965). The basis for use of methadone is that high doses alleviate craving and induce cross-tolerance to other opioids so that heroin-induced euphoria is blocked. Therefore, in theory, opioid-dependent individuals would have no need to use heroin or to be involved with the various maladaptive behaviors needed to maintain heroin addiction. Results with more psychologically disturbed and less-motivated patients than those of Dole and Nyswander were less dramatic than they had originally demonstrated (Sells 1979). Nevertheless, methadone maintenance does reduce heroin use, nonopioid use, health problems, and crime (e.g., Ball et al. 1987; Gerstein and Harwood 1990; Senay 1985). Despite the benefits of methadone maintenance, some addicts have a negative attitude toward methadone maintenance client and are often misinformed about methadone itself, factors that may lead to reluctance to enter into this form of treatment (Hunt et al. 1985-86). It is also a controversial treatment among health professionals and the general public. Despite its proven success, some believe its primary purpose is crime reduction; others see it as merely a substitution of one addiction for another.

Methadone is a mu-receptor agonist with special properties that make it particularly useful as a maintenance agent. Reliably absorbed orally, it does not reach peak concentration until about 4 hours and maintains a large extravascular reservoir (Kreek 1979). These properties minimize acute euphoric effects. The reservoir results in a plasma half-life of 1–2 days, so there are usually no rapid blood level drops that could lead to withdrawal syndromes between daily doses. Effective blood levels are in the range of 150–600 ng/ml (Dole 1988). There is wide variability among individuals in blood levels with identical doses (Kreek 1979), and some have inadequate levels even with doses as high as 80–100 mg/day (Tennant 1987a). Since methadone is metabolized in the liver, hepatic enzyme-inducing drugs such as phenobarbital, phenytoin, and rifampin may markedly reduce serum methadone concentrations (Bell et al. 1988; Kreek 1979). Even with adequate plasma levels, some patients continue to abuse drugs, such as sedatives, possibly because they are seeking some form of intoxication rather than relief of opioid hunger (Bell et al. 1990).

Although tolerance develops as with all opioids, some pharmacologic effects of methadone may persist (Kreek 1983; see pharmacology above). Euphoria and drowsiness are generally more pronounced in the first weeks of treatment or at a later date if the dosage is rapidly increased. Some slight but measurable mood elevation occurs at about the time of peak plasma levels in those on chronic methadone and may be one reason why some patients stay in treatment (McCaul et al. 1982). Effects to which tolerance may not develop fully include constipation, increased perspiration, and complaints of sexual dysfunction and decreased libido. (Opioid-induced endocrine effects usually resolve after a few months, but chronic opioids may lower testosterone and follicle-stimulating hormone levels. However, there is not a strong correlation between these levels and sexual dysfunction.) During the early months of treatment, there may be altered electroencephalogram sleep patterns and insomnia. Although electroencephalograms appear to normalize, sleep disturbance may persist. There is no evidence for long-term organ damage with methadone.

Methadone maintenance programs usually are staffed by a part-time physician, nurse, and counselors of varying levels of training. Federal, state, and sometimes local regulations govern each program. Federal requirements regulate areas such as standards for admission, frequency of urine testing, methadone dosage, quantity of take-home medication, and treatment of pregnant addicts. Regulations include the following. Clients must be at least 18 years old (with some exceptions), be addicted for most of the prior year, and have 1 year of "physiologic dependence." Only after patients have adhered to program rules for 3 months are they eligible to receive up to a 2-day take-home supply; if adherent for 3 consecutive years, they may be eligible for up to a 6-day take-home supply. Maximum first-day dosage is 40 mg (unless such a dosage does not suppress opioid abstinence symptoms). Physiologic dependence is not a requirement for those persons recently released from prison or a chronic care institution provided they would have been eligible prior to institutionalization or incarceration, or for selected patients who had previously been treated with methadone maintenance. There is no maximum allowable dose, but doses of greater than 100 mg/day must be justified in the patient's record (National Institute on Drug Abuse and Food and Drug Administration 1987).

Patients initially return daily for each dose of methadone. Treatment is monitored by counselors, and since opioid addicts often underreport their drug use (Magura et al. 1987), urine testing is a standard element of most programs. Reasons for discharge from maintenance include persistent opioid or other substance use, sporadic attendance, and aggressive behavior at the clinic. Although such patients undermine the purpose of treatment and the treatment milieu, it is often difficult to discharge them because clinicians generally believe that they would likely do worse without treatment.

Although standard regulations and common underlying philosophy result in many similarities among programs, there are also a number of differences. Programs modeled after the original Dole and Nyswander (1965) model tend to use high doses (80–120 mg/day) or more flexible dosing to ensure cross-tolerance and suppression of craving. Since illicit opioid use is seen as a response to a metabolic deficiency, indefinite continuation of methadone is felt to be the only way to preclude relapse. One group (Novick et al. 1988) has had good results with outpatient "medical maintenance." Selected, highly successful methadone maintenance patients were seen in a physician's office every 28 days and given a take-home supply of methadone tablets up to 100 mg/day. The percentage relapsing to heroin use or getting into legal difficulty or dropping out of treatment was very low. Results are preliminary, and there is a potential for diversion and serious overdose (Wesson 1988).

Other programs use methadone doses in the range of 20–60 mg/day and less flexible dosing. Although lower doses may reduce drug-seeking behaviors, they often are not high enough to prevent heroin-induced euphoria. Clients are not viewed as suffering from a biological illness but rather as responsible persons who will do best if gradually shifted from maintenance to detoxification. These programs are thus less tolerant of continued drug use and are more likely to discharge clients for problem behavior. The programs using lower doses generally had lower rates of retention in treatment (Brown et al. 1982-83). In a study of six methadone clinics believed to be operating effectively, the percentage of patients who had used illicit drugs intravenously within the month before the interview ranged from 9 to 57%. Even after adjusting for differences among patients, factors associated with decreased iv drug use (in addition to higher methadone dosage) were quality of program leadership and services provided (Ball et al. 1988). There is also variability within programs. Some counselors are demonstrably more effective than others.

In addition to factors related to the treatment program, there are demographic and psychological correlates of retention. Clients who are employed, married, black, and older have longer retention times. Those persons with criminal histories and higher levels of psychopathology tend to leave treatment sooner. Severity and duration of opioid use per se do not appear to correlate with retention.

Treatment outcome is, of course, determined by multiple factors. Once again, duration and severity of use do not correlate with outcome. Many of the factors contributing to retention rate also similarly affect treatment outcome. For example, patients with serious psychopathology or criminal backgrounds do less well. This is not to say, however, that such clients never improve. In one 2.5-year follow-up study, clients with criminal backgrounds showed significant improvement in substance abuse and family, legal, and psychological problems (Kosten et al. 1987b). Maintenance programs appear to be more helpful for clients with severe psychopathology than are therapeutic communities (McLellan 1986). Opioid users with more criminality and less psychopathology appear to prefer short-term detoxification to maintenance (Kosten et al. 1986b).

Detoxification from methadone maintenance. Those factors that correlate with treatment success do not clearly apply to success after detoxification from methadone maintenance. Correlates of successful detoxification include: 1) less criminal behavior; 2) more stable family; 3) more stable employment; 4) shorter drug history; 5) long maintenance with lower dosage; and 6) detoxification, with patient and staff consensus as opposed to unilateral discharge from treatment (Dole and Joseph 1978). In one study, addicts were followed an average of 2 years after detoxification (Stimmel et al. 1977). Although only 28% of the total sample remained abstinent, 83% of those who had fully completed treatment remained abstinent. Since almost all patients maintained on methadone are ambulatory and presumably functioning well, gradual reduction of dosage is preferred, with careful monitoring of drug craving and withdrawal symptoms. As many as one-third of methadone maintenance clients have been found to have a marked fear of detoxification (Milby et al. 1986).

Clients who need to reenter treatment at a later date often are doing much better than at original treatment, showing less dependence, criminality, and physical disability (Kosten et al. 1986b). Such findings indicate that intermittent treatment appears to be beneficial. Therefore, reentry does not necessarily indicate failure and may instead be one further step to eventual recovery. On the other hand, there is a high probability that those who discontinue methadone will resume iv drug use with attendant risks for HIV infection (Ball et al. 1988).

Opioid Antagonists

Originally, behavioral principles were the basis for the use of opioid antagonists to treat addiction. In theory, drug use that was once operantly reinforced by euphoria would no longer be reinforced if the patients were maintained on high enough doses of opioid antagonist. In addition, with no regular opioid use, there would be extinction of the association between withdrawal symptoms and the addict's environment (Wickler 1980). Studies of cyclazocine, naloxone, and naltrexone showed them all to be successful in blocking opioid effects, but addicts generally stayed in treatment only for an average of 6–8 weeks (Capone et al. 1986; Fram et al. 1989; Resnick et al. 1980).

Naltrexone is the only opioid antagonist currently in use for treatment of addiction. Naloxone is used to treat opioid overdose and to test for opioid addiction but has a short half-life and is relatively ineffective orally; cyclazocine's dysphoric side effects make it unacceptable (Resnick et al. 1980). Patients who are likely to continue to use naltrexone and to benefit from treatment are those who have established careers (e.g., health professionals) and family support and are well motivated. Up to 70% of such clients are abstinent at 1-year follow-up (Washton et al. 1984). Programs that utilize additional rehabilitative services have better results than those seen in drug-only studies. Successful treatment is also associated with taking naltrexone for greater than 2 months (Capone et al. 1986). A multiclinic, double-blind study (National Research Council 1978) involving primarily heroin addicts had such a high attrition rate that conclusions could not be drawn.

Naltrexone (Trexan) is orally effective and long-acting. It may be given daily in doses of 50 mg/day or three times a week, in doses of 100 mg on weekdays and 150 mg on a weekend day. Some say naltrexone should be started slowly and only after a waiting period (e.g., maximum starting dosage of 50 mg only after the patient is 7 days heroin-free or 10 days methadone-free, confirmed by a negative naloxone challenge) (Ginzburg 1984). However, there is some relapse during such a waiting period. There has been some success in rapidly beginning naltrexone during clonidine detoxification from opioids. Naltrexone may actually reduce protracted withdrawal symptoms in part because it may accelerate return of normal central nervous sys-
· tem function (Charney et al. 1986).

At the doses used, there is blockage of the effects of as much as 25 mg of intravenous heroin. Toxicity in heroin addicts is low, but some report subtle adverse effects such as decreased energy (Hollister et al. 1981). Nonaddict obese subjects have been known to develop markedly elevated transaminase levels at doses of 300 mg/day. The inference has been drawn that high doses are potentially hepatotoxic, and the drug is contraindicated in liver failure or acute hepatitis.

LAAM

LAAM (*l*-alpha-acetylmethadol or levomethadyl acetate) is an investigational drug with pharmacologic properties similar to those of methadone. There is a great deal of individual variability in rates of conversion to its various metabolites, so treatment is more difficult for the clinician (Ling et al. 1978; Tennant et al. 1986). The two primary metabolites (nor-LAAM and di-nor-LAAM) have half-lives of 2–3 days, so LAAM may be given as infrequently as three times per week. Therefore, clients need not attend the clinic daily, and, without take-home drug, there is less likelihood of diversion. LAAM usually has been prescribed in dosages of 20–140 mg per dosage, with an average of about 60 mg per dosage (Ling et al. 1978; Tennant et al. 1986). For some patients LAAM "holds better" than methadone, and others prefer it because they can attend the clinic less often (Tennant et al. 1986; Trueblood et al. 1978). However, a few experience nervousness and stimulation.

A number of studies have demonstrated that treatment with LAAM results in reduction of opioid use and beneficial effects comparable to that achieved with methadone (Ling et al. 1978; Tennant et al. 1986; Zangwell et al. 1986). However, retention rates are higher in patients who take methadone 80–100 mg/day. It is important to realize that LAAM is not fully effective in suppressing opioid withdrawal during the first 72 hours of treatment. Therefore, other agents may need to be used during this period (Tennant et al. 1986). There is some evidence that LAAM may be helpful in some patients who do not respond to high-dose methadone because of low plasma levels (Tennant 1987b).

Therapeutic Communities

Therapeutic communities are supervised communal drug-free living situations for opioid and nonopioid abusers. Since substance abuse is viewed as a disorder of the whole person, the goal is a dramatic alteration of the addict's entire life-style (DeLeon 1985). Addicts are expected to live in these communities for 6–18 months. Therefore, they are not indicated for people who have a strong intimate relationship or stable employment. The community is a surrogate family in many ways. Treatment may include peer confrontation techniques in group and milieu settings as well as education and rehabilitation. The user is expected to be an active member of the community, whose existence depends on the involvement of all. The more responsibility one assumes, the more status, freedom, and comfortable living situation one may obtain.

Therapeutic communities vary a great deal in staffing and philosophy (Bale et al. 1984; DeLeon 1985), but all have some recovering addicts on staff. They are present not only because of some clients' belief that recovering addicts are needed to understand their situation, but also because they are role models who provide hope for those who doubt they can change their life-styles. Some therapeutic communities are becoming more aligned with a traditional psychiatric model, developing individual treatment plans and employing mental health professionals in important positions. Some are directed by psychiatrists.

At present, many clients are court-referred and thus are required to complete treatment. Another recent change has been that entrants appear to be more depressed and less intelligent and to have more behavioral problems than in the past. Even in the past, when clients had to indicate much motivation before acceptance, dropout rates were high (DeLeon 1985). About 50% of patients drop out within the first 3 months, and only about 15% of entrants complete a year of treatment.

High dropout rates notwithstanding, those who stay in treatment have excellent results. Clients remaining for 90 days or more do better than dropouts on legitimate employment, number of arrests, self-reported drug use, and antisocial behavior. These results hold true at 1- and 5-year follow-up periods (Bale et al. 1984; DeLeon 1985). However, some research shows a negative correlation between duration of residence and outcome, particularly for those clients with a great deal of psychiatric symptomatology who do comparatively poorly in therapeutic community settings (McLellan 1986).

Outpatient Drug-free Treatment and Psychotherapy

Outpatient drug-free programs, like therapeutic communities, seek to achieve abstinence without the use of psychoactive medication. They treat primarily polysubstance users. Other potential clients include new clients, who can be evaluated in this setting for the most appropriate treatment and who may not yet be eligible for methadone maintenance, and successful clients, who have returned to a life free of drug contacts but continue to need the less intensive support that an outpatient program can provide (Rounsaville and Kleber 1985a). Programs range from unstructured drop-in centers with "rap" sessions and recreational activities to organized day treatment programs. One of the only controlled evaluations has been of a group program that facilitates avoidance of conditioned stimuli associated with withdrawal, craving, and euphoria (McAuliffe and Ch'ien 1986). This self-help group approach appears to have significant value.

Individual psychotherapy in the context of other opioid addiction treatment such as methadone maintenance appears to be most helpful for patients with severe psychopathology. Methadone maintenance clients do better with individual psychotherapy than when they have only drug counseling. Individual supportive-expressive psychotherapy plus drug counseling and individual cognitive-behavioral psychotherapy plus drug counseling were both superior to counseling alone at 12-month follow-up (Woody et al. 1987). To engage patients in individual therapy, it should be considered a valued part of the program and should be started early in treatment. Once patients have been in treatment for a significant time, they often are reluctant to begin psychotherapy (Rounsaville et al. 1983).

Family therapy is often an adjunct treatment for opioid-dependent individuals (Kaufman 1986). One controlled study of patients on methadone maintenance found that there was less use of illicit drugs by those clients who received drug counseling alone (Stanton 1982).

REFERENCES

Akil H, Watson SJ, Young E, et al: Endogenous opioids: biology and function. Annu Rev Neurosci 7:223–255, 1984

American Psychiatric Association: Diagnostic and Statistical Manual of Mental Disorders, 3rd Edition. Washington, DC, American Psychiatric Association, 1980

Anglin MD: The efficacy of civil commitment in treating narcotic addiction. Natl Inst Drug Abuse Res Monogr Ser 86:8–34, 1988

Anglin MD, McGlothlin WH: Outcome of narcotic addict treatment in California. Natl Inst Drug Abuse Res Monogr Ser 51:106–128, 1984

Anglin MD, Brecht, ML, Woodward JA, et al: An empirical study of maturing out: conditional factors. Int J Addict 21:233–246, 1986

Anglin MD, Hser Y, Booth MW: Sex differences in addict careers, 4: treatment. Am J Drug Alcohol Abuse 13:253–280, 1987

Arndt I, Dorozynsky L, McLellan AT, et al: Desipramine treatment of cocaine abuse in methadone maintenance patients. NIDA Res Monogr Ser 95:322–323, 1990

Bale RN, Zarcone VP, VanStone WW, et al: Three therapeutic communities: a prospective controlled study of narcotic addiction treatment; process and two-year follow-up results. Arch Gen Psychiatry 41:185–191, 1984

Ball J, Corty E, Bond H, et al: The reduction of intravenous heroin use, nonopiate use and crime during methadone maintenance treatment: further findings. Natl Inst Drug Abuse Res Monogr Ser 81:224–230, 1987

Ball JC, Lange WR, Myers CP, et al: Reducing the risk of AIDS through methadone maintenance treatment. J Health Soc Behav 29:214–226, 1988

Barr HL, Cohen A: Abusers of alcohol and narcotics: who are they? Int J Addict 22:525–541, 1987

Baum C, Hsu JP, Nelson RC: The impact of the addition of naloxone on the use and abuse of pentazocine. Public Health Rep 102:426–429, 1987

Bell J, Seres V, Bowron P, et al: The use of serum methadone levels in patients receiving methadone maintenance. Clin Pharmacol Ther 43:623–629, 1988

Bell J, Bowron P, Lewis J, et al: Serum levels of methadone in maintenance clients who persist in illicit drug use. Br J Addict 85:1599–1602, 1990

Bickel WK, Johnson RE, Stitzer ML, et al: A clinical trial of buprenorphine, I: comparison with methadone in the detoxification of heroin addicts, II: examination of its opioid blocking properties. Natl Inst Drug Abuse Res Monogr Ser 76:182–188, 1987

Brown BS, Watters JK, Iglehart AS: Methadone maintenance dosage levels and program retention. Am J Drug Alcohol Abuse 9:129–139, 1982-83

Callahan P, Pasternak GW: Opiate receptor multiplicity: evidence for multiple mu receptors. Monogr Neural Sci 13:121–131, 1987

Capone T, Brahen L, Condren R, et al: Retention and outcome in a narcotic antagonist treatment program. J Clin Psychol 42:825–833, 1986

Charney DS, Sternberg DE, Kleber HD, et al: The clinical use of clonidine in abrupt withdrawal from methadone. Arch Gen Psychiatry 38:1273–1277, 1981

Charney DS, Heninger GR, Kleber HD: The combined use of clonidine and naltrexone as a rapid, safe, and effective treatment of abrupt withdrawal from methadone. Am J Psychiatry 143:831–837, 1986

Childress AR, McLellan AT, Ehrman R, et al: Classically conditioned responses in opioid and cocaine dependence: a role in relapse? Natl Inst Drug Abuse Res Monogr Ser 84: 25–43, 1988

Ciraulo DA, Ciraulo AN: Substance abuse, in Handbook of Clinical Psychopharmacology. Edited by Tupin JP, Shader RI, Harnett DS. Northvale, NJ, Jason Aronson, 1988, p 143

Clayton RR, Voss HL: Young men and drugs in Manhattan: a causal analysis. Natl Inst Drug Abuse Res Monogr Ser 39:1–187, 1981

Cushman P, Dole VP: Detoxification of rehabilitated methadone-maintained patients. JAMA 226:747–752, 1973

DeLeon G: The therapeutic community: status and evolution. International Journal of the Addictions 20:823–844, 1985

Dole VP: Implications of methadone maintenance for theories of narcotic addiction. JAMA 260:3025–3029, 1988

Dole VP, Joseph H: Long-term outcome of patients treated with methadone. Ann NY Acad Sci 311:181–189, 1978

Dole VP, Nyswander MN: A medical treatment for diacetylmorphine (heroin) addiction. JAMA 193:646–650, 1965

Dole VP, Nyswander MN: Heroin addiction: a metabolic disease. Arch Intern Med 120:19–24, 1967

Finnegan LP, Michael H, Leifer B, et al: An evaluation of neonatal abstinence treatment modalities. Natl Inst Drug Abuse Res Monogr Ser 49:282–288, 1984

Fram DH, Marmo J, Holden R: Naltrexone treatment: the problem of patient acceptance. J Subst Abuse Treat 6:119–122, 1989

Fudala PJ, Jaffe JH, Dax EM, et al: Use of buprenorphine in the treatment of opioid addiction, II: physiologic and behavioral effects of daily and alternate-day administration and abrupt withdrawal. Clin Pharmacol Ther 47:525–534, 1990a

Fudala PJ, Johnson RE, Jaffe JH: Outpatient comparison of buprenorphine and methadone maintenance, II: effects on cocaine use, retention time in study, and missed clinic visits. Paper presented at the scientific meeting of the Committee on Problems of Drug Dependence, Richmond, VA, June 1990b

Gerstein DR, Harwood HJ (eds): Treating Drug Problems, Vol 1: A Study of the Evolution, Effectiveness, and Financing of Public and Private Drug Treatment Systems. Washington, DC, National Academy Press, 1990

Ginzburg HM: Naltrexone: its clinical utility (NIDA Treatment Research Report ADM-84-1358). Washington, DC, U.S. Government Printing Office, 1984

Ginzburg HM, Allison M, Hubbard RL: Depressive symptoms in drug abuse treatment clients: correlates, treatment and changes. Natl Inst Drug Abuse Res Monogr Ser 49:313–319, 1984

Gold MS, Redmond DE, Kleber HD: Clonidine in opiate withdrawal. Lancet 1:929–930, 1978

Goldstein A: Opioid peptides: function and significance, in Opioids: Past, Present, and Future. Edited by Collier HDJ, Hughes J, Rance MJ, et al. London, Taylor and Frances, 1984, pp 127–143

Gossop M, Bradley B, Phillips GT: An investigation of withdrawal symptoms shown by opiate addicts during and subsequent to a 21-day inpatient methadone detoxification procedure. Addict Behav 12:1–6, 1987

Green J, Jaffe JH: Alcohol and opiate dependence. J Stud Alcohol 38:1274–1293, 1977

Green L, Gossop M: Effects of information on the opiate withdrawal syndrome. Br J Addict 83:305–309, 1988

Hartog J, Tusel DJ: Valium use and abuse by methadone maintenance clients. Int J Addict 22:1147–1154, 1987

Herrington RE, Benzer DG, Jacobson GR, et al: Treating substance use disorders among physicians. JAMA 247:2253–2257, 1982

Heishman SJ, Stitzer ML, Bigelow GE, et al: Acute opioid physical dependence in postaddict humans: naloxone dose effects after brief morphine exposure. J Pharmacol Exp Ther 248:127–134, 1989

Himmelsbach CK: The morphine abstinence syndrome, its nature and treatment. Ann Intern Med 15:829–839, 1941

Hollister LE, Johnson K, Bowkhabza, et al: Aversive effects of naltrexone in subjects not dependent on opiates. Drug Alcohol Depend 8:37–41, 1981

Hubbard RL, Marsden ME, Rachal JV, et al: Drug Abuse Treatment: A National Study of Effectiveness. Chapel Hill, University of North Carolina Press, 1989

Hunt DE, Lipton DS, Goldsmith DS, et al: "It takes your heart": the image of methadone maintenance in the addict world and its effect on recruitment into treatment. Int J Addict 20:1751–1771, 1985-86

Jaffe JH: Drug dependence: opioids, nonnarcotics, nicotine (tobacco), and caffeine, in Comprehensive Textbook of Psychiatry, 5th Edition, Vol 1. Edited by Kaplan HI, Sadock BJ. Baltimore, Williams & Wilkins, 1989, pp 642–686

Jaffe JH: Drug addiction and drug abuse, in Goodman and Gilman's The Pharmacological Basis of Therapeutics, 8th Edition. Edited by Gilman AG, Rall TW, Nies AS, et al. New York, Pergamon, 1990, pp 522–573

Jaffe JH, Martin WR: Opioid analgesics and antagonists, in Goodman and

Gilman's The Pharmacological Basis of Therapeutics, 8th Edition. Edited by Gilman AG, Rall TW, Nies AS, et al. New York, Pergamon, 1990, pp 485–521

Jasinski DR, Pevnick JS, Griffith JD: Human pharmacology and abuse potential of the analgesic buprenorphine. Arch Gen Psychiatry 35:501–516, 1978

Jasinski DR, Johnson RE, Kocher TR: Clonidine in morphine withdrawal: differential effects on signs and symptoms. Arch Gen Psychiatry 42:1063–1066, 1985

Joe GW, Simpson DD: Mortality rates among opioid addicts in a longitudinal study. Am J Public Health 77:347–348, 1987

Johnson RE, Fudala PJ, Jaffe JH: Outpatient comparison of buprenorphine and methadone maintenance, I: effects on opiate use and subject-reported side effects and withdrawal symptoms. Paper presented at the scientific meeting of the Committee on Problems of Drug Dependence, Richmond, VA, June 1990

Jones RT: Dependence in non-addict humans after a single dose of morphine, in Endogenous and Exogenous Opiate Agonists and Antagonists Edited by Way EL. New York, Pergamon, 1979, pp 557–560

Joseph H, Appel P: Alcoholism and methadone treatment: consequences for the patient and program. Am J Drug Alcohol Abuse 11:37–53, 1985

Kandel D, Faust R: Sequence and stages in patterns of adolescent drug use. Arch Gen Psychiatry 32:923–932, 1975

Kaufman E: A contemporary approach to the family treatment of substance abuse disorders. Am J Drug Alcohol Abuse 12:199–211, 1986

Khantzian EJ, Schneider RJ: Treatment implications of a psychodynamic understanding of opioid addicts, in Psychopathology and Addictive Disorders. Edited by Meyer RE. New York, Guilford, 1986, pp 323–333

Khantzian EJ, Treece T: DSM-III psychiatric diagnosis of narcotic addicts: recent findings. Arch Gen Psychiatry 42:1067–1071, 1985

Kleber HD: Detoxification from narcotics, in Substance Abuse: Clinical Problems and Perspectives. Edited by Lowinson J, Ruiz P. Baltimore, Williams & Wilkins, 1981, pp 317–338

Kleber HD, Kosten TR: Naltrexone induction: psychologic and pharmacologic strategies. J Clin Psychiatry 45:29–38, 1984

Kleber HD, Weissman MM, Rounsaville BJ, et al: Imipramine as treatment for depression in addicts. Arch Gen Psychiatry 40:649–653, 1983

Kleber HD, Riordan CE, Rounsaville B, et al: Clonidine in outpatient detoxification from methadone maintenance. Arch Gen Psychiatry 42:391–394, 1985

Kleber HD, Topazian M, Gaspari J, et al: Clonidine and naltrexone in the outpatient treatment of heroin withdrawal. Am J Drug Alcohol Abuse 13:1–17, 1987

Kosten TR, Kleber HD: Buprenorphine detoxification from opioid dependence: a pilot study. Life Sci 42:635–641, 1988

Kosten TR, Rounsaville BJ, Kleber HD: A 2.5 year follow-up of depression, life crises, and treatment effects on abstinence among opioid addicts. Arch Gen Psychiatry 43:733–738, 1986a

Kosten TR, Rounsaville BJ, Kleber HD: A 2.5 year follow-up of treatment retention and reentry among opioid addicts. J Subst Abuse Treat 3:181–189, 1986b

Kosten TR, Rounsaville BJ, Kleber HD. Multidimensionality and prediction of treatment outcome in opioid addicts: 2.5 year follow-up. Compr Psychiatry 28:3–13, 1987a

Kosten TR, Rounsaville BJ, Kleber HD. Predictors of 2.5 year outcome in opioid addicts: pretreatment source of income. Am J Drug Alcohol Abuse 13:19–32, 1987b

Kosten TR, Rounsaville BJ, Kleber HD: A 2.5 year follow-up of cocaine use among treated opioid addicts. Arch Gen Psychiatry 44:281–284, 1987c

Kosten TR, Gawin F, Schumann B: Treating cocaine abusing methadone maintenance patients with desipramine. Natl Inst Drug Abuse Res Monogr Ser 81:237–241, 1987d

Kosten TR, Morgan C, Kosten TA: Depressive symptoms during buprenorphine treatment of opioid abusers. J Subst Abuse Treat 7:51–54, 1990

Kreek MJ: Methadone in treatment: physiological and pharmacological issues, in Handbook on Drug Abuse. Edited by Dupont RL, Goldstein A, O'Donnell J. Washington, DC, U.S. Government Printing Office, 1979, pp 57–86

Kreek MJ: Health consequences associated with the use of methadone, in Research on the Treatment of Narcotic Addiction: State of the Art. NIDA Research Monograph ADM-83-1281. Edited by Cooper JR, Altman R, Brown BS, et al. Washington, DC, U.S. Government Printing Office, 1983, pp 456–482

Ling W, Klett CJ, Gillis RD: A cooperative clinical study of methadyl acetate. Arch Gen Psychiatry 35:345–353, 1978

Ling W, Weiss DG, Charuvastra VC, et al: Use of disulfiram for alcoholics in methadone maintenance programs. Arch Gen Psychiatry 40:851–854, 1983

Maany I, Dhopesh V, Arndt IO, et al: Increase in desipramine serum levels associated with methadone treatment. Am J Psychiatry 146:1611–1613, 1989

Magura S, Goldsmith D, Casriel C, et al: The validity of methadone clients' self-reported drug use. Int J Addict 22:727–749, 1987

Martin WA: Pharmacology of opioids. Pharmacol Rev 35:283–323, 1983

Martin WR, Jasinski DR, Haertzen CA, et al: Methadone: a reevaluation. Arch Gen Psychiatry 28:286–295, 1973

McAuliffe WE, Ch'ien JMN: Recovery training and self help: a relapse-prevention program for treated opiate addicts. J Subst Abuse Treat 3:9–20, 1986

McCaul ME, Bigelow GE, Stitzer ML, et al: Short-term effects of oral methadone in methadone maintenance subjects. Clin Pharmacol Ther 31:753–761, 1982

McLellan AT: "Psychiatric severity" as a predictor of outcome from substance abuse treatments, in Psychopathology and Addictive Disorders. Edited by Meyer RE. New York, Guilford, 1986, pp 97–139

McLellan AT, Luborsky L, Woody GE, et al: Predicting responses to alcohol and drug abuse treatments: role of psychiatric severity. Arch Gen Psychiatry 40:620–625, 1983

McLellan AT, Childress AR, Ehrman R, et al: Extinguishing conditioned responses during opiate dependence treatment; turning laboratory findings into clinical procedures. J Subst Abuse Treat 3:33–40, 1986

Mello NK, Mendelson JH: Buprenorphine suppresses heroin use by heroin addicts. Science 207:657–659, 1980

Mello NK, Mendelson JH, Bree MT, et al: Buprenorphine and naltrexone affects on cocaine self-administration by rhesus monkeys. J Pharmacol Exp Ther 254:926–939, 1990

Menk EJ, Baumgarten RK, Kingsley CP, et al: Success of reentry into anesthesiology training programs by residents with a history of substance abuse. JAMA 263:3060–3062, 1990

Meyer RE, Mirin SM: The Heroin Stimulus: Implication for a Theory of Addiction. New York, Plenum, 1979

Milby JB, Gurwitch RH, Wiebe DJ, et al: Prevalence and diagnostic reliability of methadone maintenance detoxification fear. Am J Psychiatry 143:739–743, 1986

Mirin SM, Weiss RD, Michael J: Family pedigree of psychopathology in substance abusers, in Psychopathology and Addictive Disorders. Edited by Meyer RE. New York, Guilford, 1986, pp 57–77

Mirin SM, Weiss RD, Michael J: Psychopathology in substance abusers: diagnosis and treatment. Am J Drug Alcohol Abuse 14:139–157, 1988

Misra AL: Metabolism of opiates, in Factors Affecting the Action of Narcotics. Edited by Adler ML, Mangra L, Samanin R. New York, Raven, 1978, pp 297–343

National Institute on Drug Abuse and Food and Drug Administration: Methadone in maintenance and detoxification: joint proposed reissue of conditions for use. Federal Register Part II, October 2, 1987, pp 37046–37061

National Institute on Drug Abuse: National Household Survey on Drug Abuse: Main Findings 1985. Rockville, MD, National Institute on Drug Abuse, 1988

National Research Council: Clinical evaluation of naltrexone treatment of opiate-dependent individuals: report of the National Research Council Committee on Clinical Evaluation of Narcotic Antagonists. Arch Gen Psychiatry 35:335–340, 1978

Novick DM, Pascarelli EF, Joseph H, et al: Methadone maintenance patients in general medical practice: a preliminary report. JAMA 259:3299–3302, 1988

Nurco DN, Shaffer JW, Ball JC, et al: Trends in the commission of crime among narcotic addicts over successive periods of addiction and nonaddiction. Am J Drug Alcohol Abuse 10:481–489, 1984

Nurco DN, Kinlock TW, Hanlon TE, et al: Nonnarcotic drug use over an addiction career: a study of heroin addicts in Baltimore and New York City. Compr Psychiatry 29:450–459, 1988

O'Brien CP, Terenius L, Wahlstrom A, et al: Endorphin levels in opioid-dependent human subjects: a longitudinal study. Ann NY Acad Sci 398:377–387, 1982

Peyrot M: Narcotics Anonymous: its history, structure, and approach. Int J Addict 20:1509–1522, 1985

Portenoy RK, Foley KM: Chronic use of opioid analgesics in non-malignant pain: report of 38 cases. Pain 25:171–186, 1986

Redmond DE, Krystal JH: Multiple mechanisms of withdrawal from opioid drugs. Annu Rev Neurosci 7:443–478, 1984

Reed DA, Schnoll SH: Abuse of pentazocine-naloxone combination. JAMA 256:2562–2564, 1986

Regier DA, Farmer ME, Rae DS, et al: Comorbidity of mental disorders with alcohol and other drug abuse. JAMA 264:2511–2518, 1990

Resnick RB, Schuyten-Resnick E, Washton AM: Assessment of narcotic antagonists in the treatment of opioid dependence. Annu Rev Pharmacol Toxicol 20:463–474, 1980

Robins LN, Helzer JE, Davis DH: Narcotic use in Southeast Asia and afterwards. Arch Gen Psychiatry 32:955–961, 1975

Roehrich H, Gold MS: Propranolol as adjunct to clonidine in opiate detoxification. Am J Psychiatry 144:1099–1100, 1987

Rosen TS, Johnson HL: Long-term effects of prenatal methadone maintenance. Natl Inst Drug Abuse Res Monogr Ser 59:73–83, 1985

Rounsaville BJ, Kleber HD: Psychotherapy/counseling for opiate addicts: strategies for use in different treatment settings. Int J Addict 20:869–896, 1985a

Rounsaville BJ, Kleber HD: Untreated opiate addicts. Arch Gen Psychiatry 42:1072–1077, 1985b

Rounsaville BJ, Weissman MM, Kleber HD, et al: Heterogeneity of psychiatric diagnosis in treated opiate addicts. Arch Gen Psychiatry 39:161–166, 1982

Rounsaville BJ, Glazer W, Wilber CH, et al: Short-term interpersonal psychotherapy in methadone-maintained opiate addicts. Arch Gen Psychiatry 40:629–636, 1983

Rounsaville BJ, Kosten TR, Kleber HD: Long-term changes in current psychiatric diagnoses of treated opiate addicts. Compr Psychiatry 27:480–498, 1986a

Rounsaville BJ, Kosten TR, Weissman MM, et al: Prognostic significance of psychopathology in treated opiate addicts. Arch Gen Psychiatry 43:739–745, 1986b

Rounsaville BJ, Kosten TR, Kleber HD: The antecedents and benefits of achieving abstinence in opioid addicts: a 2.5 year follow-up study. Am J Drug Alcohol Abuse 13:213–229, 1987

Rounsaville J, Kosten TR, Weissman MM, et al: Psychiatric disorders in relatives of probands with opiate addiction. Arch Gen Psychiatry 48:33–42, 1991

Seecof R, Tennant FS: Subjective perceptions to the intravenous "rush" of heroin and cocaine in opioid addicts. Am J Drug Alcohol Abuse 12:79–87, 1987

Sells SB: Treatment effectiveness, in Handbook on Drug Abuse. Edited by Dupont RL, Goldstein A, O'Donnell J. Washington, DC, U.S. Government Printing Office, 1979, pp 105–118

Senay EC: Methadone maintenance treatment. Int J Addict 20:803–821, 1985

Senay EC, Dorus W, Goldberg F, et al: Withdrawal from methadone maintenance: rate of withdrawal and expectation. Arch Gen Psychiatry 34:361–367, 1977

Simpson DD, Marsh KL: Relapse and recovery among opioid addicts 12 years after treatment. Natl Inst Drug Abuse Res Monogr Ser 72:86–103, 1986

Simpson DD, Joe GW, Bracy SA: Six-year follow-up of opioid addicts after admission to treatment. Arch Gen Psychiatry 39:1318–1323, 1982

Simpson DD, Joe GW, Lehman WEK: Addiction careers: summary of studies based on the DARP 12-year follow-up (NIDA Treatment Research Report ADM-86-1420). Washington, DC, U.S. Government Printing Office, 1986

Spitzer RL, Endicott J, Robins E: Research Diagnostic Criteria: rationale and reliability. Arch Gen Psychiatry 35:773–782, 1978

Stanton MD: The Family Therapy of Drug Abuse and Addiction. New York, Guilford, 1982

Stimmel B, Goldberg J, Rotkopf E, et al: Ability to remain abstinent after methadone detoxification: a six year study. JAMA 237:1216–1220, 1977

Stimson GV, Oppenheimer E: Heroin Addiction: Treatment and Control in Britain. London, Tavistock, 1982

Tennant FS: Inadequate plasma concentrations in some high-dose methadone maintenance patients. Am J Psychiatry 144:1349–1350, 1987a

Tennant FS: LAAM maintenance for opioid addicts who cannot maintain with methadone. Natl Inst Drug Abuse Res Monogr Ser 81:294, 1987b

Tennant FS, Rawson RA, Pumphrey E, et al: Clinical experiences with 959 opioid-dependent patients treated with levo-alpha-acetylmethadol (LAAM). J Subst Abuse Treat 3:195–202, 1986

Trueblood B, Judson BA, Goldstein A: Acceptability of methadyl acetate (L-AAM) as compared with methadone in a treatment program for heroin addicts. Drug Alcohol Depend 3:125–132, 1978

Vining E, Kosten TR, Kleber H: Clinical utility of rapid clonidine-naltrexone detoxification for opioid abusers. Br J Addict 83:567–575, 1988

Washton AM, Resnick RG: Clonidine in opiate withdrawal: review and appraisal of clinical findings. Pharmacotherapy 1:140–146, 1981

Washton AM, Pottash AC, Gold MS: Naltrexone in addicted business executives and physicians. J Clin Psychiatry 45:39–41, 1984

Way EL: Distribution and metabolism of morphine and its surrogates. Res Publ Assoc Res Nerv Ment Dis 46:13–31, 1968

Way EL: Sites and mechanisms of basic narcotic receptor function based on current research. Ann Emerg Med 15:1021–1025, 1986

Wesson DR: Revival of medical maintenance in the treatment of heroin dependence (editorial). JAMA 259:3314–3315, 1988

Wikler A: Opioid Dependence: Mechanisms and Treatment. New York, Plenum, 1980

Woody GE, O'Brien CP, Rickels K: Depression and anxiety in heroin addicts: a placebo-controlled study of doxepin in combination with methadone. Am J Psychiatry 132:447–450, 1975

Woody GE, Luborsky L, McLellan AT, et al: Psychotherapy for opiate addicts: does it help? Arch Gen Psychiatry 40:639–645, 1983

Woody GE, McLellan AT, Luborsky L, et al: Severity of psychiatric symptoms as a predictor of benefits from psychotherapy: the Veterans Administration-Penn study. Am J Psychiatry 141:1172–1177, 1984

Woody GE, McLellan AT, Luborsky L, et al: Twelve-month follow-up of psychotherapy for opiate dependence. Am J Psychiatry 144:590–596, 1987

Wurmser L: The Hidden Dimensions: Psychotherapy of Compulsive Drug Use. Northvale, NJ, Jason Aronson, 1979

Zangwell BC, McGahan P, Dorozynsky L, et al: How effective is LAAM treatment? clinical comparison with methadone. Natl Inst Drug Abuse Monogr Ser 67:249–255, 1986

Chapter 3

Anxiolytics

Domenic A. Ciraulo, M.D.
Brian F. Sands, M.D.
Richard I. Shader, M.D.
David J. Greenblatt, M.D.

Benzodiazepines

Diagnosis

The diagnosis and treatment of benzodiazepine dependence is an important issue for both the generalist and the substance dependence specialist. There is now a large body of literature on this subject, consideration of which requires some clarity of thought and language. Terminology has changed substantially in the past 20 years, imposing the need to understand the nosologic assumptions of individual studies to interpret their findings. The most recent redaction is DSM-III-R (American Psychiatric Association 1987), where the substance abuse disorders are renamed psychoactive substance dependence disorders (Rounsaville et al. 1986). Dependence is here defined along the lines of the World Health Organization (WHO) memorandum on nomenclature and classification of drug- and alcohol-related problems: "a syndrome manifested by a behavioral pattern in which the use of a given psychoactive drug, or class of drugs, is given a much higher priority than other behaviors that once had higher value" (World Health Organization 1981, p. 240). The "old" definition of dependence was simply that a discontinuation syndrome could be demonstrated when drug ingestion ceased. The condition of "drug addiction" may exist in the presence of either dependence or tolerance.

The distinction between the old and the new definition of dependence is particularly important in attempting to interpret the now considerable literature on benzodiazepines. When these drugs were originally introduced, they were thought not to cause dependence (in the old sense, henceforth we refer to this as physiologic dependence to distinguish it from DSM-III-R dependence). This was heralded as a pharmacologic advance, in contradistinction to the barbiturates. It was therefore of considerable interest when Hollister et al. (1961) demonstrated physiologic dependence after very large doses of chlordiazepoxide for many months. This and other work led to the perspective that physiologic dependence did occur at high doses but not in regular, therapeutic clinical use. As concern grew over the staggering growth in sales of benzodiazepines in the 1960s, attention was paid to the potential of these drugs to be "addicting." Tolerance to the antianxiety effect has not been convincingly demonstrated, although it does develop to the sedative and psychomotor effects. Research in benzodiazepine dependence has, as a consequence, relied on the abstinence syndrome as an objective marker of addictiveness.

As new information became available, the concept of the dose and exposure time needed to produce physiologic dependence changed. Busto et al. (1986a, 1986b) demonstrated a withdrawal syndrome following chronic use of several benzodiazepines at therapeutic doses, and an abstinence syndrome has been demonstrated in cats after a single dose of diazepam using the benzodiazepine antagonist Ro 15-1788 (Rosenberg and Chiu 1985). Thus the presence of a discontinuation syndrome is not uncommon following chronic treatment and is not sufficient evidence for DSM-III-R substance dependence. This distinction is crucial in considering both the literature and the clinical situations where benzodiazepine use may come under our scrutiny.

Diagnostic criteria are those for psychoactive substance dependence as listed in DSM-III-R. Patients who do not meet all the criteria may qualify for the diagnosis of psychoactive substance abuse.

Of the patients who are referred for assessment of benzodiazepine use, some meet criteria for substance dependence while others are using the medication appropriately. In the first group, patients may be dependent on benzodiazepines alone, or benzodiazepines may be part of a picture of mixed substance dependence. When benzodiazepines are part of mixed substance dependence, the doses tend to be higher and the patients younger than in "pure" benzodiazepine dependence (Busto et al. 1986a, 1986b). High-dose use may be correlated with high levels of caffeine use, male sex, and youth (Perera and Jenner 1987). For the group of patients taking legitimately prescribed medication, it is necessary to consider the indications for the benzodiazepine, the presence of adverse effects, and whether a trial at a lower dose or medication free is appropriate.

Several events can trigger intervention: 1) self-referral of a patient who is concerned about the inability to stop taking legitimately prescribed medication; 2) detection of benzodiazepines or benzodiazepine metabolites in serum or urine of a patient who is not prescribed benzodiazepines (indicating a nonmedical source); 3) observation of a physiologic withdrawal syndrome in a patient who, when admitted for other reasons, denied benzodiazepine use; 4) evidence of strange or dangerous behavior because of benzodiazepine intoxication; or 5) allegation of benzodiazepine dependence when in treatment for another substance. As usual, the clinician's best diagnostic "tool" is a good, detailed history, from both the patient and the family.

Prevalence

Benzodiazepine dependence case reports peaked between 1969 and 1973, approximately 10 years after their introduction (Petursson and Lader 1981a). Changing medical opinion has had an effect: after years of steady growth, benzodiazepine prescribing declined in the Federal Republic of Germany in 1983 and 1984 (Müller-Oerlinghausen 1986). Since 1985, prescriptions for anxiolytic benzodiazepines in the United States have remained constant at about 61 million annually (American Psychiatric Association 1990). However, lorazepam and alparzolam have steadily increased their market share; by 1987 alprazolam was the most widely prescribed anxiolytic benzodiazepine (American Psychiatric Association 1990). Public attitudes about benzodiazepines have also shifted (Clinthorne et al. 1986).

Marks (1978) reviewed published reports of benzodiazepine dependence in the literature from 1961 to 1977 and estimated that benzodiazepine dependence occurred in one case per 50 million patient months of use. His assessment of risk has been criticized, however, because published case reports tend to occur less frequently than the phenomenon they describe.

Estimates of prevalence may be more appropriately based on several national and cross-national surveys of use in the general population and on surveys of use in medical clinics, psychiatric clinics, and chemical dependency treatment units.

A national survey in 1971 showed that 15% (20% of women and 8% of men) had taken at least one dose of a minor tranquilizer in the past year (Parry et al. 1973). A second survey conducted by the same group in 1979 (Mellinger and Balter 1981) demonstrated the use of a tranquilizing agent in 14.1% of women and 7.5% of men (11.1% for both men and women). A multinational survey done in 1981 showed prevalence of 17.6% in Belgium, 12.9% in the United States, and 7.4% in the Netherlands (Balter et al. 1984). Results between these studies are not completely comparable because of differences in the way that medications are defined. A 1984 survey evaluated chronic anxiolytic use in the United States and found that long-term users tend to be older and female, with high levels of emotional distress and chronic somatic health problems (Mellinger et al. 1984). That study also concluded that women are more likely than men to use anxiolytics, but once men become users, they are at least as likely to become long-term users.

Greenblatt et al. (1975) reported results of the Boston Collaborative Drug Surveillance Program, which showed that of 24,633 consecutive admissions to general medical or surgical wards of 24 Boston hospitals, 14% of patients remembered having taken an antianxiety agent at least once in the preceding 3 months. Interestingly, no cases of physiologic withdrawal symptoms were reported.

One would expect that the prevalence of benzodiazepine use among psychiatric patients would be higher than in the general population. Gottschalk et al. (1971) compared 65 adults presenting for the first time to a mental health crisis center with 48 presenting for the first time to a general medical clinic and found that 36.9% of the mental health patients versus 14.5% of the general medical patients were using minor tranquilizers. A study of psychiatric outpatients in a behaviorally oriented adult clinic in the United Kingdom reported that 38% of patients used minor tranquilizers (Samarasinghe et al. 1984).

In an effort to determine whether persons chronically treated with benzodiazepines would become dependent (old definition), Hallstrom and Lader (1982) contacted members of the Phobics Society (a voluntary self-help organization in the United Kingdom for phobia sufferers) through their newsletter. Eighty-five members volunteered to take part in a survey, and 71 returned the survey with enough information to be included in the study. Of these, 80% were female. Of the 71 respondents, 72% took only benzodiazepines, and the remainder took them in combination with other medications. Of the 71, 58 had tried to reduce or discontinue their medication at some time; 22 of these (38%) experienced the emergence of new symptoms (not present before the start of treatment). A prospective study by Garvey and Tollefson (1986) followed 71 patients with either an anxiety disorder or major depression who were prescribed benzodiazepines for an average of 8 months. No patient abused a benzodiazepine but misuse was reported in 5 (7%).

Among the cases of benzodiazepine dependence collected by Marks (1978), 151 were within the framework of multiple substance abuse, with 250 less definite cases. Abusers take benzodiazepines when other, more desirable drugs are unavailable, to "come down" from stimulants; or to potentiate the effects of opiates. Use in terminating an amphetamine or cocaine binge is fairly common.

Urinary evidence of benzodiazepines was found in 69 (9.2%) of 750 consecutive persons entering a chemical dependence treatment hospital (Cushman and Benzer 1980). Of these, all but one admitted to abuse of multiple drugs or alcohol. In another study, of 176 consecutive patients referred for assessment and treatment of benzodiazepine abuse in 1982 and 1983, 44% also abused other drugs (Busto et al. 1986a, 1986b).

In a unique and valuable study (Fleischhacker et al. 1986), a chart review of 10,861 inpatients and outpatients of the Innsbruck University Department of Psychiatry seen between January 1978 and September 1981, 1,743 inpatients and 2,130 outpatients were dependent on a psychotropic substance by ICD-9 criteria (World Health Organization 1977). Although benzodiazepines were abused in 57 inpatients and 73 outpatients, in most of these cases, the benzodiazepine dependence was part of polysubstance dependence. Benzodiazepine dependence alone was found in only 9 inpatients and 21 outpatients.

In summary, 7.4–17.6% of the general population appears to use a benzodiazepine at least once during any given year. This compares to a 17–36.9% usage rate among psychiatric outpatients. Of patients in treatment for substance dependence, 1.3–9.2% included benzodiazepines among their multiple substances, but only a very small number (on the order of 0.2%) were dependent on benzodiazepines only. Studies of benzodiazepine use in alcoholics indicate that between 3% and 41% are taking these drugs (Ashley et al. 1978; Bell et al. 1984; Busto et al. 1983; Kania and Kofoed 1984; Kryspin-Exner 1966; Kryspin-Exner and Demel 1975; Rothstein et al. 1976; Schuckit and Morrissey 1979; Sokolow et al. 1981; Wiseman and Spencer-Peet 1985). The liability of alprazolam dependence is greater among alcoholics than nonalcoholics (Ciraulo et al. 1988a, 1988b) and likely for other benzodiazepines although differences in abuse potential exist between individual benzodiazepines (Griffiths and Wolf 1990; Jaffe et al. 1983). There is also evidence that oxazepam and halazepam have lower potential for abuse than diazepam (Griffiths et al. 1984; Jaffe et al. 1983). Alprazolam, diazepam, and lorazepam appear to have approximately the same potential for abuse; to the extent that acute euphoric effects predict abuse potential, they present the greatest risk. The actual risk of benzodiazepine dependence among alcoholics is unclear because methodological deficiencies of existing studies are substantial, but risk is probably higher in them as well as in the opiate addict (Ciraulo et al. 1988b).

Pharmacology

The term *benzodiazepine* refers to drugs with a structural core consisting of a benzene ring fused to a diazepine ring. All benzodiazepines in clinical use also contain a 5-aryl substituent ring and a 1,4-diazepine ring; and so the term has come to mean the 5-aryl-1,4-benzodiazepines (Greenblatt et al. 1983a, 1983b; Harvey 1985). A novel 1,5-benzodiazepine, clobazam (Divoll et al. 1982), is currently being studied. In the United States, 13 variations on the benzodiazepine core are approved for clinical use, and they all are sedative, hypnotic, anxiolytic, muscle relaxant, and anticonvulsant. Two benzodiazepines (alprazolam and clonazepam) also are efficacious in panic disorder, and one of these (alprazolam) has antidepressant properties. Alprazolam and triazolam are unique in that they contain a triazolo ring and are thus called triazolobenzodiazepines; adinazolam is another triazolobenzodiazepine that may have antidepressant properties and is now in premarketing clinical trials.

High-affinity binding sites for the benzodiazepines were first discovered in animal and human brain tissue in 1977 (Braestrup and

Squires 1977; Braestrup et al. 1977; Möhler and Okada 1977). Although benzodiazepine binding sites have been identified outside of the central nervous system (CNS), their function is not clear. Binding of benzodiazepines to CNS receptors is stereospecific and saturable and correlates to benzodiazepine potency as anxiolytics and anticonvulsants (Braestrup and Squires 1978). Benzodiazepines exert their pharmacodynamic action through facilitation of the inhibitory neurotransmitter, gamma-aminobutyric acid (GABA), at an allosterically linked site (Tallman et al. 1980). Binding at the receptor occurs at a macromolecular membrane complex containing four chloride-dependent, allosterically linked receptor sites: benzodiazepine, picrotoxin/convulsant, barbiturates, and GABA-A (Olsen et al. 1986). The macromolecular complex appears to consist of two alpha subunits, two beta subunits (which contain GABA-A binding sites), and a gamma 2 unit (which contains the benzodiazepine binding site). Recent evidence suggests heterogeneity of all three subunits (Zorumsky and Isenbeg 1991).

Two major groups of benzodiazepine binding sites have been identified: type I and type II (Zorumsky and Isenberg 1991). Type I receptors predominate in the CNS and have a higher affinity for CL 218872. Type II receptors are concentrated in the striatum, hippocampus, superior colliculus, and neocortex. CL 218872 appears in animals to be anxiolytic but not sedating, which suggests that different receptors may mediate sedative and anxiolytic effects. It is intriguing to speculate that abuse liability might relate to relative affinity for type I and type II receptors or that substance abuse prone individuals might express different receptor subunits.

Evidence also links ethanol to this macromolecular complex. It has been shown to stimulate chloride uptake in cell-free preparations of rat brain, an effect that was markedly inhibited by GABA antagonists picrotoxin and bicuculline (Suzdak et al. 1986). Ethanol may influence GABA-dependent chloride flux at a point beyond the binding sites for benzodiazepines or GABA. Benzodiazepine antagonists have been shown to block anticonflict actions of ethanol in rats (Liljequist and Engel 1984). The fact that benzodiazepines, barbiturates, and ethanol all impact on chloride flux is consistent with clinically demonstrated cross-tolerance between the three drugs and suggests potentially helpful, new pharmacotherapies. In an animal study, rats decreased their voluntary intake of ethanol when given homotaurine, a GABA agonist (Boismare et al. 1984). In a human study, homotaurine prevented relapse in some abstinent alcoholics (Lhuintre et al. 1985). This is an interesting development, but it has yet to be replicated.

A number of benzodiazepine receptor ligands have been characterized and can be considered in three overlapping groups (Braestrup et al. 1983): 1) agonists, which are ligands with benzodiazepine-like effects, such as muscimol; 2) antagonists, which bind to benzodiazepine receptors and inhibit receptor-mediated effects, such as B-carboline-3-carboxylate and 1,4-benzodiazepine-3-carboxylate (Ro 15-1788); and 3) inverse agonists, which bind to benzodiazepine receptors but have effects that are opposite those of agonists. Four examples of the last group are methyl B-carboline-3-carboxylate, methyl 6,7-dimethoxy-4-ethyl-B-carboline-3-carboxylate, Ro 15-4513, and CGS 8216. A classification scheme proposed by Nutt and Linnoila (1988) divides ligands into agonists or inverse agonists and then subclassifies each as full, partial, or antagonist.

Pharmacodynamic tolerance to the psychomotor effects of benzodiazepine has been demonstrated after single or multiple doses (File 1985; Greenblatt and Shader; 1978; Rosenberg and Chiu 1985). Pharmacodynamic tolerance to the anxiolytic effect (over a 6-month period) has not been demonstrated (Rickels et al. 1983), but replication from a larger number of investigators is lacking. An important clinical consequence of tolerance is observed in benzodiazepine overdoses, in which the patient may initially be somnolent, but may wake up and recover while the serum level of benzodiazepine active metabolite is very high and still rising.

Tolerance to the psychomotor impairment of lorazepam in mice (as demonstrated by a decrease in rotorod ataxia) has been correlated with a decrease in CNS benzodiazepine receptor binding, attributed to a decrease in receptor number (Miller et al. 1988a, 1988b). The greatest decrease in both ataxia and receptor binding occurred between days 4 and 7 of treatment. When lorazepam administration in mice was terminated after 7 days of treatment, receptor binding remained lower than baseline (before lorazepam administration) for 24 hours but had increased over baseline by 4 days posttermination (Miller et al. 1988a, 1988b). Binding returned to control levels by 7 days posttermination. Tolerance and withdrawal may therefore be mediated by changes in benzodiazepine receptor binding.

Pharmacokinetics

Absorption of benzodiazepines by the oral route is essentially complete, except for clorazepate, which is decarboxylated in gastric secretions to N-desmethyldiazepam, which is absorbed. Diazepam and N-desmethyldiazepam are the fastest absorbed and will reach a peak in serum soonest after ingestion (Greenblatt et al. 1983a, 1983b). Prazepam and halazepam are inactive or only slightly active prodrugs that are converted slowly to the active form. The appearance in serum of desmethyldiazepam from prazepam is the slowest among the benzodiazepines.

Some patients have reported sublingual use (particularly of lorazepam and alprazolam) to obtain a "high," presumably on the basis of faster absorption. While one group has found faster absorption of lorazepam by the sublingual route (Caille et al. 1983), a rigorous kinetic comparison of intravenous, intramuscular, oral, and sublingual routes failed to reveal significant differences between sublingual and oral administration in the fasted state (Greenblatt et al. 1982). It might be that sublingual absorption does offer an increased rate of absorption in the postprandial state. Alprazolam and triazolam may reach higher peak levels via the sublingual route. While benzodiazepines are all highly lipophilic, the lipophilicity varies more than 50-fold among individual benzodiazepines (Harvey 1985). Although the more lipophilic drugs tend to enter the cerebrospinal fluid most rapidly, in a study of diazepam, desmethyldiazepam, midazolam, lorazepam, alprazolam, flunitrazepam, and clobazam, all attained peak cerebrospinal fluid concentrations within 15 minutes of intravenous administration (Arendt et al. 1983). Benzodiazepines and their active metabolites all bind to plasma proteins, and this correlates with lipophilicity—from 70% for alprazolam to 99% for diazepam (Harvey 1985).

Benzodiazepines are metabolized via the hepatic microsomal system. Renal clearance is slight and of negligible clinical importance. All benzodiazepines ultimately undergo glucuronidation and some require prior oxidative metabolism, either N-dealkylation or aliphatic hydroxylation. Oxidative metabolism is relatively more susceptible to impairment from certain population characteristics (old age), coadministration of other drugs (cimetidine, disulfiram), or disease states (cirrhosis) than is glucuronidation. The metabolism of those drugs

that require only glucuronidation (oxazepam, lorazepam, temaze-
pam) is less susceptible to these influences than those drugs that require oxidation (chlordiazepoxide, diazepam, clorazepate, prazepam,
halazepam, flurazepam, triazolam, and alprazolam).

Benzodiazepines do not induce their own metabolism, and there
is no evidence for the development of pharmacokinetic tolerance
(Greenblatt and Shader 1986). The behavioral tolerance seen with
chronic dosing is explicable entirely on the basis of pharmacodynamic
tolerance (as described above).

Etiologic Theories

The genesis of benzodiazepine dependence is usually seen in one of
three quite different contexts: 1) sole benzodiazepine dependence in a
recreational drug setting (rare), 2) multiple substance dependence, or
3) dependence developing from medically sanctioned use. In the first
two cases, the drugs are usually illicitly obtained, and doses are commonly supratherapeutic. In the third case, benzodiazepines are more
likely to be obtained from one or several medical sources and may be
used at therapeutic or supratherapeutic doses. The common etiologic
thread derives from adherence to the concept of substance dependence, and hence the implication that the value of obtaining and ingesting the substance occupies a very high priority in the life of the
patient (World Health Organization 1981). The factors that could
contribute to the development of such dependence are 1) individual
genetic and developmental vulnerability; 2) the sociocultural-eco-
nomic setting; and 3) the reinforcing properties of the particular substance, both positive (drug effect) and negative (discontinuation syndrome).

Various models exist to explain individual developmental vulnerability. Psychoanalytic explanations began with a focus on fixation
at primitive developmental stages, as in Rado's (1926) concept of
"pharmacogenic orgasm" or oral eroticism. Glover (1928) postulated
partial fixation of the ego at oral and anal stages of development, with
a primitive conscience and a tendency to regress to narcissistic ego
organization. Then, in a transition that seemed to anticipate object
relations theory by many years, Glover (1931) wrote that the abused
substance was the symbolic embodiment of a necessary external love-
object that could not be internalized. This was further developed by
Krystal (1977), who explained the specific disturbance of drug-depen-

dent individuals as "the 'walling-off' of the maternal object-representation, and within it self-helping and comforting modes" (p. 93). The best modern psychodynamic synthesis is probably that of Khantzian (1986), who emphasized the role of substances for dependent patients in "regulating their internal emotional life and adjustment to external reality" (p. 213).

The issues of social, cultural, and economic influences are beyond the scope of this chapter. The last element, then, is the capacity of individual psychoactive agents to induce dependence. This can be divided into a positive, behavior-reinforcing aspect of taking the drug ("getting high"), and attempts to self-medicate an abstinence syndrome (physical dependence).

The positive behavioral reinforcement of substances has been examined in animal models but has been inconclusive for benzodiazepines (Griffiths and Ator 1980). Studies in humans have commonly involved choice paradigms. In subjects with a history of sedative drug abuse given a choice between pentobarbital, diazepam, chlorpromazine, and placebo, pentobarbital was preferred over diazepam, and both were preferred over chlorpromazine and placebo (Griffiths et al. 1979). Preference of pentobarbital over diazepam was replicated by the same group (Griffiths et al. 1980) and comparisons between other benzodiazepines made. Diazepam was preferred to halazepam (Jaffe et al. 1983) and to oxazepam (Griffiths et al. 1984). These results suggest that benzodiazepines differ from each other in reinforcement but as a group are less reinforcing than barbiturates. An explanation for why barbiturates are preferred in choice paradigms is lacking, but an interesting hypothesis is suggested by the results of a study by Yu et al. (1988) looking at modulation of GABA-gated chloride ion flux in rat brain microsacs. When chloride ion flux is plotted against GABA concentration, midazolam shifted the curve to the left without increasing the maximum response, whereas pentobarbital both shifted the curve leftward and increased the maximal response.

There is now ample evidence that benzodiazepines induce physiologic dependence. An abstinence syndrome was first demonstrated in patients receiving very high doses for long periods of time (Hollister et al. 1961), but has more recently been demonstrated with lower doses (Busto et al. 1986b). There is a relationship in animal models of the ability of some drugs to induce physiologic dependence and their ability to act as a reinforcer of drug administration behavior (Schuster and Thompson 1969), but this relationship is complex.

Differences in euphorigenic potential of benzodiazepines have been documented by several investigators. Those that induce euphoria most rapidly, and by inference have the highest abuse liability, are diazepam, alprazolam, lorazepam, and triazolam. Drugs that have a slow onset of activity, such as halazepam, do not produce euphoria.

Clinical Signs and Symptoms of Intoxication, Chronic Use, and Abstinence Syndrome

Intoxication. Benzodiazepines produce few pathognomonic signs of intoxication. Sedation, behavioral disinhibition, and occasional paradoxical excitation may all be seen. Toxicity can occur after large single doses (as in some cases of abuse or in deliberate overdose) or by drug accumulation in persons with impaired metabolism. Three cardinal features of benzodiazepine toxicity are ataxia, diplopia, and impaired gag reflex. Level of consciousness may vary from light sedation to obtundation. Unless combined with other drugs (such as alcohol), morbidity is slight. Tolerance develops rapidly and it is not uncommon following single, large doses to see an initial period of sedation followed by apparent recovery while serum levels of active metabolites are still rising (Greenblatt et al. 1979). The competitive benzodiazepine antagonist Ro 15-1788 (available in Europe under the name flumazenil) has been used to reverse benzodiazepine-induced sedation following surgery or diagnostic procedures (Brogden and Goa 1988). Use of flumazenil would not likely be required in benzodiazepine-only overdoses, but could be useful in mixed intoxication.

Chronic use. There are no consistent signs in chronic dependence on benzodiazepines alone. Such dependence generally comes to medical attention either because of withdrawal phenomena unexpected by the clinician or by consequences of obtaining the drug.

Abstinence syndrome. An abstinence syndrome after prolonged, high-dose administration was demonstrated with chlordiazepoxide (Hollister et al. 1961) and with diazepam (Hollister et al. 1963). This high-dose abstinence syndrome has been repeatedly confirmed and has been categorized by Smith and Wesson (1983) into either a minor withdrawal syndrome consisting of "anxiety, insomnia, and nightmares," or a major withdrawal syndrome consisting of "grand mal seizures, psychosis, hyperpyrexia, and possibly death" (p. 87).

An abstinence syndrome after long-term, low-dose treatment has also been described (Busto et al. 1986b; Covi et al. 1973; Petursson and Lader 1981b; Tyrer et al. 1981). Symptoms reported include: muscle twitching, abnormal perception of movement, depersonalization or derealization, anxiety, headache, insomnia, diaphoresis, difficulty concentrating, tremor, fear, fatigue, lowered threshold to perception of sensory stimuli, and dysphoria.

A rebound sleep disturbance has been found after only 7–10 days of treatment with therapeutic doses of triazolam (Greenblatt et al. 1987). Additionally, a withdrawal syndrome has also been described after substitution of a short-acting benzodiazepine for a long-acting benzodiazepine (Conell and Berlin 1983).

The clinician must be cautious in interpreting some of the above symptoms (especially anxiety) in patients withdrawing from benzodiazepines. Anxiety, fearfulness, and dysphoria may represent symptoms that were treated by the benzodiazepine and unmasked on withdrawal.

Protocols for Detoxification

Clinical situations where detoxification is indicated can be grouped into three categories: 1) patients who have been maintained on therapeutic dosages for moderate to long periods of time and for whom a trial off their medication is warranted; 2) patients taking supratherapeutic doses (usually benzodiazepine dependence); and 3) patients who use benzodiazepines as part of mixed substance dependence. Detoxification should be approached differently in each category.

Therapeutic doses. Patients may have been prescribed benzodiazepines for an acute problem that has since resolved but prescriptions were nonetheless renewed, for ill-defined reasons, or for a diagnosed anxiety disorder. The unifying features in this group are that patients have been using benzodiazepines at stable, therapeutic doses; they have been obtaining them from legitimate sources; and they may or may not still be deriving clinical benefit from the medication. Determining continued benefit may be difficult and may require periodic tapering or discontinuation of the benzodiazepine. Return of symptoms during the taper may support continued treatment, but the clinician should also consider the possibility of a discontinuation syndrome.

Detoxification can usually be accomplished using the same benzodiazepine that the patient is taking. Switching from a benzodiazepine with a short elimination half-life to one with a long elimination half-life may not be necessary if the tapering program is sufficiently long. If difficulty is encountered in tapering one benzodiazepine, however, then switching to one with a longer elimination half-life may be helpful. Substituting a medication with a shorter elimination half-life for one with a longer one is not advised (Conell and Berlin 1983). Approximate dosage equivalencies of benzodiazepines are listed in Table 3-1.

A consensus exists that tapering the first 50% of the dose may be done relatively quickly; the next 25% more slowly; and the last 25% even more slowly (American Psychiatric Association 1990). This should be individually adjusted based on the emergence of discontinuation symptoms.

Clinical experience suggests that alprazolam can be particularly difficult to taper when lower doses are reached (e.g., from 1 to 0 mg) (Ciraulo et al. 1990). One possible explanation for this is suggested by data in an animal model showing that alprazolam at doses of .02–.05 mg/kg increases benzodiazepine receptor number above baseline (Miller et al. 1987). When difficulty is encountered in tapering the last 1–2 mg of alprazolam, the rate of dose reduction can be decreased to .25 mg/week, and/or adjunctive medication strategies using clonazepam or carbamazepine may be employed.

Table 3-1. Approximate benzodiazepine dose equivalency

Generic name	Dose (mg)
Chlordiazepoxide	25
Diazepam	10
Lorazepam	2
Alprazolam	1
Triazolam	0.25
Clonazepam	0.5
Oxazepam	30
Temazepam	20
Clorazepate	15
Flurazepam	30
Prazepam	10

High doses. Patients requiring detoxification from high or supratherapeutic doses of benzodiazepines constitute a smaller number of patients, but they are at greater risk for life-threatening discontinuation symptoms, such as seizures, delirium, and psychoses. There has been more experience with inpatient detoxification in this group, but outpatient detoxification is possible if conducted slowly (5% reduction per week), with frequent contact, and in the context of a therapeutic alliance with the patient. Often, such an alliance proves unworkable because the patient's impoverished control results in supplementation from outside sources or early exhaustion of prescribed supplies meant to be tapered. In these cases, as in those with a history of seizures, delirium, or psychoses during previous detoxification attempts, inpatient detoxification is indicated.

A protocol for tapering high-dose benzodiazepines has been developed (Harrison et al. 1984) based on previous work by the same group that demonstrated barbiturate withdrawal symptoms did not develop if the t ½ β was greater than 60 hours. Based on this model, the authors devised a tapering schedule for diazepam with an initial dose equivalent to 40% of reported daily consumption and subsequent doses tapered by 10% per day to obtain an apparent t ½ β of 64.6 hours. In the study, 23 subjects who abused high doses of benzodiazepines (median equivalent diazepam dose, 150 mg) were treated according to this protocol. Of 16 subjects completing the program, 1 became paranoid and confused on day 7, and the rest reported only minor withdrawal symptoms. On further evaluation, it turned out that the patient who became paranoid and confused had been treated with less benzodiazepine than was called for by the model. The high dropout rate is likely an indicator that withdrawal symptoms, although "minor," were distressing enough for 7 patients to leave the study. For this reason, we recommend a more gradual schedule.

In high-dose detoxification, the risk of major adverse consequences requires that a smooth decline in plasma benzodiazepine levels be achieved. Here, switching from the substance of abuse to diazepam or other long-acting benzodiazepine is indicated. Patients should be switched to an equivalent dose of long-acting benzodiazepine given in divided daily doses (see Table 3-1) and stabilized on this for the first day. Then a 30% cut is made in dose on day 2, followed by a 5% cut on each day thereafter. This will result in complete detoxification in about 2 weeks for most patients, but the rate of tapering should be slowed even further in the presence of diaphoresis, tremulousness, or elevated vital signs. Hyperpyrexia is a grave sign and should prompt aggressive management. Supplemental benzodiazepine and supportive medical care are necessary in these instances. This protocol should serve only as a guideline because individual patients will vary in their sensitivity to withdrawal. True withdrawal is best distinguished from recurrence of anxiety by the development of new symptoms and/or the appearance of perceptual disturbance (e.g., ringing in ears, sensitivity to sounds, and dizziness). Whenever possible, doses should be adjusted to keep patients comfortable. Clonidine or beta-blockers, such as propranolol, can be helpful adjuncts in withdrawal (see below). Close monitoring for the week following detoxification is prudent because some symptoms may not be evident until then, as the desmethyldiazepam level continues to fall.

Benzodiazepines in mixed substance abuse. Sporadic use (as in the induction of sleep following a psychostimulant binge) does not require specific detoxification. Sustained use can be treated as described above for low or high doses but with added caution. In mixed opiate and benzodiazepine abuse, the patient should be stabilized on methadone and a benzodiazepine. Either drug may be tapered first; however, sedative-hypnotic withdrawal is the more medically serious procedure, and we usually taper the benzodiazepine first. In multiple CNS depressant abuse (benzodiazepines, barbiturates, ethanol, and propanediols), coverage can be achieved by a single medication, and a benzodiazepine is probably the safest choice.

Adjunctive medication strategies. Blockade of beta-adrenergic receptors by propranolol (60–120 mg/day) attentuates some withdrawal symptoms (Tyrer et al. 1981) and it, or other beta blockers, can be used as an adjunct to a program of dose tapering. Reduction of adrenergic transmission by use of clonidine (an alpha$_2$ agonist) has also been used with moderate success (Ashton 1984; Fyer et al. 1988). Clonidine can be started at .1 mg bid and can be increased to .2 mg tid if adequate blood pressure is sustained. It must be stressed that neither propranolol nor clonidine raises the seizure threshold and is therefore not, by itself, sufficient to cover benzodiazepine withdrawal. Buspirone is not cross-tolerant to benzodiazepines and is not helpful in relieving withdrawal symptoms (Lader and Olajide 1987).

Two medication strategies have been shown to be of benefit in assisting alprazolam tapering. Clonazepam can be substituted gradu-ally over the course of a week at an alprazolam-to-clonazepam equivalency ratio of 2:1 (Herman et al. 1987) and the clonazepam tapered as described above. It is important to note that diazepam may not block alprazolam withdrawal symptoms in some patients, either because of insufficient doses of diazepam or because of different pharmacodynamic actions of alprazolam. Carbamazepine has also been used to facilitate alprazolam withdrawal (Klein et al. 1986). The optimal dose to help with withdrawal has yet to be experimentally verified. In practice, once the alprazolam has been tapered to the lowest level tolerable for the patient, carbamazepine 200 mg bid can be added. The carbamazepine dose is adjusted to obtain a serum level found therapeutic in seizure disorders (4–10 μg/ml) and then the alprazolam tapered over 1–2 weeks. The carbamazepine can then be rapidly tapered, but while it is being administered, the usual laboratory indices (liver function tests and complete blood count) should be monitored.

Psychological adjuncts. A number of techniques have been designed to enable an individual to reduce anxiety using internal resources. These include progressive muscular relaxation, meditation, autogenic training, biofeedback, and hypnotically induced relaxation. (Klajner et al. 1984; Roszell and Chaney 1982). These techniques (as a group called "relaxation training") have been advocated in the treatment of substance dependence in general and would seem particularly appropriate in the treatment of benzodiazepine dependence. Although there is evidence of some modest success with these techniques, study attrition rates are high (Nathan et al. 1986), and, on the whole, results have been less than encouraging. In particular, patients who meet criteria for generalized anxiety disorder are probably poor candidates for relaxation training. In one study of 10 outpatients with generalized anxiety disorder treated with "applied anxiety management training," no patient was able to discontinue benzodiazepine use, and only three decreased their use by more than 25% (Laughren et al. 1986). Extant studies have suffered from difficult recruitment of subjects, with consequently small sample sizes. Larger studies may identify subgroups for whom these techniques are valuable adjuncts to reducing benzodiazepine use.

Relaxation techniques have been employed as part of "cognitive

restructuring" in a program designed to allow patients a "graded exposure" to their benzodiazepine withdrawal symptoms (Higgitt et al.
1987).

In one study, benzodiazepines were tapered slowly, and patients
were taught cognitive coping strategies for withdrawal symptoms in
either group or individual sessions (Tyrer et al. 1985). Patients
treated in group settings showed lower attrition rates and better long-
term outcome. A key element is that patients use coping strategies in
response to distressing symptoms, without necessarily labeling them
as withdrawal symptoms. The investigators suggest that if distressing
symptoms that occur during benzodiazepine withdrawal are labeled
specifically as withdrawal symptoms, then patients feel that they
have less control over them (Tyrer et al. 1985).

From a solely psychopharmacologic approach, most authorities
recommend gradual reduction of dose to minimize withdrawal symptoms. The effectiveness of this approach was investigated in a double-
blind outpatient trial in which patients were either tapered gradually
from their medication ($n=23$) or abruptly discontinued by substitution with a placebo ($n=19$) (Sanchez-Craig et al. 1987). The mean
($\pm$ SD) daily doses in diazepam equivalents were 16.2 ± 11.5 and
13.9 ± 8.1, respectively, for gradual taper versus placebo groups,
with respective mean time of use 72 and 75 months. Attrition during
the study period and abstinence at the end were not significantly different, but those treated with placebo were significantly more likely
to be abstinent at 1-year follow-up. The authors suggested that some
distress experienced during treatment (when the patient has support
from the treatment team) may be beneficial in later coping. This is an
arguable point and is certainly not appropriate for patients on higher
doses, where withdrawal symptoms can include delirium, psychoses,
or seizures.

Medical and Psychological Consequences of Abuse

There is no convincing evidence to suggest adverse medical consequences of chronic benzodiazepine dependence. In one European
study (Piesiur-Strehlow et al. 1986), patients with isolated benzodiazepine dependence showed a mortality rate greater than the general
population, but equivalent to the control group (nondependent patients with comparable psychiatric illnesses). Virtually all reported
morbidity and mortality result from combination with other CNS de-

pressants in individual occurrences; for example, a person chronically abusing diazepam in high doses who then drinks alcohol may encounter severe CNS depression resulting in respiratory depression or coma.

Anterograde amnesia has been well documented with a variety of benzodiazepines, and decrement in learning probably represents the single most significant drawback to medically indicated, chronic use. In persons with preexisting deficits in learning or orientation, the effect is magnified and may be a contraindication to use. The mechanism for memory impairment is unclear, but may become further elucidated using animal models. Preliminary data suggest that the benzodiazepine inverse agonists may enhance learning and memory (Venault et al. 1986). No studies have convincingly shown cognitive impairment that persisted after drug discontinuation and a reasonable period for withdrawal. Similarly, although there are concerns about structural CNS changes occurring with chronic benzodiazepine treatment, no adequately designed studies exist. In particular, alcohol intake has often been ignored.

Summary of Benzodiazepine Dependence Issues

Anxiety is a normal part of mental life and plays a crucial role in human psychological development and other forms of learning. While systematic studies are lacking, suppression of normal levels of anxiety could impair the development of adaptive coping mechanisms. On the other hand, disabling anxiety impairs adaptation as well and is associated with significant morbidity and mortality.

Patients with specifically diagnosed anxiety disorders often require psychopharmacologic treatment. There are little data to suggest to the clinician an appropriate length of treatment, but the prudent clinician should periodically assess the need for continued pharmacotherapy. It is well established that the longer the period of therapy and the higher the benzodiazepine dose, the more severe the discontinuation syndrome. Most withdrawal symptoms are easily managed by slow taper or adjunctive therapy with propranolol or carbamazepine.

Benzodiazepines have a low risk for abuse in anxiety disorder patients without a history of alcoholism or drug abuse. Among the benzodiazepines there is a spectrum of abuse liability, with halazepam and oxazepam having the least potential for abuse. Other slow-onset benzodiazepines such as clorazepate and chlordiazepoxide probably also have lower abuse potential than diazepam.

GLUTETHIMIDE DEPENDENCE

Glutethimide (3-ethyl-3-phenyl-2, 6-piperidinedione) is a sedative-hypnotic drug rarely used therapeutically today because of wide variation in gastrointestinal absorption, fast development of pharmacodynamic tolerance, a fairly severe discontinuation syndrome, and high potential for abuse. Reports of glutethimide dependence had declined pari passu with a decline in physician prescribing but have increased in the past 10 years, probably because of combination use. The drug is taken along with codeine orally ("a load" in street parlance), which is reported to be euphorigenic in a manner resembling parenteral opiates (Khajawall et al. 1982; Sramek and Khajawall 1981).

Patients with glutethimide intoxication may present with CNS depression, widely dilated and fixed pupils, less respiration depression than barbiturates (although sudden apnea may occur), and a waxing and waning course that may persist for up to 120 hours (Maher et al. 1962). It has recently been suggested that such fluctuations may actually represent superimposed withdrawal phenomena (Bauer et al. 1988). The abstinence syndrome may include tremulousness, nausea, tachycardia, fever, tonic muscle spasms, and generalized convulsions (Harvey 1985). There has been one report of catatonia-like symptoms and dyskinesias associated with withdrawal (Campbell et al. 1983; Good 1975).

Detoxification may be accomplished with phenobarbital (60 mg phenobarbital for 500 mg glutethimide). If concomitant codeine dependency is present (and this should be strongly suspected), then methadone can be used adjunctively (10 mg of methadone for 120 mg of codeine) (Khajawall et al. 1982). Approximate sedative-hypnotic dosage equivalencies are listed in Table 3-2. Table 3-3 provides data on dosage and duration of withdrawal symptoms of nonbarbiturate sedative-hypnotics.

Table 3-2. Sedative-hypnotic dose equivalency (equal to 30 mg phenobarbital)

Generic name	Dose (mg)
Secobarbital	100
Pentobarbital	60
Chloral hydrate	250
Glutethimide	250
Meprobamate	200
Diazepam	5

Source. Adapted from Shader (1975).

Table 3-3. Nonbarbiturate sedative-hypnotic agents: dosage and duration associated with withdrawal symptoms

Generic name	Dose (g)	Duration
Ethchlorvynol	2.0–4.0	7–8 months
Glutethimide	2.5	3 months
	5.0	several weeks
Methaqualone	0.6–0.9	1 to several months
Meprobamate	2.4	9 months
	3.2–6.4	40 days
Chlordiazepoxide	0.3–0.6	5–6 months
Diazepam	0.1–1.5	several months

Note. Derived from case reports.
Source. Reprinted with permission from Shader (1975).

BARBITURATES

Prevalence of Dependence

Dependence on barbiturates has declined in recent years as physicians have substituted benzodiazepines for the treatment of many of the conditions for which barbiturates were formerly used. Clinicians will still see cases of abuse and dependence in medical patients receiving barbiturates or barbiturate combination products (e.g., Fiorinal) and in substance abusers. Tables 3-4, 3-5, and 3-6 present data on the use of sedatives in the general population and on mentions of barbiturates in emergency rooms and by medical examiners.

Table 3-4. Trends in percentage of persons reporting sedative/ tranquilizer use in past year: 1974–1985, selected years

Ages	Drug	1974 (N=952)	1976 (986)	1977 (1,272)	1979 (2,156)	1982 (1,581)	1985 (2,246)
12–17	Sedatives	2.0	1.2	2.0	2.2	3.7	2.9
	Tranquilizers	2.0	1.8	2.9	2.7	3.3	3.4
18–25	Sedatives	4.2	5.7	8.2	7.3	8.7	5.0
	Tranquilizers	4.6	6.2	7.8	7.1	5.9	6.4
26 and	Sedatives	<0.5	0.6	<0.5	0.8	1.4	2.0
up	Tranquilizers	<0.5	1.2	1.1	0.9	1.1	2.8

Note. Ns are unweighted.
Source. National Institute on Drug Abuse (1988).

Pharmacology

Harvey (1985), Matthew (1971), and Wesson and Smith (1977) have discussed the pharmacology of barbiturates. Barbiturates are derived from barbituric acid, which is the product of the fusion of malonic acid and urea. Barbituric acid lacks CNS activity. The two main classes of barbiturates are the highly lipid soluble thiobarbiturates, in which sulfur replaces oxygen at C2 of the barbituric acid ring, and the less soluble oxybarbiturates, with oxygen at C2 (see Tables 3-7 and 3-8). Lipid soluble barbiturates have a more rapid onset, a shorter duration of action, and greater potency than those with lower lipid solubility.

The ultra-short-acting barbiturates include methohexital sodium (Brevital), thiamylal sodium (Surital), and thiopental sodium (Pentothal). These are used as anesthetics and are administered intravenously.

Barbiturates with short to intermediate duration of action are used for their sedative-hypnotic effect in the treatment of anxiety. These include amobarbital (Amytal), butabarbital (Butisol), sodium pentobarbital (Nembutal), secobarbital (Seconal), and vinbarbital (Delvinal).

Long-acting barbiturates used as sedative-hypnotics and also for their anticonvulsant effects include phenobarbital (Luminal), mephobarbital (Mebaral), and metharbital (Gemonil).

Although these divisions are of historical interest, duration of action, especially with a single dose, depends more on distribution ef-

Table 3-5. Barbiturates and selected other drugs mentioned most frequently in emergency rooms in 1989

Generic name	Number of mentions	Total emergency room drug mentions (%)
Acetaminophen	6,456	4.20
Alcohol (in combination)	46,735	30.42
Alprazolam	3,567	2.32
Amobarbital	11	0.01
Aspirin	5,048	3.29
Belladonna/phenobarbital	22	0.01
Butabarbital combinations	265	0.17
Butalbital combinations	789	0.52
Chloral hydrate	98	0.06
Chlordiazepoxide	861	0.56
Clonazepam	584	0.38
Clorazepate	449	0.29
Cocaine	61,665	40.13
Diazepam	4,874	3.17
Flurazepam	724	0.47
Glutethimide	197	0.13
Heroin/morphine	20,566	13.38
Lorazepam	1,518	0.99
Marijuana/hashish	9,867	6.42
Methadone	1,609	1.05
Methamphetamine/speed	2,715	1.77
Methaqualone	178	0.12
Over-the-counter sleep aids	1,766	1.15
Oxazepam	132	0.09
Pentobarbital	39	0.03
Phenobarbital	1,067	0.69
Prazepam	98	0.06
Phencyclidine combinations	4,899	3.19
Secobarbital/amobarbital	59	0.04
Secobarbital	115	0.07
Temazepam	641	0.42
Theophylline/ephedrine/ phenobarbital	41	0.03
Triazolam	1,194	0.78
Unspecified benzodiazepines	955	0.62

Source. National Institute on Drug Abuse (1990).

fects than elimination half-life. Furthermore, as the dose increases, duration of action is prolonged.

Barbiturates produce CNS depression, which ranges from seda-

Table 3-6. Barbiturates and selected other drugs mentioned most frequently by medical examiners in 1989

Rank	Generic name	Number of mentions	Total drug episodes (%)
1	Cocaine	3,618	50.52
2	Alcohol (in combination)	2,778	38.79
3	Heroin/morphine	2,743	38.30
4	Codeine	840	11.73
5	Methadone	450	6.28
6	Diazepam	428	5.98
7	Amitriptyline	382	5.33
8	Nortriptyline	304	4.24
9	*d*-Propoxyphene	282	3.94
10	Marijuana/hashish	246	3.43
18	Unspecified benzodiazepines	177	2.47
19	Phenobarbital	173	2.42
24	Secobarbital	89	1.24
26	Chlordiazepoxide	72	1.01
27	Alprazolam	61	0.85
29	Butabital	55	0.77
31	Glutethimide	50	0.70
33	Amobarbital	41	0.57
35	Flurazepam	40	0.57
37	Temazepam	35	0.49
41	Triazolam	33	0.46
46	Pentobarbital	22	0.31
52	Oxazepam	18	0.25
57	Lorazepam	15	0.21

Source. National Institute on Drug Abuse (1990).

tion to general anesthesia. Action is through suppression of the mesencephalic reticular activating system. Barbiturates enhance GABA-induced inhibition; the site of inhibition may be presynaptic in the spinal cord, or postsynaptic in the cortical and cerebellar pyramidal cells, substantia nigra, and thalamic relay neurons. Studies show barbiturates potentiate GABA-induced increases in chloride ion conductance in spinal neurons while reducing glutamate-induced depolarization. In high concentrations, barbiturates depress calcium-dependent action and aid chloride ion conductance in the absence of GABA. Although barbiturates decrease the frequency of chloride channel openings, this is more than compensated for by their ability to increase the length of time the channels remain open. Benzodiazepines,

Table 3-7. Barbiturates

Duration of action	Generic name	Brand name(s)
Ultra-short acting (15 minutes to 3 hours)	Thiamylal	Surital
	Thiopental	Pentothal
Short acting (3–6 hours)	Pentobarbital	Nembutal Wigraine-PB suppositories
	Secobarbital	Seconal Tuinal (with amobarbital)
Intermediate acting (6–12 hours)	Amobarbital	Amytal Tuinal (with secobarbital)
	Aprobarbital	Alurate
	Butabarbital	Butisol Pyridium Plus Quibron Plus
	Butalbital	Many combination products, such as ABC Compound with Codeine, Axotal, Bucet, Buff-A Comp, Esgic, Fiorinal, G-1, G-2, G-3 Pacaps, Phrenilin, Repan, Sedapap, Tencet, Tencon
	Talbutal	Lotusate
Long acting (12–24 hours)	Barbital	Veronal
	Phenobarbital	Luminal, many combination products, such as antispasmodic drugs, Antrocol, Arco-Lase Plus, Bronkolixir, Bronkotabs, Chardonna-2, Levsin/Phenobarbital, Levsinex/Phenobarbital, Mudrane GG, Phazyme PB, Primatene P-Formula, Quadrinal, Solfoton, Donnatal, Kinesed, Tedral SA
	Mephobarbital	Mebaral

it will be recalled, increase the frequency of chloride channel openings without affecting the duration of each opening.

In addition to the CNS effect, barbiturates depress autonomic ganglia and nicotinic excitation. This may explain drops in blood pressure in cases of barbiturate intoxication.

Table 3-8. Short-acting barbiturates: brand and street names

Generic name	Brand name (manufacturer)	Street name
Amobarbital	Amytal (Lilly)	blue angels bluebirds blue bullets blue devils blue dolls blue heavens blues blue tips
Pentobarbital	Nembutal (Abbott)	nebbies nembies yellow bullets yellow dolls yellow jackets yellows
Secobarbital	Seconal (Lilly)	F-40s Mexican reds M & Ms R.D.s red birds red bullets red devils red dolls red lillies reds seccies seggies
Equal parts of secobarbital and amobarbital	Tuinal (Lilly)	double trouble gorilla pills rainbows reds and blues tootsies trees tuies

Source.   From data presented in Wesson and Smith (1977).

Psychological effects.   Barbiturates create a sense of relaxation and reduce tensions and induce euphoria as measured by standardized scales. Concentration is greatly reduced, as is judgment, and irritability often results. Chronic use slurs speech and leads to incoherency, staggered gait, and tremors.

CNS effects. As already mentioned, all barbiturates produce general CNS depression. Barbiturates have been used to treat anxiety. Barbiturates with a 5-phenyl substituent (phenobarbital and mephobarbital) have an anticonvulsant effect as well. The effects of barbiturates are largely nonselective, and general CNS depression is required to produce a particular effect, although pain sensitivity is unaffected by barbiturates until the subject loses consciousness.

Barbiturates alter characteristics of sleep. Body movement and the number of awakenings per night are reduced. Rapid-eye-movement (REM) activity is reduced, although in the last third of the night some REM compensation occurs. Slow-wave sleep (stages 3 and 4) are shortened, although phenobarbital may increase stage 4 sleep.

Effects on other organs. Respiratory drive and rhythm are depressed by barbiturates. Coughing, sneezing, hiccuping, and laryngospasm may occur during anesthesia with barbiturates. Sedative or hypnotic doses of barbiturates reduce heart rate and blood pressure to levels found in normal sleep. Anesthetic doses produce more pronounced effects. Barbiturates cross the placenta; when used in labor, they can cause respiratory depression in neonates. With respect to pregnant women, anesthetic doses decrease force and frequency of uterine contractions.

Pharmacokinetics

The pharmacokinetics of barbituates have been discussed by Harvey (1985). When used as hypnotics or antianxiety agents, the barbiturates are administered orally. As anticonvulsants, they may be used either orally or intravenously, although the latter route of administration may be problematic because these drugs are very alkaline and necrosis and pain occur at the site of injection.

Barbiturates are primarily absorbed in the intestine and bind to plasma albumin in varying degrees based on their lipid solubility (the more lipid soluble, the more highly bound). The most lipid soluble barbiturates (e.g., thiopental) reach the gray matter of the brain in a flow-limited uptake within 30 seconds, inducing sleep shortly thereafter. Because they are highly vascular, the heart, liver, and kidney also quickly reach their equilibrium concentrations. In contrast, barbiturates with low lipid solubility like barbital or phenobarbital take up to 20 minutes to induce sleep because permeability, and not flow, is the limitation on uptake. In both cases, the drug then redistributes to the less vascular brain areas and to smooth muscle and skin within about 30 minutes and to fat after 60 minutes. With short-acting barbiturates, this redistribution reduces gray matter levels of the drug by up to 90% and is responsible for termination of drug effect after a single dose.

Elimination of barbiturates depends on their lipid solubility. Lipid soluble barbiturates are highly bound; these are poorly filtered by the kidneys and reabsorbed from the lumen and tubule. Less lipid soluble barbiturates, such as phenobarbital, may have appreciable amounts (e.g., 25%) excreted unchanged in the urine. Both urine alkalinization and osmotic diuresis increase renal excretion of phenobarbital or other less lipid soluble barbiturates. Oxybarbiturates are metabolized exclusively in the liver; thiobarbiturates are also metabolized in the kidney and brain. Metabolites are more polar than parent compounds and are easily excreted. Because of long elimination half-lives, oral doses of barbiturates will accumulate during chronic administration, requiring dosage adjustment to avoid toxicity. There is some evidence that enantiomers of barbiturates have different clinical effects and kinetic characteristics.

Tolerance

Pharmacodynamic tolerance to barbiturates develops over weeks to months, whereas pharmacokinetic tolerance occurs in a period of days. At maximum tolerance, the dosage of a barbiturate may be six times the original dosage.

Detoxification

Ciraulo and Ciraulo (1988) have discussed barbiturate detoxification. Tolerance to the clinical effects of barbiturates and an abstinence syndrome occurring on abrupt discontinuation of administration is well recognized. The oxybarbiturates, with short to intermediate elimination half-lives such as butalbital, amobarbital, secobarbital, and pentobarbital, are most likely to produce a withdrawal syndrome. Table 3-9 describes the signs and symptoms of the barbiturate abstinence syndrome occurring after the abrupt withdrawal of secobarbital or pentobarbital following chronic intoxication at oral doses of 0.8–2.2 g/day for 6 weeks or more. According to Wikler's classifica-

Table 3-9. Signs and symptoms of barbiturate withdrawal

Signs and symptoms	Day of onset	Duration (days)
Apprehension and uneasiness	1	3–14
Muscular weakness	1	3–14
Coarse tremors	1	3–14
Postural faintness, orthostatic hypotension	1	3–14
Anorexia and vomiting	1	3–14
Twitches, myoclonic jerks	1	3–14
Grand mal seizures	2–3	8
Delirium	3–8	3–14

Source. Reprinted with permission from Ciraulo and Ciraulo (1988).

tion (1968), minor symptoms (apprehension, muscular weakness, tremors, postural hypotension, twitches, insomnia, diaphoresis, paroxysmal discharges in the electroencephalogram, and anorexia) appear within 24 hours of the last barbiturate dose and persist up to 2 weeks. Major abstinence phenomena include clonic-tonic seizures and delirium. Two-thirds of patients with seizures have more than one, and they may have as many as four. The interictal electroencephalogram shows recurrent 4-per-second spike-wave discharges. The delirium may be accompanied by hyperthermia, which can be fatal. Chronic intoxication with pentobarbital at daily doses of 0.6–0.8 g for periods of 35–57 days produces a clinically significant withdrawal syndrome; daily doses of 0.2–0.4 g for 90 days or more rarely leads to withdrawal symptoms.

There are two common protocols for barbiturate detoxification. In both, the goal is to prevent the occurrence of major symptoms and to minimize the development of intolerable minor symptoms. The first procedure is based on protocols described by several authors (Ewing and Bakewell 1967; Isbell 1950; Wikler 1968). The first step is determination of the severity of tolerance. If the patient is intoxicated, no additional barbiturate should be given until these symptoms have resolved. If there is substantial evidence or strong suspicion of chronic barbiturate use, it is not necessary or desirable to wait until withdrawal symptoms appear prior to the first dose. A 200-mg oral dose of pentobarbital is given on an empty stomach to a sober patient (i.e., one who is not exhibiting signs of barbiturate intoxication), and the effects are observed at 1 hour. The patient's condition 1 hour after the test is done is used to determine the daily dose for stabilization (see Table 3-10).

If no physical changes are observed after 1 hour, the test is repeated 3 hours later using 300 mg. If there is no response to the 300-mg dose, the probable 24-hour requirement is above 1,600 mg/day. The daily dose is given every 4–6 hours for a 2–3-day stabilization period. Withdrawal regimens must be individualized, but the initial reduction is usually 10% of the daily stabilization dose. Some clinicians recommend the use of phenobarbital for stabilization and withdrawal since it is longer acting and may provide a smoother course of withdrawal. Phenobarbital doses are one-third those suggested for pentobarbital and may be adapted to the above schedule. The barbiturate withdrawal protocol can also be used for other sedative-hypnotic abstinence syndromes (e.g., chloral hydrate, glutethimide, and meprobamate).

The second protocol for barbiturate withdrawal has been proposed by Sellers (1988). Citing uncertainties regarding dosage, reinforcement of drug-taking behavior by repeated administration, and

Table 3-10.   Guidelines for barbiturate detoxification

Symptoms after test dose of 200 mg oral pentobaribital	Estimated 24-hour oral pentobarbital dose (mg)	Estimated 24-hour oral phenobarbital dose (mg)
Asleep, but can be aroused	0	0
Sedated, drowsy, slurred speech, nystagmus, ataxia, positive Romberg sign	500–600	150–200
Few signs of intoxication, patient is comfortable, may have lateral nystagmus	800	250
No drug effect	1,000–1,200	300–400

Note.   Maximum phenobarbital dose is 600 mg.
Source.   Modified from Ewing and Bakewell (1967).

difficulties assessing the clinical state as shortcomings of the older protocol, he proposed a loading dose strategy. With this protocol, 120-mg doses of phenobarbital are given every 1–2 hours until 3 of 5 signs—nystagmus, drowsiness, ataxia, dysarthria, and emotional lability—are present or, if patients are symptomatic, withdrawal signs disappear. Patients are assessed for therapeutic or toxic effects prior to each dose. Sellers reported that the median loading dose was 1,440 mg. In some cases, hourly doses are required for 15–20 hours. In medically ill patients, phenobarbital may be infused intravenously (0.3 mg/kg/minute). Under this protocol, medical supervision is necessary for 3 days. Those who require less than 7 mg/kg (usually about 480 mg) are not sufficiently dependent to require further detoxification.

Clinical Uses

Although benzodiazepines have largely replaced the barbiturates in the treatment of anxiety and insomnia, the barbiturates still have many therapeutic uses (Cooper 1977; Harvey 1985). In psychiatry, they are used to treat agitated psychotic patients who are unresponsive to neuroleptics alone or to neuroleptics with benzodiazepines. Occasionally, patients withdrawing from alcohol will be resistant to benzodiazepines yet be responsive to barbiturates. The barbiturates are also used in catatonia ("Amytal interview") to temporarily relieve symptoms, permitting the patient to eat, bathe, and give historical information to the staff.

As a provocative drug challenge, barbiturates may evoke latent abnormalities in the electroencephalogram.

In other areas of medicine, barbiturates are sometimes used as sedatives for ill children, in seizure disorders, as preanesthetic agents, and to induce anesthesia.

Toxicity

The most common unwanted effects of the barbiturates are oversedation and psychomotor impairment, which may persist well into the next day following an hypnotic dose. Paradoxical excitement, hypersensitivity reactions, and muscle or joint pain may occur in rare cases. Drug-drug interactions occur with the CNS sedatives, and a number of drugs have enhanced metabolism when coadministered with barbiturates (Barnhill et al. 1989).

Death from overdose of barbiturates may occur and is more likely when more than 10 times the hypnotic dose is ingested. The barbiturates with high lipid solubility and short half-lives are the most toxic. Thus the lethal dose of phenobarbital is 6–10 g, whereas that of secobarbital, pentobarbital, or amobarbital is 2–3 g. Symptoms of barbiturate poisoning include depression of the CNS, coma, depressed reflex activity, a positive Babinski reflex, contracted pupils (with hypoxia there may be paralytic dilation), altered respiration, hypothermia, depressed cardiac function, hypotension, shock, pulmonary complications, and renal failure.

Treatment of barbiturate poisoning centers on supportive measures and close monitoring of patients in the intensive care unit. Adequate ventilation is a priority and may require endotracheal intubation (Gary and Tresnewsky 1983). In alert patients, emesis may be induced by apomorphine 0.06 mg/kg. It is usually effective within a few minutes, and its effect is partially reversed by naloxone. Alternatively, ipecac syrup 15–30 ml orally is given. Although it is usually effective within 15 minutes, it may take longer in some patients. If a patient loses consciousness during this period, attempts should be made to remove the ipecac by lavage to avoid aspiration of vomitus. Charcoal will inactivate ipecac. Gastric lavage with a cuffed tube to prevent aspiration may also be of value. After 4 hours, little drug remains in the stomach, but many clinicians will perform lavage up to 24 hours after ingestion. Emesis presents a risk of aspiration in patients with impaired consciousness, convulsions, or absent gag reflex. A saline cathartic may be used when bowel sounds are present and a slurry of activated charcoal may also help to adsorb residual drug. In patients with intact renal and cardiovascular function, osmotic diuresis and urine alkalinization may significantly increase renal excretion of barbital, phenobarbital, aprobarbital, and allobarbital since these drugs rely on this mechanism for a significant portion of their total elimination. Guidelines for forced alkaline diuresis have been presented by Olson et al. (1983) and include 1) check baseline electrolytes and urine and arterial blood pH values; 2) administer 1,000 ml of 5% dextrose in one-third normal saline solution iv with 20 mEq of KCl and 44 mEq of NaHCO$_3$ (1 ample, 50 ml) at a rate of 500 ml/ hour with hourly adjustments to maintain urine flow at 300–500 ml/ hour; 3) measure urine volume via indwelling catheter; 4) observe for pulmonary edema or congestive heart failure; and 5) maintain urine pH above 7.0 by adding $NaHCO_3$ to the infusion if urinary pH falls below this level. Dialysis or hemoperfusion may also be necessary, especially if renal failure has occurred. Hemodialysis is most effective with long-acting drugs because they are water soluble and not highly bound to proteins. For the short-acting lipid soluble drugs, the use of a lipid-containing dialysate or hemoperfusion through activated charcoal, acrylic hydrogel-coated carbon, or ion-exchange resins has been recommended (Harvey 1985). Pulmonary function, blood gases, body temperature, and cardiovascular effects should also be monitored.

REFERENCES

American Psychiatric Association: Diagnostic and Statistical Manual of Mental Disorders, 3rd Edition, Revised. Washington, DC, American Psychiatric Association, 1987

American Psychiatric Association: Benzodiazepine Dependence, Toxicity, and Abuse. Washington, DC, American Psychiatric Association, 1990

Arendt RM, Greenblatt DJ, DeJong RH, et al: In vitro correlates of benzodiazepine cerebrospinal fluid uptake, pharmacodynamic action, and peripheral distribution. J Pharmacol Exp Ther 277:98–106, 1983

Ashley MJ, Harding le Riche W, Olin JS, et al: 'Mixed' (drug abusing) and 'pure' alcoholics: a socio-medical comparison. Br J Addict 73:19–34, 1978

Ashton H: Benzodiazepine withdrawal: an unfinished story. Br Med J 288: 1135–1140, 1984

Balter MB, Manheimer DI, Mellinger GD, et al: A cross-national comparison of anti-anxiety/sedative drug use. Curr Med Res Opin 8 (suppl 4):5–20, 1984

Barnhill JG, Ciraulo AM, Ciraulo DA: Interactions of importance in chemical dependence, in Drug Interactions in Psychiatry. Edited by Ciraulo DA, Shader RI, Greenblatt DJ, et al. Baltimore, MD, Williams & Wilkins, 1989, pp 234–237

Bauer MS, Fus AF, Hanich RF, et al: Glutethimide intoxication and withdrawal [letter]. Am J Psychiatry 145:530–531, 1988

Bell R, Havlicek P, Roncek D, et al: Sex differences in the use of alcohol and tranquilizers: testing a role convergence hypothesis. Am J Drug Alcohol Abuse 10:551–561, 1984

Boismare F, Daoust M, Moore N, et al: A homotaurine derivative reduces the voluntary intake of ethanol by rats: are cerebral GABA receptors involved? Pharmacol Biochem Behav 21:787–789, 1984

Braestrup C, Squires RF: Benzodiazepine receptors in rat brain. Nature 266:732–734, 1977

Braestrup C, Squires RF: Pharmacologic characterization of benzodiazepine receptors in the brain. Eur J Pharmacol 48:263–270, 1978

Braestrup C, Albrechten R, Squires RF, et al: High densities of benzodiaze-
    pine receptors in human cortical areas. Nature 269:702–704, 1977
Braestrup C, Nielsen M, Honore T, et al: Benzodiazepine receptor ligands
    with positive and negative efficacy. Neuropharmacology 22:1451–
    1457, 1983
Brogden RN, Goa KL: Flumazenil: a preliminary review of its benzo-
    diazepine antagonist properties, intrinsic activity, and therapeutic use.
    Drugs 35:448–467, 1988
Busto U, Simpkins MA, Sellers EM, et al: Objective determination of
    benzodiazepine use and abuse in alcoholics. Br J Addict 78:429–435,
    1983
Busto U, Sellers EM, Naranjo CA, et al: Patterns of benzodiazepine abuse
    and dependence. Br J Addict 81:87–94, 1986a
Busto U, Sellers EM, Naranjo CA, et al: Withdrawal reaction after long-
    term therapeutic use of benzodiazepines. N Engl J Med 315:854–859,
    1986b
Caille G, Spenard J, Lacasse Y, et al: Pharmacokinetics of two lorazepam
    formulations, oral and sublingual, after multiple doses. Biopharm Drug
    Dispos 4:31–42, 1983
Campbell R, Schaffer CB, Tupin J: Catatonia associated with glutethimide
    withdrawal. J Clin Psychiatry 44:32–33, 1983
Ciraulo DA, Ciraulo AM: Substance abuse, in Handbook of Clinical Psy-
    chopharmacology. Edited by Tupin JP, Shader RI, Harnett DS.
    Northvale, NJ, Jason Aronson, 1988
Ciraulo DA, Barnhill JG, Greenblatt DJ, et al: Abuse liability and clinical
    pharmacokinetics of alprazolam in alcoholic men. J Clin Psychiatry
    49:333–337, 1988a
Ciraulo DA, Sands BF, Shader RI: Abuse liability of benzodiazepines in
    alcoholics: a critical review. Am J Psychiatry 145:1501–1506, 1988b
Ciraulo DA, Antal EJ, Smith RB, et al: The relationship of alprazolam dose
    to steady state plasma concentrations. J Clin Psychopharmacol
    10:27–32, 1990
Clinthorne JK, Cisin IH, Balter MB, et al: Changes in popular attitudes
    and beliefs about tranquilizers. Arch Gen Psychiatry 43:527–532,
    1986
Conell LJ, Berlin RM: Withdrawal after substitution of a short-acting for a
    long-acting benzodiazepine. JAMA 250:2838–2840, 1983
Cooper JR (ed): Sedative-hypnotic drugs: risks and benefits (DHEW Publ
    No ADM-78-592). Rockville, MD, National Institute on Drug Abuse,
    1977
Covi L, Lipman RS, Pattison JH, et al: Length of treatment with anxiolytic
    sedatives and response to their sudden withdrawal. Acta Psychiatr
    Scand 49:51–64, 1973
Cushman P, Benzer D: Benzodiazepines and drug abuse: clinical observa-
    tions in chemically dependent persons before and during abstinence.
    Drug Alcohol Depend 6:365–371, 1980
Divoll M, Greenblatt DJ, Ciraulo DA, et al: Clobazam kinetics: inter-
    subject variability and effect of food on absorption. J Clin Pharmacol
    22:69–73, 1982

Ewing JA, Bakewell WE: Diagnosis and management of depressant drug dependence. Am J Psychiatry 123:909–917, 1967

File SE: Tolerance to the behavioral actions of benzodiazepines. Neurosci Biobehav Rev 9:113–121, 1985

Fleischhacker WW, Barnas C, Hackenberg B: Epidemiology of benzodiazepine dependence. Acta Psychiatr Scand 74:80–83, 1986

Fyer AJ, Liebowitz MR, Gorman JM, et al: Effects of clonidine on alprazolam discontinuation in panic patients: a pilot study. J Clin Psychopharmacol 8:270–274, 1988

Garvey MJ, Tollefson GD: Prevalence of misuse of prescribed benzodiazepines in patients with primary anxiety disorder or major depression. Am J Psychiatry 143:1601–1603, 1986

Gary NE, Tresnewsky O: Clinical aspects of drug intoxication: barbiturates and a potpourri of other sedatives, hypnotics, and tranquilizers. Heart Lung 12:122, 1983

Glover E: The etiology of alcoholism. Proceedings of the Royal Society of Medicine 21:1351–1386, 1928

Glover E: The prevention and treatment of drug addiction. British Journal of Inebriety 29:13–18, 1931

Good MI: Catatonia-like symptomatology and withdrawal dyskinesias. Am J Psychiatry 133:1454–1456, 1975

Gottschalk LA, Bates DE, Fox RA, et al: Psychoactive drug use: patterns found in samples from a mental health clinic and a general medical clinic. Arch Gen Psychiatry 25:395–397, 1971

Greenblatt DJ, Shader RI: Dependence, tolerance, and addiction to benzodiazepines: clinical and pharmacokinetic considerations. Drug Metab Rev 8:13–28, 1978

Greenblatt DJ, Shader RI: Long-term administration of benzodiazepines: pharmacokinetic versus pharmacodynamic tolerance. Psychopharmacol Bull 22:416–423, 1986

Greenblatt DJ, Shader RI, Koch-Weser J: Psychotropic drug use in the Boston area: a report from the Boston Collaborative Drug Surveillance Program. Arch Gen Psychiatry 32:518–521, 1975

Greenblatt DJ, Shader RI, Harmatz JS, et al: Self-rated sedation and plasma concentrations of desmethyldiazepam following single doses of clorazepate. Psychopharmacology 66:289–290, 1979

Greenblatt DJ, Divoll M, Harmatz JS, et al: Pharmacokinetic comparison of sublingual lorazepam with intravenous, intramuscular, and oral lorazepam. J Pharm Sci 71:248–252, 1982

Greenblatt DJ, Shader RI, Abernethy DR: Drug therapy: current state of the benzodiazepines, Part 1. N Engl J Med 309:354–358, 1983a

Greenblatt DJ, Shader RI, Abernethy DR: Drug therapy: current state of the benzodiazepines, Part 2. N Engl J Med 309:410–416, 1983b

Greenblatt DJ, Harmatz JS, Zinny MA, et al: Effect of gradual withdrawal on the rebound sleep disorder after discontinuation of triazolam. N Engl J Med 317:722–727, 1987

Griffiths RR, Ator NA: Benzodiazepine self-administration in animals and humans: a comprehensive literature review. Natl Inst Drug Abuse Res Monogr 33:22–36, 1980

Griffiths RR, Wolf B: Relative abuse liability of different benzodiazepines in drug abusers J Clin Psychopharmacol 10:237–243, 1990

Griffiths RR, Bigelow GE, Liebson I: Human drug self-administration: double-blind comparison of pentabarbital, diazepam, chlorpromazine, and placebo. J Pharmacol Exp Ther 210:301–310, 1979

Griffiths RR, Bigelow GE, Liebson I, et al: Drug preference in humans: double-blind choice comparison of pentabarbital, diazepam, and placebo. J Pharmacol Exp Ther 215:649–661, 1980

Griffiths RR, McLeod DR, Liebson I, et al: Comparison of diazepam and oxazepam: preference, liking, and extent of abuse. J Pharmacol Exp Ther 229:501–508, 1984

Hallstrom C, Lader M: The incidence of benzodiazepine dependence in long-term users. Journal of Psychiatric Treatment and Evaluation 4:293–296, 1982

Harrison M, Busto U, Naranjo CA, et al: Diazepam tapering in detoxification for high-dose benzodiazepine abuse. Clin Pharmacol Ther 36:527–533, 1984

Harvey SC: Hypnotics and sedatives, in The Pharmacologic Basis of Therapeutics, 7th Edition. Edited by Gilman AG, Goodman LS, Rall TW, et al. New York, Macmillan, 1985, pp 339–371

Herman JB, Rosenbaum JF, Brotman AW: The alprazolam to clonazepam switch for the treatment of panic disorder. J Clin Psychopharmacol 7:175–178, 1987

Higgitt A, Golombok S, Fonagy P, et al: Group treatment of benzodiazepine dependence. Br J Addict 82:517–532, 1987

Hollister LE, Motzenbecker FP, Degan RO: Withdrawal reactions from chlordiazepoxide. Psychopharmacologia 2:63–68, 1961

Hollister LE, Bennet JL, Kimbell L Jr, et al: Diazepam in newly admitted schizophrenics. Diseases of the Nervous System 24:746–750, 1963

Isbell H: Manifestations and treatment of addiction to narcotic drugs and barbiturates. Med Clin North Am 34:425–438, 1950

Jaffe JH, Ciraulo DA, Nies A, et al: Abuse potential of halazepam and of diazepam in patients recently treated for acute alcohol withdrawal. Clin Pharmacol Ther 34:623–630, 1983

Kania J, Kofoed L: Drug use by alcoholics in outpatient treatment. Am J Drug Alcohol Abuse 10:529–534, 1984

Khajawall AM, Sramek JJ Jr, Simpson GM: 'Loads' alert. West J Med 137:166–168, 1982

Khantzian EJ: A contemporary psychodynamic approach to drug abuse treatment. Am J Drug Alcohol Abuse 13:213–222, 1986

Klajner F, Hartman LM, Sobell MB: Treatment of substance abuse by relaxation training: a review of its rationale, efficacy and mechanisms. Addict Behav 9:41–55, 1984

Klein E, Uhde TW, Post PM: Preliminary evidence for the utility of carbamazepine in alprazolam withdrawal. Am J Psychiatry 143:235–236, 1986

Kryspin-Exner K: Missbrauch von Benzodiazepinderivaten bei Alkoholkranken (misuse of benzodiazepine derivatives by alcoholics). Br J Addict 61:283–290, 1966

Kryspin-Exner K, Demel I: The use of tranquilizers in the treatment of mixed drug abuse. International Journal of Clinical Pharmacology and Biopharmacy 12:13–18, 1975

Krystal H: Self and object representation in alcoholism and other drug dependence: implications for therapy. Natl Inst Drug Abuse Res Monogr Ser 12:88–100, 1977

Lader M, Olajide D: A comparison of buspirone and placebo in relieving benzodiazepine withdrawal syndromes. J Clin Psychopharmacol 7:11–15, 1987

Laughren TP, Dias AM, Keene C, et al: Can chronically anxious patients learn to cope without medications? McLean Hospital Journal 11:72–78, 1986

Liljequist S, Engel JA: The effects of GABA and benzodiazepine receptor antagonists on the anti-conflict actions of diazepam or ethanol. Pharmacol Biochem Behav 21:521–525, 1984

Lhuintre JP, Daoust M, Moore ND, et al: Ability of calcium bis acetyl homotaurine, a GABA agonist, to prevent relapse in weaned alcoholics. Lancet 1:1014–1016, 1985

Maher J, Scheiner G, Westervelt F: Acute glutethimide intoxication, I: clinical experience (twenty-two patients) compared to acute barbiturate intoxication (sixty-three patients). Am J Med 33:70–82, 1962

Marks J: The Benzodiazepines: Use, Overuse, Misuse, Abuse. Baltimore, MD, University Park Press, 1978

Matthew H: Acute Barbiturate Poisoning. Amsterdam, Excerpta Medica, 1971

Mellinger GD, Balter MB: Prevalence and patterns of use of psychotropic drugs: results from a 1979 national survey of American adults, in Epidemiological impact of psychotropic drugs: proceedings of the International Seminar on Psychotropic Drugs. Edited by Tognoni G, Bellantuono C, Lader M. Amsterdam, North Holland Publishing, 1981, pp 117–135

Mellinger GD, Balter MB, Uhlenhuth EH: Prevalence and correlates of the long-term regular use of anxiolytics. JAMA 251:375–379, 1984

Miller LG, Greenblatt DJ, Barnhill JG, et al: Benzodiazepine receptor binding of triazolobenzodiazepines in vivo: increased receptor number with low-dose alprazolam. J Neurochem 49:1595–1601, 1987

Miller LG, Greenblatt DJ, Barnhill JG, et al: Chronic benzodiazepine administration, I: tolerance is associated with benzodiazepine receptor downregulation and decreased gamma-aminobutyric acid A receptor function. J Pharmacol Exp Ther 246:170–176, 1988a

Miller LG, Greenblatt DA, Roy RB, et al: Chronic benzodiazepine administration, II: discontinuation syndrome is associated with upregulation of gamma-aminobutyric acid receptor complex binding and function. J Pharmacol Exp Ther 246:177–182, 1988b

Möhler H, Okada T: Benzodiazepine receptor demonstration in the central nervous system. Science 198:849–851, 1977

Müller-Oerlinghausen: Prescription and misuse of benzodiazepines in the Federal Republic of Germany. Pharmacopsychiatry 19:8–13, 1986

Nathan RG, Robinson D, Cherek DR, et al: Alternative treatments for withdrawing the long-term benzodiazepine user: a pilot study. Int J Addict 21:195–211, 1986

National Institute on Drug Abuse: National Household Survey on Drug Abuse: Main Findings 1985 (DHHS Publ No ADM–88–1586). Rockville, MD, National Institute on Drug Abuse, 1988

National Institute on Drug Abuse: Drug Abuse Warning Network (data file). Rockville, MD, National Institute on Drug Abuse, 1990

Nutt DJ, Linnoila M: Neuroreceptor science: a clarification of terms. J Clin Psychopharmacol 8:387–389, 1988

Olsen RW, Yang J, King RG, et al: Current topics: benzodiazepine function, V: barbiturate and benzodiazepine modulation of GABA receptor binding and function. Life Sci 39:1969–1976, 1986

Olson E, McErue J, Greenbaum DM: Recognition, general considerations, and techniques in the management of drug intoxication. Heart Lung 12:110, 1983

Parry HJ, Balter MB, Mellinger GD, et al: National patterns of psychotherapeutic drug use. Arch Gen Psychiatry 28:769–783, 1973

Perera KMH, Jenner FA: Some characteristics distinguishing high and low dose users of benzodiazepines. Br J Addict 82:1329–1334, 1987

Petursson H, Lader MH: Benzodiazepine dependence. Br J Addict 76:133–145, 1981a

Petursson H, Lader MH: Withdrawal from long term benzodiazepine treatment. Br J Med 283:643–645, 1981b

Piesiur-Strehlow B, Strehlow U, Poser W: Mortality of patients dependent on benzodiazepines. Acta Psychiatr Scand 73:330–335, 1986

Rado S: The psychic effects of intoxicants. Int J Psychoanal 7:396, 1926

Rickels K, Case W, Downing RW, et al: Long-term diazepam therapy and clinical outcome JAMA 250:767–771, 1983

Rosenberg HC, Chiu TH: Time course for development of benzodiazepine tolerance and physical dependence. Neurosci Behav Rev 9:123–131, 1985

Roszell DK, Chaney EF: Autogenic training in a drug abuse program. Int J Addict 17:1337–1349, 1982

Rothstein E, Cobble JC, Sampson N: Chlordiazepoxide: long term use in alcoholism. Ann NY Acad Sci 273:381–384, 1976

Rounsaville BJ, Spitzer RL, Williams JBW: Proposed changes in DSM-III substance use disorders: description and rationale. Am J Psychiatry 143:463–468, 1986

Samarasinghe DS, Tilley S, Marks IM: Alcohol and sedative drug use in neurotic outpatients. Br J Psychiatry 145:45–48, 1984

Sanchez-Craig M, Cappel H, Busto U, et al: Cognitive-behavioural treatment for benzodiazepine dependence: a comparison of gradual versus abrupt cessation of drug intake. Br J Addict 82:1317–1327, 1987

Schuckit M, Morrissey E: Drug abuse among alcoholic women. Am J Psychiatry 136:607–611, 1979

Schuster CR, Thompson T: Self administration of and behavioral dependence on drugs. Annual Review of Pharmacology 9:483–502, 1969

Sellers EM: Alcohol, barbiturate and benzodiazepine withdrawal syndromes: clinical management. Can Med Assoc J 139:113, 1988

Shader RI: Manual of Psychiatric Therapeutics. Boston, MA, Little, Brown, 1975

Smith DE, Wesson DR: Benzodiazepine dependency syndromes. J Psychoactive Drugs 15:85–95, 1983

Sokolow JD, Welte J, Hynes BA, et al: Multiple substance abuse by alcoholics. Br J Addict 76:147–158, 1981

Sramek J, Khajawall AM: "Loads" (letter). N Engl J Med 305:231, 1981

Suzdak PD, Schwartz RD, Skolnick P, et al: Ethanol stimulates gamma-aminobutyric acid receptor-mediated chloride transport in rat brain synaptoneurosomes. Proc Natl Acad Sci USA 83:4071–4075, 1986

Tallman JF, Paul SM, Skolnick P, et al: Receptors for the age of anxiety: pharmacology of the benzodiazepines. Science 207:274–281, 1980

Tyrer P, Rutherford D, Huggett T: Benzodiazepine withdrawal syndromes and propranolol. Lancet 1:520–522, 1981

Tyrer P, Murphy S, Oates G: Psychological treatment for benzodiazepine dependence. Lancet 1:1042–1043, 1985

Venault P, Chapoutier G, de Carvalho LP: Benzodiazepine impairs and beta carboline enhances performance in learning and memory. Nature 321:864–866, 1986

Wesson DR, Smith DE: Barbiturates: Their Use, Misuse, and Abuse. New York, Human Sciences Press, 1977

Wikler A: Diagnosis and treatment of drug dependence of the barbiturate type. Am J Psychiatry 125:758–765, 1968

Wiseman SM, Spencer-Peet J: Prescribing for alcoholics: a survey of drugs taken prior to admission to an alcoholism unit. Practitioner 229:88–89, 1985

World Health Organization: International Classification of Diseases, 9th Revision. Geneva, World Health Organization, 1977

World Health Organization: Nomenclature and classification of drug and alcohol related problems: a WHO memorandum. Bull WHO 59:225–242, 1981

World Health Organization Review Group: Use and abuse of benzodiazepines. Bull WHO 61:551–562, 1983

Yu O, Chiu TH, Rosenberg HC: Modulation of chloride ion flux in rat brain by acute and chronic benzodiazepine administration. J Pharmacol Exp Ther 256:107–113, 1988

Zorumsky CF, Isenberg KE: Insights into the structure and function of GABA-benzodiazepine receptors: ion channels and psychiatry. Am J Psychiatry 148:162–173, 1991

Chapter 4

Marijuana

Jack H. Mendelson, M.D.
Nancy K. Mello, Ph.D.

DIAGNOSIS, PREVALENCE, AND ETIOLOGIC THEORIES

Data reported by the Division of Epidemiology and Statistical Analysis of the National Institute on Drug Abuse highlight that marijuana is the most widely abused illegal drug in the United States (Kozel and Adams 1986). The major data resource for assessing incidence and prevalence of marijuana use in America is the National Household Survey on Drug Abuse. This general population survey of persons age 12 and above has been carried out every 2–3 years since 1971. The survey does not include persons in institutional settings (e.g., colleges, military bases, or prisons) or nonresidential and transient populations. Because of these exclusions, it is highly likely that the survey yields a lower than actual estimate of drug abuse. Nevertheless, the 1982 survey revealed that approximately 56 million people in the United States had used marijuana at least on a single occasion and that more than 20 million persons had used the drug during the month prior to the survey (National Institute on Drug Abuse 1983a, 1983b). Data obtained during the 1985 survey indicated that the lifetime prevalence rate of marijuana use in the United States increased to 62 million persons (National Institute on Drug Abuse 1988).

Table 4-1 shows the trend in estimated prevalence of marijuana use among persons 12–17 years old, those 18–25 years old, and those of 26 years and older. These estimates represent a substantial percentage of the national population, but the lifetime (ever used), annual, and past month prevalence trends show a decline or leveling among all age groups during the most recent measurement points. The increase in those 26 years and older was found to be the result of a cohort effect; that is, the entry of the 23–25-year-old age cohort into the 26 and older age group between 1979 and 1982. The net change in the older adult group was not statistically significant (Adams et al. 1986).

These national household trends are reflected in data from high school senior classes, which reached their apex in marijuana use with the classes of 1978 and 1979 and have since declined through 1984 and leveled off in 1985 (Table 4-2). A clue to the reasons underlying the surge in marijuana abuse during the 1970s and its subsequent decline also may be garnered from the high school senior survey. The point at which marijuana abuse had reached its peak was the same point at which perceived harmfulness was at its nadir. In 1978, for example, the monthly prevalence of use among high school seniors was at 37%; almost 11% used marijuana daily. At the same time, only 12% of seniors nationwide believed that there was great risk of harm associated with occasional use, and 35% perceived great risk with regular use. By 1985, monthly prevalence declined to 26% and daily use to below 5%, whereas perceived risk rose to 25% for occasional use and to 70% for regular use.

Thus the belief that marijuana use, even once or twice, poses no great risk is highly correlated with an increase in prevalence trends and probably had its genesis in the social status afforded the drug during the 1960s and early 1970s and the lack at that time of conclusive findings regarding short- or long-term health consequences (National Commission on Marijuana and Drug Abuse 1972). Now it is clear that marijuana has a serious impact on social functioning as well as on health. Behaviorally, use of marijuana, especially long-term heavy use, has been directly related to subsequent abuse of other illicit drugs (Clayton and Voss 1981). Marijuana has been called a "gateway" drug, and indeed the single best predictor of cocaine use is frequent use of marijuana during adolescence (Kandel et al. 1985).

Table 4-1. Trend in estimated prevalence of marijuana use among three age groups, 1972–1985, selected years

Prevalence	Marijuana use (%)						
	1972	1974	1976	1977	1979	1982	1985
12–17 years old							
N	880	952	986	1,272	2,165	1,581	2,287
Ever used	14.0	23.0	22.4	28.0	30.9	26.7	23.7
Used in past year	NA	18.5	18.4	22.3	24.1	20.6	20.0
Used in past month	7.0	12.0	12.3	16.6	16.7	11.5	12.3
18–25 years old							
N	772	849	882	1,500	2,044	1,283	1,804
Ever used	47.9	52.7	52.9	59.9	68.2	64.1	60.5
Used in past year	NA	34.2	35.0	38.7	46.9	40.4	37.0
Used in past month	27.8	25.2	25.0	27.4	35.4	27.4	21.9
26 years and older							
N	1,613	2,221	1,708	1,822	3,015	2,760	3,947
Ever used	7.4	9.9	12.9	15.3	19.6	23.0	27.2
Used in past year	NA	3.8	5.4	6.4	9.0	10.6	9.5
Used in past month	2.5	2.0	3.5	3.3	6.0	6.6	6.2

Note. NA = not available.
Source. From Kozel and Adams (1986). Used with permission.

Table 4-2. Trend in estimated prevalence of marijuana use among high school senior classes, 1975–1985

						Marijuana use (%)					
Prevalence	1975	1976	1977	1978	1979	1980	1981	1982	1983	1984	1985
N	9,400	15,400	17,100	17,800	15,500	15,900	17,500	17,700	16,300	15,900	16,000
Ever used	47.3	52.8	56.4	59.2	60.4	60.3	59.5	58.7	57.0	54.9	54.2
Used in past year	40.0	44.5	47.6	50.2	50.8	48.8	46.1	44.3	42.3	40.0	40.6
Used in past month	27.1	32.2	35.4	37.1	36.5	33.7	31.6	28.5	27.0	25.2	25.7
Used daily in past month	6.0	8.2	9.1	10.7	10.3	9.1	7.0	6.3	5.5	5.0	4.9

Source. From Kozel and Adams (1986). Used with permission.

PHARMACOLOGY AND PHARMACOKINETICS

The most common mode of marijuana self-administration is via smoking and inhalation. Marijuana smoke contains more than 400 compounds in addition to delta^9-tetrahydrocannabinol (THC), the major psychoactive agent of the drug. The most common type of marijuana cigarette smoked in the United States contains approximately .5–1 g of leaves and flowering tops of *Cannabis sativa*. The average amount of THC found in most marijuana cigarettes is approximately 10 mg, but forensic reports have indicated that THC in concentrations as high as 100 mg have been detected in some cigarettes. In 1980 there was increasing evidence that higher potency marijuana cigarettes were becoming available in many parts of the United States (Novak 1980; Petersen 1980) and that health benefits associated with the later age of onset of marijuana smoking by young men and women may be offset by the higher concentrations of THC present in marijuana cigarettes. There is also evidence that often the concentration of THC in marijuana cigarettes is enhanced by the addition of "hash oil." This material is prepared by extracting plant materials in lipid solvents that yield 25–60% THC concentrations.

The process of pyrolysis of plant materials in the marijuana cigarette produces an additional 150 compounds, which are volatilized in smoke and fumes. Thus inhalation of smoked marijuana results in pulmonary absorption and transfer of an extremely large number of complex and potentially hazardous organic compounds.

Volatilized THC produced by pyrolysis of marijuana is quickly absorbed from the lungs following inhalation and is subsequently rapidly sequestered from blood into body tissues. The pharmacokinetic properties of THC and THC metabolites are very complex in humans (Hunt and Jones 1980). Since THC and THC metabolites are highly lipid soluble, it is perhaps not surprising that it has been difficult to establish correlations between peak levels of drug effects and peak levels of THC in blood plasma. The metabolism of THC is also affected as a consequence of the high lipid solubility of the drug. The very rapid decline of THC in plasma following inhalation of the volatilized drug is not due to metabolism of THC but is associated with a very rapid intake of the drug into tissue compartments. For example, following intravenous administration of THC, more than 70% of the drug rapidly enters tissue compartments, and only 30% is metabolized over a period of several hours. Most THC is metabolized in the liver. The major metabolite is 11-hydroxy-THC, but there are at least 20 other metabolites, some of which have psychoactive and physiologic effects. The majority of THC metabolites are slowly excreted via the feces.

THC and THC metabolites may be detected in blood plasma and tissue samples for many days following cessation of marijuana smoking. This is due to the prolonged sequestration of THC and THC metabolites in body lipid pools. Hunt and Jones (1980) showed that after approximately 6 hours, the rate-limiting step for elimination of THC is the slow return to plasma of THC sequestered in tissues and not the rate of THC metabolism.

It has been postulated that long-term physiologic consequences of inhalation of THC may be due to progressive accumulation of a major THC metabolite, 11-nor-COOH THC (9-carboxy THC) (Wall et al. 1983). The accumulation of this THC metabolite may explain in part the difficulty in finding significant positive correlations between peak behavioral effects following marijuana smoking and peak plasma THC levels (Barnett et al. 1982; Galanter et al. 1972; Ohlsson et al. 1980, 1982; Perez-Reyes et al. 1982; Reeve et al. 1983). As noted previously, this phenomenon may be due also to the rapid sequestration and slow release of THC from lipid fractions in body tissues. The relevance of this process for the central nervous system would be especially important because of the critical role of lipid fractions in brain structural components (e.g., neural membranes).

CLINICAL SIGNS AND SYMPTOMS OF INTOXICATION

The intoxicating properties of marijuana have been described as similar to those of moderate alcohol intoxication. The principal salient features of such intoxication are the induction of subjective feeling states of relaxation and euphoria. However, aversive aspects of marijuana use have also been reported, and these effects are similar to the unpleasant subjective states following alcohol intake (i.e., nausea, vertigo, and dysarthria). Many regular heavy marijuana users have reported that their first experience with the drug was aversive.

Acute and chronic marijuana use may cause undesirable effects on cognitive processes and perception. There have been reports of marijuana-induced distortion in object size and object distance perception (Isbell et al. 1967). Marijuana smoking has also been reported to impair accurate color discrimination (Adams et al. 1975), to increase visual reaction time (Moskowitz 1976), and to decrease accuracy in ocular motor-tracking ability (Adams et al. 1975). A particularly severe behavioral impairment associated with marijuana smoking is a decrease in accurate detection of light stimuli in the peripheral visual field (Moskowitz et al. 1972). This impairment is believed to be due to a direct effect of marijuana smoking on ocular motor control (Moskowitz et al. 1972). Decreased perception of peripheral light stimuli may enhance risk of automobile accidents by persons who have smoked marijuana recently.

Many studies have shown that marijuana use may result in a distortion of time sense. The subjective determination of elapsed time may either increase or decrease following marijuana smoking, and these events have been linked with more generalized disturbances of ideational states following marijuana use (Melges et al. 1970; Meyer 1975). Marijuana-related changes in time sense perception may also be a factor associated with increased risk for automobile driving impairment.

Significant dose-effect relationships between marijuana use and driving impairment have been reported in a number of studies (Klonoff 1974; Le Dain et al. 1972; Sharma and Moskowitz 1972). It is of considerable interest that marijuana-related impairment of automobile driving may persist for long periods of time following acute marijuana use. For example, it has been shown that marijuana may impair driving ability for more than 2 hours following acute marijuana use. There is also considerable evidence that marijuana use can adversely affect aircraft pilot performance. Studies utilizing simulated instrument flying devices have demonstrated that acute marijuana use is associated with decrements in pilots' ability to make adequate judgments and use appropriate motor skills for safe aircraft operation (Blaine et al. 1976; Janowsky et al. 1976a, 1976b). There is also evidence that residual or "hangover" effects after marijuana smoking may also adversely affect aircraft pilots' functioning. Studies of marijuana effects on pilots' performance utilizing simulated flight devices have shown that adverse effects of the drug may last for as long as 24 hours following acute use. It therefore appears that marijuana use, similar to alcohol use, may cause protracted adverse effects following cessation of use.

Acute and chronic marijuana use may significantly affect cognitive function. Marijuana smoking produces impairment in performance of complex cognitive tasks (Butler et al. 1976; Ray et al.

1978). However, in general, adverse affects of marijuana on cognitive function are related to degree of familiarity or practice with the task as well as task complexity and difficulty. Low doses of marijuana may impede solution of difficult cognitive tasks, whereas high doses of marijuana may not impair tasks that are simple and not difficult to perform. Perhaps the most significant degree of marijuana-related impairment in cognitive performance is associated with learning new information. Marijuana use impairs performance that is dependent on systematic study and practice recall of information (Abel 1975; Rickles et al. 1973; Smith and Seymour 1982; Voth 1980). This may be due to marijuana's effect on short-term memory function (Belmore and Miller 1980; Clark et al. 1979; Clopton et al. 1979; Lantner 1982; Melges et al. 1970; Roth et al. 1977).

McGlothlin and West (1968) reported the occurrence of an "amotivational syndrome" following marijuana use. Since publication of this report, there has been considerable controversy about the specificity of marijuana for inducing changes in human motivation. Some investigators have found that amotivation and loss of interest in conventional social goals is not a direct effect of marijuana use (Negrete 1973). Other studies suggest a direct relationship between marijuana use and decreases in motivation and achievement (Cohen 1982; Creason and Goldman 1981; Johnston et al. 1980; Manno et al. 1974). A number of experimental laboratory studies of human motivation have examined the effects of marijuana smoking on operant acquisition of marijuana and money. Most of these studies (Mello and Mendelson 1985, 1987; Mendelson et al. 1974b, 1976a, 1976b) did not reveal any significant direct effect of marijuana on operant performance. It is important to point out, however, that all of the operant studies (Mello and Mendelson 1985, 1987; Mendelson et al. 1974b, 1976a, 1976b; Miles et al. 1974) involved relatively easy task performance. Since it is very difficult to define and assess normal motivational processes in humans, it is highly likely that the purported marijuana-induced amotivational syndrome will continue to remain a subject of great controversy.

A number of psychiatric disorders, such as anxiety, depersonalization, and dissociative episodes, have been reported to occur as a consequence of marijuana smoking (Chopra and Smith 1974: Isbell et al. 1967; Jones and Stone 1970; Melges et al. 1970; Negrete 1973; Tart 1970). At present, it appears as if marijuana per se does not cause specific psychiatric illness but that marijuana smoking may increase risk for decompensation among those individuals who have preexisting psychiatric disorders. There is evidence that affective disorders and paranoia may be exacerbated after marijuana smoking (Chopra 1973; Harmatz et al. 1972; Naditch 1974; Tart 1970). Persons with a past history of anxiety disorders have reported panic reactions following marijuana smoking (Meyer 1975; Novak 1980; Weil et al. 1968).

TOLERANCE AND PHYSICAL DEPENDENCE

There are considerable data showing that significant tolerance to marijuana effects may develop rapidly following initiation of use of the drug. Tolerance appears to be more closely related to adaptations in central nervous system sensitivity rather than to changes in the metabolism of cannabis compounds. Development of tolerance has been correlated with the increased dose and amount of marijuana use by both occasional and heavy users of the drug (Mello and Mendelson 1985, 1987; Mendelson et al. 1974b, 1976b, 1976c).

Signs and symptoms of overt physical dependence following administration of cannabis in all preparations to otherwise healthy males have been documented in carefully controlled studies (Jones et al. 1976, 1981). The marijuana abstinence syndrome consists of insomnia, anorexia, agitation, restlessness, irritability, depression, and tremor. In studies of chronic marijuana smoking by men carried out under controlled research ward conditions, mild abstinence syndromes (e.g., insomnia, anorexia, mild nausea, and irritability) were reported following cessation of marijuana smoking (Mendelson et al. 1974a, 1974b, 1976a, 1976b, 1976c).

Physical dependence has also been demonstrated to occur following chronic marijuana smoking in studies of women who self-administered marijuana on a controlled research ward. Following 21 days of heavy smoking, abrupt cessation of marijuana use was associated with an abstinence syndrome consisting of tremor of the tongue and extremities, insomnia, anorexia, anxiety, dysphoria, sweating, lateral gaze nystagmus, and exaggerated deep tendon reflexes. Onset of abstinence signs and symptoms occurred 10 hours following cessation of marijuana smoking. The intensity of withdrawal signs and symptoms progressed rapidly and were at maximal levels 48 hours following smoking. Symptoms decreased 72 hours following smoking, and complete remission of all withdrawal signs and symptoms was noted by the fifth day after marijuana withdrawal. Based on the amount and frequency of marijuana smoked, it was concluded that a THC dose of 3.2 mg/kg of body weight per day for 3 consecutive weeks would induce physical dependence (Mendelson et al. 1984).

ADVERSE PHYSIOLOGIC EFFECTS ASSOCIATED WITH MARIJUANA USE

One of the most consistent physiologic effects that occurs following marijuana smoking is tachycardia (Aronow and Cassidy 1974; Beaconsfield et al. 1972; Clark et al. 1974; Galanter et al. 1973; Johnson and Domino 1971; Jones 1977). Associated with tachycardia is electrocardiographic evidence of inversion or flattening of the T wave, elevations of the ST segment, and increase in amplitude of the P wave (Beaconsfield et al. 1972; Cohen 1976; Kochar and Hosko 1973; Roth et al. 1973; Wendkos 1973). It has also been reported that high-dose marijuana use or chronic marijuana smoking may cause premature ventricular contractions (Kochar and Hosko 1973). Although there have been no specific reports of marijuana-induced fatal arrhythmias, there is evidence that chronic marijuana smoking may produce exacerbations of cardiac disorders in persons who have heart disease (National Institute on Drug Abuse 1974).

Marijuana smoking may cause major disorders of respiratory function. In part, this is due to the most frequent mode of self-administration of marijuana via inhalation of pyrolized THC and cannabis compounds plus smoke and fumes. Decreased exercise tolerance has been found in heavy marijuana smokers (Henderson et al. 1972). Chronic cough and bronchitis have also been frequently observed in marijuana smokers (Abramson 1974; Tennant 1980). Impairments in vital capacity and ventilatory function have been found in pulmonary function studies of persons who regularly use marijuana (Henderson et al. 1972; Mendelson et al. 1972; Moss and Friedman 1976; Tashkin et al. 1976). Marijuana use adversely affects pulmonary function in part by impairing gas fusion across the surface of lung-cell membranes (Tilles et al. 1986). Marijuana-related impairments of pulmonary function are greater in persons who also smoke tobacco cigarettes. However, marijuana smoking alone, even in the absence of tobacco cigarette use, can produce significant damage to pulmonary function (Tilles et al. 1986).

A number of studies have shown that marijuana may adversely affect reproductive system function. There are controversial data concerning marijuana effects on plasma testosterone levels in healthy males. Some researchers have reported marijuana-related decrements in plasma testosterone levels (Cohen 1976; Kolodny 1975; Kolodny et al. 1974); however, other studies have failed to confirm these observations (Cushman 1975; Hembree et al. 1976; Mendelson et al. 1974b, 1975, 1978; Schaefer et al. 1974). Marijuana smoking may cause a decrease in sperm cell count and motility (Hembree et al. 1979) as well as abnormalities of sperm cell morphology (Hembree et al. 1979; Issidorides 1979; Morishima 1984).

Adverse effects of marijuana on reproductive hormone function in females have been detected following acute THC administration to experimental animals (Asch et al. 1979a, 1979b; Chakravarty et al. 1975; Hughes and Tyrey 1982; Kramer and Ben-David 1974, 1978; Marks 1973; Nir et al. 1973; Smith et al. 1979a, 1979b). However, tolerance for THC disruption of anterior pituitary and gonadal hormone function occurs when the drug is administered chronically. Different effects of marijuana on reproductive hormone function in women have been found as a function of specific phases of the menstrual cycle (Mendelson et al. 1985a, 1985b, 1985c). Acute marijuana smoking appears to stimulate the luteinizing hormone surge at mid cycle. In contrast, acute marijuana smoking during the luteal phase of the menstrual cycle is associated with a suppression of luteinizing hormone (Mendelson et al. 1985a). It has been postulated that marijuana-induced changes in reproductive hormone function in women may contribute to defects in newborns whose mothers were chronic users of marijuana (Linn et al. 1983).

Women who chronically smoke marijuana during pregnancy often have children whose birth weight is lower than normal (Tennes 1984). There appears to be a significant negative correlation between the frequency of marijuana use and birth weight; lowest birth weight of newborns was observed in women who were the heaviest marijuana smokers. There has also been one interesting report that signs and symptoms associated with fetal alcohol syndrome were also found in the newborns of women who smoked marijuana heavily (Hingson et al. 1982). In addition, infants whose mothers reported a history of heavy marijuana smoking had a high frequency of startle responses and tremor (Linn et al. 1983).

DETOXIFICATION AND TREATMENT ISSUES

No specific detoxification procedures for chronic marijuana use have been developed and subjected to controlled clinical trials as of this writing. Although physical dependence may develop following chronic marijuana smoking, the withdrawal syndromes observed to date do not appear to require specific pharmacologic intervention. It should be cautioned, however, that as higher potency cannabis compounds become available, more severe withdrawal signs and symptoms may occur. Based on existing data, such withdrawal syndromes are likely to resemble those commonly associated with ethanol withdrawal.

Sustained drug-seeking behavior and psychological dependence are commonly found following chronic marijuana use. However, no specifically unique interventions or treatment programs have been devised to attenuate this process. Since many chronic marijuana users also have concurrent psychological and social problems, a number of psychosocial treatment procedures ranging from psychotherapy to membership in peer self-help groups may be of value for certain individuals.

Because of the widespread use of marijuana, psychological and physiologic disorders associated with chronic use of the drug may be underestimated or ignored. Persons who use cannabis compounds on a regular basis are at a high risk for other serious physical illnesses (such as pulmonary disease) and are also at high risk for developing concomitant polydrug abuse problems. The adequate treatment of such persons is crucially dependent on thorough evaluation of psychological, sociocultural, and interpersonal function. A rational decision for treatment assignment can be made only after a careful and perceptive diagnostic evaluation. Often multimodal treatment and intervention procedures have to be utilized and recrudescence of drug use may occur during treatment. Chronic marijuana use should never be regarded as a benign phenomenon. As with chronic alcohol abuse, no single treatment panacea has been achieved, but combined efforts by persons from a number of disciplines (e.g., physicians, social workers, self-help groups, counselors, and clergy) have contributed to either recovery from, or long-lasting remissions of, chronic marijuana abuse.

REFERENCES

Abel EL: Marihuana, learning, and memory. Int Rev Neurobiol 18:329–356, 1975

Abramson HA: Respiratory disorders and marijuana use. The Journal of Asthma Research 11:97, 1974

Adams AJ, Brown B, Flom MC, et al: Alcohol and marijuana effects on static visual acuity. Am J Optom Physiol Opt 52:729–735, 1975

Adams EH, Gfroerer JC, Rouse BA, et al: Trends in prevalence and consequences of cocaine use. Advances in Alcohol and Drug Abuse 6:49–71, 1986

Aronow WS, Cassidy J: Effect of marihuana and placebo-marihuana smoking on angina pectoris. N Engl J Med 291:65–67, 1974

Asch RH, Smith CG, Siler-Khodr TM, et al: Acute decreases in serum prolactin concentrations caused by delta-9-tetrahydrocannabinol in nonhuman primates. Fertil Steril 32:571–575, 1979a

Asch RH, Fernandez EO, Smith CG, et al: Blockage of the ovulatory reflex in the rabbit with delta-9-tetrahydrocannabinol. Fertil Steril 31:331, 1979b

Barnett G, Chiang CN, Perez-Reyes M, et al: Kinetic study of smoking marijuana. J Pharmacokinet Biopharm 10:495–506, 1982

Beaconsfield P, Ginsburg J, Rainsbury R: Cardiovascular effects in man and possible mechanisms. N Engl J Med 287:209–212, 1972

Belmore SM, Miller LL: Levels of processing and acute effects of marijuana on memory. Pharmacol Biochem Behav 13:199–203, 1980

Blaine JD, Meacham MP, Janowsky DS, et al: Marijuana smoking and simulated flying performance, in Pharmacology of Marijuana. Edited by Braude MC, Szara S. New York, Raven, 1976, pp 445–447

Butler JL, Gaines LS, Lenox JR: Effects of marijuana expectation and "suggestibility" on cognitive functioning. Percept Mot Skills 42:1059–1065, 1976

Chakravarty I, Shah PG, Sheth AR, et al: Effect of acute delta⁹-tetrahydrocannabinol treatment on serum luteinizing hormone and prolactin levels in adult female rats. Fertil Steril 26:947–948, 1975

Chopra GS: Studies on psychoclinical aspects of long-term marihuana use in 124 cases. Int J Addict 8:1015–1026, 1973

Chopra GS, Smith JW: Psychotic reaction following cannabis use in East Indians. Arch Gen Psychiatry 30:24–27, 1974

Clark SC, Greene C, Karr GW, et al: Cardiovascular effects of marihuana in man. Can J Physiol Pharmacol 52:706–719, 1974

Clark WC, Goetz RR, McCarthy RH, et al: Effects of marihuana on pain and verbal memory: a sensory decision theory analysis, in Marihuana: Biological Effects: Analysis, Metabolism, Cellular Responses, Reproduction and Brain. Edited by Nahas GG, Paton WDM. New York, Pergamon, 1979, pp 665–680

Clayton RR, Voss HL: Young men and drugs in Manhattan: a causal analysis. Natl Inst Drug Abuse Res Monogr Ser 39:1–187, 1981

Clopton PL, Janowsky DS, Clopton JM, et al: Marijuana and the perception of affect. Psychopharmacology 61:203–206, 1979

Cohen S: The 94-day cannabis study. Ann NY Acad Sci 282:211–220, 1976

Cohen S: Cannabis: effects upon adolescent motivation, in Marijuana and Youth: Clinical Observations on Motivation and Learning (NIDA, DHHS Publication No ADM-82-1186). Washington, DC, U.S. Government Printing Office, 1982, pp 2–11

Creason CR, Goldman M: Varying levels of marijuana use by adolescents and the amotivational syndrome. Psychol Rep 48:447–454, 1981

Cushman P: Plasma testosterone levels in healthy male marijuana smokers. Am J Drug Alcohol Abuse 2:269–276, 1975

Galanter M, Wyatt RJ, Lemberger L, et al: Effects on humans of delta⁹-tetrahydrocannabinol administered by smoking. Science 176:934–936, 1972

Galanter M, Weingartner H, Vaughan TB, et al: Delta⁹-tetrahydrocannabinol and natural marihuana: a controlled comparison. Arch Gen Psychiatry 28:278–281, 1973

Harmatz JS, Shader RI, Salzman C: Marihuana users and non users: personality test differences. Arch Gen Psychiatry 26:108–112, 1972

Hembree WC, Nahas GG, Zeidenberg P, et al: Marihuana effects on the human testes. Clin Res 24:272a, 1976

Hembree WC, Nahas GG, Zeidenberg P, et al: Changes in human spermatozoa associated with high dose marihuana smoking, in Marihuana: Biological Effects: Analysis, Metabolism, Cellular Responses, Reproduction and Brain. Edited by Nahas GG, Paton WDM. New York, Pergamon, 1979, pp 429–439

Henderson RL, Tennant FS, Guerry R: Respiratory manifestations of hashish smoking. Archives of Otolaryngology 92:248–251, 1972

Hingson R, Alpert J, Day N, et al: Effects of maternal drinking and marihuana use on fetal growth and development. Pediatrics 70:539–546, 1980

Hughes CL Jr, Tyrey L: Effects of (-)-trans-delta-9-tetrahydrocannabinol on serum prolactin in the pseudopregnant rat. Endocrine Research Communications 9:25–36, 1982

Hunt CA, Jones RT: Tolerance and disposition of tetrahydrocannabinol in man. J Pharmacol Exp Ther 215:35–44, 1980

Isbell H, Gorodetzsky CW, Jasinski DR, et al: Effects of (-)-trans-tetrahydrocannabinol in man. Psychopharmacologia 11:184–188, 1967

Issidorides MR: Observations in chronic hashish users: nuclear aberrations in blood and sperm and abnormal acrosomes in spermatozoa, in Marihuana: Biological Effects: Analysis, Metabolism, Cellular Responses, Reproduction and Brain. Edited by Nahas GG, Paton WDM. New York, Pergamon, 1979, pp 377–388

Janowsky DS, Meacham MP, Blaine JD, et al: Marijuana effects on simulated flying ability. Am J Psychiatry 133:383–388, 1976a

Janowsky DS, Meacham MP, Blaine JD, et al: Simulated flying performance after marihuana intoxication. Aviat Space Environ Med 47:124–128, 1976b

Johnson S, Domino EF: Some cardiovascular effects of marihuana smoking in normal volunteers. Clin Pharmacol Ther 12:762–768, 1971

Johnston LD, Bachman JG, O'Malley P: Highlights from Student Drug Use in America 1975–1980 (NIDA, DHHS Publication No ADM-81-1066). Washington, DC, U.S. Government Printing Office, 1980

Jones RT: Human effects in Marihuana Research Findings: 1976. Natl Inst Drug Abuse Res Monogr Ser 14:128–178, 1977

Jones RT, Stone G: Psychological studies of marijuana and alcohol in man. Psychopharmacologia 18:108–117, 1970

Jones RT, Benowitz N, Bachman J: Clinical studies of cannabis tolerance and dependence. Ann NY Acad Sci 282:221–239, 1976

Jones RT, Benowitz NL, Herning RI: Clinical relevance of cannabis tolerance and dependence. J Clin Pharmacol 21:143S–152S, 1981

Kandel DB, Murphy D, Karus D: Cocaine use in young adulthood: patterns of use and psychosocial correlates. Natl Inst Drug Abuse Res Monogr Ser 61:76–110, 1985

Klonoff H: Marijuana and driving in real-life situations. Science 1986:317–324, 1974

Kochar MS, Hosko MJ: Electrocardiographic effects of marihuana. JAMA 225:25–27, 1973

Kolodny RC: Research issues in the study of marijuana and male reproductive physiology in humans, in Marijuana and Health Hazards: Methodological Issues in Current Research. Edited by Tinklenberg JR. New York, Academic, 1975, pp 71–81

Kolodny RCF, Masters WH, Kolodny RM, et al: Depression of plasma testosterone levels after chronic intensive marihuana use. N Engl J Med 290:872–874, 1974

Kozel NJ, Adams EH: Epidemiology of drug abuse: an overview. Science 234:970–974, 1986

Kramer J, Ben-David M: Suppression of prolactin secretion by acute administration of delta-9-THC in rats. Proc Soc Exp Biol Med 147:484, 1974

Kramer J, Ben-David M: Prolactin suppression by (-) delta-9-tetrahydrocannabinol (THC): involvement of serotonergic and dopaminergic pathways. Endocrinology 103:452–457, 1978

Lantner IL: Marijuana abuse by children and teenagers: a pediatrician's view, in Marijuana and Youth: Clinical Observations on Motivation and Learning (NIDA, DHHS Publication No ADM-82-1186). Washington, DC, U.S. Government Printing Office, 1982, pp 84–92

Le Dain G, Campell IL, Lehmann H, et al: Cannabis: A Report of the Commission of Inquiry into the Non-Medical Use of Drugs. Ottawa, Information Canada, 1972

Linn S, Shoenbaum S, Monson RR, et al: The association of marijuana use with outcome of pregnancy. Am J Public Health 73:1161–1164, 1983

Manno JE, Manno BR, Kiplinger GF, et al: Motor and mental performance with marijuana: relationship to administered dose of delta⁹-tetrahydrocannabinol and its interactions with alcohol, in Marijuana: Effects on Human Behavior. Edited by Miller LL. New York, Academic, 1974, pp 46–72

Marks BH: Delta⁹-THC and luteinizing hormone secretion, in Progress in Brain Research/Drug Effects on Neuroendocrine Regulation, Vol 10.

Edited by Gispin WH, Marks BH, DeWied D. Amsterdam, Elsevier, 1973, pp 331–338

McGlothlin WH, West LJ: The marihuana problem: an overview. Am J Psychiatry 125:370–378, 1968

Melges FT, Tinklenberg JR, Hollister LE, et al: Marihuana and temporal disintegration. Science 168:1118–1120, 1970

Mello NK, Mendelson JH: Operant acquisition of marihuana by women. J Pharmacol Exp Ther 235:162–171, 1985

Mello NK, Mendelson JH: Operant analysis of human drug self-administration: marihuana, alcohol, heroin and polydrug use, in Methods of Assessing the Reinforcing Properties of Abused Drugs. Edited by Bozarth MA. New York, Springer Verlag, 1987, pp 525–558

Mendelson JH, Meyer RE, Rossi AM, et al: Behavioral and biological concomitants of chronic marihuana smoking by heavy and casual users, in Marihuana: A Signal of Misunderstanding. Technical Papers, Vol 1. Washington, DC, U.S. Government Printing Office, 1972, pp 68–246

Mendelson JH, Kuehnle J, Ellingboe J, et al: Plasma testosterone levels before, during and after chronic marihuana smoking. N Engl J Med 291:1051–1055, 1974a

Mendelson JH, Rossi AM, Meyer RE (eds): The Use of Marihuana: A Psychological and Physiological Inquiry. New York, Plenum, 1974b

Mendelson JH, Kuehnle JC, Ellingboe J, et al: Effects of marihuana on plasma testosterone, in Marihuana and Health Hazards: Methodological Issues in Current Research. Edited by Tinklenberg JR. New York, Academic, 1975, pp 83–93

Mendelson JH, Babor TF, Kuehnle JC, et al: Behavioral and biological aspects of marihuana use. Ann NY Acad Sci 282:186–210, 1976a

Mendelson JH, Kuehnle JC, Greenberg I, et al: The effects of marihuana use on human operant behavior: individual data, in The Pharmacology of Marihuana. Edited by Braude MC, Szara S. New York, Raven, 1976b, pp 643–653

Mendelson JH, Kuehnle JC, Greenberg I, et al: Operant acquisition of marihuana in man. J Pharmacol Exp Ther 198:42–53, 1976c

Mendelson JH, Ellingboe J, Kuehnle JC, et al: Effects of chronic marihuana use on integrated plasma testosterone and luteinizing hormone levels. J Pharmacol Exp Ther 207:611–617, 1978

Mendelson JH, Mello NK, Lex BW, et al: Marijuana withdrawal syndrome in a woman. Am J Psychiatry 141:1289–1290, 1984

Mendelson JH, Cristofaro P, Ellingboe J, et al: Acute effects of marihuana on luteinizing hormone in menopausal women. Pharmacol Biochem Behav 23:765–768, 1985a

Mendelson JH, Mello NK, Cristofaro P, et al: Acute effects of marijuana on pituitary and gonadal hormones during the periovulatory phase of the menstrual cycle. Natl Inst Drug Abuse Res Monogr Ser 55:24–31, 1985b

Mendelson JH, Mello NK, Ellingboe J: Acute effects of marihuana smoking on prolactin levels in human females. J Pharmacol Exp Ther 232:220–222, 1985c

Meyer RE: Psychiatric consequences of marijuana use: state of the evidence, in Marijuana and Health Hazards. Edited by Tinklenberg JR. New York, Academic, 1975, pp 133–152

Miles CG, Congreve GRS, Gibbins RJ, et al: An experimental study of the effects of daily cannabis smoking on behaviour patterns. Acta Pharmacol Toxicol 34:1–43, 1974

Morishima A: Effects of cannabis and natural cannabinoids on chromosomes. Natl Inst Drug Abuse Res Monogr Ser 44:25–45, 1984

Moskowitz H: Cannabis and experimental studies of driving skills, in Research Advances in Alcohol and Drug Problems, Vol 3. Edited by Gibbons RJ, Israel Y, Kalant H, et al. New York, John Wiley, 1976, pp 283–399

Moskowitz H, Sharma S, McGlothlin W: Effect of marihuana upon peripheral vision as a function of the information processing demands in central vision. Percept Mot Skills 35:875–882, 1972

Moss IR, Friedman E: Delta⁹-tetrahydrocannabinol: depression of ventilator regulation; other respiratory and cardiovascular effects. Life Sci 19:99–104, 1976

Naditch MP: Acute adverse reactions to psychoactive drugs, drug usage and psychopathology. J Abnorm Psychol 83:394–403, 1974

National Commission on Marihuana and Drug Abuse: Marihuana: A Signal of Misunderstanding, Appendix, Vol 1. Washington, DC, U.S. Government Printing Office, 1972

National Institute on Drug Abuse: Marijuana and Health, Fourth Annual Report to the U.S. Congress from the Secretary of Health, Education and Welfare (National Institute on Drug Abuse). Washington, DC, U.S. Government Printing Office, 1974

National Institute on Drug Abuse: National Household Survey on Drug Abuse: Main Findings 1982. Rockville, MD, National Institute on Drug Abuse, 1983a

National Institute on Drug Abuse: Population Projections: Based on the National Survey on Drug Abuse 1982, Rockville, MD. National Institute on Drug Abuse, 1983b

National Institute on Drug Abuse: National Household Survey on Drug Abuse: Main Findings 1985 (DHHS Publ No ADM–88–1586). Rockville, MD, National Institute on Drug Abuse, 1988

Negrete JC: Psychological adverse effects of cannabis smoking: a tentative classification. Can Med Assoc J 108:195–196, 1973

Nir I, Ayalon D, Tsafriri A, et al: Suppression of the cyclic of luteinizing hormone secretion and of ovulation in the rat by delta-9-tetrahydrocannabinol. Nature 243:470, 1973

Novak W (ed): High Culture: Marijuana in the Lives of Americans. New York, Knopf, 1980

Ohlsson A, Lindgren J-E, Wahlen A, et al: Plasma delta-9-tetrahydrocannabinol concentrations and clinical effects after oral and intravenous administration and smoking. Clin Pharmacol Ther 28:409–416, 1980

Ohlsson A, Lindgren J-E, Wahlen A, et al: Single dose kinetics of deuterium labelled delta⁹-tetrahydrocannabinol in heavy and light cannabis users. Biomedical Mass Spectrometry 9:6–120, 1982

Perez-Reyes M, DiGuiseppi S, Davis KH, et al: Comparison of effects of marihuana cigarettes of three different potencies. Clin Pharmacol Ther 31:617–624, 1982

Petersen RC: Marijuana and health: 1980, in Marijuana Research Findings: 1980. Natl Inst Drug Abuse Res Monogr Ser 31:1–53, 1980

Ray R, Prabhu GG, Mohan D, et al: The association between chronic cannabis use and cognitive function. Drug Alcohol Depend 3:365–368, 1978

Reeve VC, Grant JD, Robertson W, et al: Plasma concentrations of delta[9]-tetrahydrocannabinol and impaired motor function. Drug Alcohol Depend 11:167–175, 1983

Rickles WH, Cohen MJ, Whitaker CA, et al: Marijuana induced state-dependent verbal learning. Psychopharmacologia 30:349–354, 1973

Roth WT, Tinklenberg JR, Kopell BS, et al: Continuous electrocardiographic monitoring during marihuana intoxication. Clin Pharmacol Ther 14:533–540, 1973

Roth WT, Tinklenberg JR, Kopell BS: Ethanol and marihuana effects on event-related potenials in a memory retrieval paradigm. Electroencephalog Clin Neurophysiol 42:381–388, 1977

Schaefer DF, Gun CG, Dubowski KM: Normal plasma testosterone concentrations after marihuana smoking. N Engl J Med 292:867–868, 1974

Sharma S, Moskowitz H: Effect of marihuana on the visual autokinetic phenomenon. Percept Mot Skills 35:891–894, 1972

Smith CG, Besch RG, Smith RG, et al: Effects of tetrahydrocannabinol on the hypothalamic-pituitary axis in the ovariectomized rhesus monkey. Fertil Steril 31:335, 1979a

Smith CG, Smith MT, Besch NF, et al: The effects of delta-9-tetrahydrocannabinol (THC) on female reproductive function, in Marihuana: Biological Effects: Analysis, Metabolism, Cellular Responses, Reproduction and Brain. Edited by Nahas GG, Paton WDM. New York, Pergamon, 1979b, pp 449–467

Smith DE, Seymour RB: Clinical perspectives on the toxicity of marijuana: 1967, 1981, in Marijuana and Youth: Clinical Observations on Motivation and Learning (NIDA, DHHS Publication No ADM-82-1186). Washington, DC, U.S. Government Printing Office, 1982, pp 61–72

Tart CT: Marijuana intoxication: common experiences. Nature 226:701–704, 1970

Tashkin DP, Shapiro BJ, Lee YE, et al: Subacute effects of heavy marihuana smoking on pulmonary function in healthy men. N Engl J Med 294:125–129, 1976

Tennant FS Jr: Histopathologic and clinical abnormalities of the respiratory system in chronic hashish smokers. Natl Inst Drug Abuse Res Monog Ser 27:309–315, 1980

Tennes K: Effect of marijuana on pregnancy and fetal development in the human. Natl Inst Drug Abuse Res Monogr Ser 44:115–123, 1984

Tilles DS, Goldenheim PD, Johnson DC, et al: Marijuana smoking as cause of reduction in single-breath carbon monoxide diffusing capacity. Am J Med 80:601–606, 1986

Voth HM: How to Get Your Child Off Marijuana. Stamford, CT, Patient Care Publications Inc. for Citizens for Informed Choices on Marijuana, 1980

Wall ME, Sadler BM, Brine D, et al: Metabolism, disposition and kinetics of delta-9-tetrahydrocannabinol in men and women. Clin Pharmacol Ther 34:352–363, 1983

Weil AT, Zinberg NE, Nelson JM: Clinical and psychological effects of marijuana in man. Science 162:1234–1242, 1968

Wendkos MH: Electrocardiographic effects of marihuana. JAMA 226:789, 1973

Chapter 5

Cocaine

Herb Roehrich, M.D.
Mark S. Gold, M.D.

DIAGNOSIS

Both clinical suspicion and laboratory confirmation are required for a firm diagnosis of cocaine abuse. Clinically, patients may present with intoxication, abstinence symptoms, overdose, or medical or psychiatric disturbance (Gold and Washton 1985). Additionally, diagnostic consideration must be given to relevant psychosocial correlates of cocaine abuse. Job loss, marital problems, financial problems, automobile accidents, fights, suicide attempts, and legal problems are concomitants of cocaine abuse in adults (Kandel et al. 1985; Washton and Gold 1984). Among adolescents, use of alcohol, marijuana, or tobacco should heighten suspicion of cocaine abuse (Clayton 1985; O'Malley et al. 1985). Additionally, cocaine-abusing adolescents are more likely to have histories of running away from home, changing friends, skipping or being expelled from school, having a decline in their academic performance, being involved in motor vehicle accidents, attempting suicide, exhibiting violent behavior (Washton et al. 1984b), and running away and being delinquent (Smith et al. 1989; Washington 1984a). Because adolescent patients will often be unwilling to discuss their psychosocial situation honestly, family or friends must often be asked for information to assist in the diagnosis.

Whether all people who test positive for or admit to using cocaine are abusers is not as clear. Although all cocaine users are at a very high risk for becoming addicts, there appears to be a small group whose use of cocaine is circumscribed to specific self-defined "recreational" situations (O'Malley et al. 1985; Siegel 1984). Whether these people can self-limit their use of the drug and do not progress to abuse of the drug will take a detailed longitudinal study. (This would be inconsistent with monkey and rodent data, however.) These are people who clinically should lack psychosocial problems correlated with cocaine and who evidence stable emotional maturity and psychosocial growth.

Laboratory confirmation of cocaine abuse is achieved by serum or urine drug testing. It must be emphasized that one negative drug screen does not rule out cocaine abuse. A urine test may be negative while the blood is positive and vice versa. The sensitivity of the testing procedure may also bias the results toward more negatives (Cone et al. 1989). Random, serial screens may be needed to confirm or refute clinical impressions. Additionally, family or friends may need to retrieve the patient's drugs or drug paraphernalia, which may also be analyzed.

There are two methods of testing for the presence of cocaine or its metabolites: competitive binding assays and chromatographic assays; both have diagnostic utility (Lehrer and Gold 1987). Competitive binding assays such as the radioimmunoassay (RIA) or enzyme immunoassay (EIA) are often used as initial screens for the presence of the cocaine metabolite benzoylecgonine in urine. The urine sample should be collected under urethral supervision, and specific gravity of the urine sample should be measured to ensure validity. A first-morning void urine provides an optimum sample. The RIA can generally detect benzoylecgonine for 3–4 days and EIA for up to 48 hours after cocaine ingestion (Van Dyke et al. 1977). However, immunoassay and enzyme multiplied immunoassay technique (EMIT®) assays have detected cocaine and its metabolites up to 10 and 22 days after last use, respectively (Cone and Weddington 1989; Weiss and Gawin 1988). RIA testing is slightly more costly and time-consuming than EIA testing. False positives on RIA testing may be obtained through cross-reaction with tropane alkaloids or thioridazine (Mule et al. 1977).

Both RIA and EIA techniques are designed as screening tests. A negative test in the face of a high index of clinical suspicion may be followed up with a more sensitive chromatographic screening procedure. Any positive screen should be chromatographically confirmed.

Chromatographic screens for cocaine include thin-layer chromatography (TLC), high-pressure liquid chromatography (HPLC), gas-liquid chromatography (GLC), and gas chromatograph-mass spectrometry (GCMS) (Jatlow et al. 1978; Kogan et al. 1977; Tindal et al. 1978; Valanzi et al. 1973; Van Dyke et al. 1976). TLC has several drawbacks. It is a qualitative test with the least reliability of all screening methods, having a sensitivity level of 1,000–2,000 ng/ml of drug or metabolite so that benzoylecgonine is detectable for only 12–24 hours after a large dose of cocaine (Hansen et al. 1985). TLC also suffers from poor specificity compounded by intertechnician variability in interpretation. Thus TLC screens are not adequate screens for cocaine use (Lehrer and Gold 1987).

Either HPLC or GLC provide greater sensitivity and specificity than EIA or RIA. Like other chromatography methods, they can be applied to blood or urine samples. Gas chromatography can also be used to detect cocaine in saliva (Cone et al. 1988). However, we commonly choose GCMS assay of urine. This test can provide "fingerprint" certain identification of the drug at low (<100 ng/ml) concentrations. This level of certainty is important because of legal, social, and economic consequences that may accompany a diagnosis of cocaine use or abuse. GCMS can be used to confirm positive EIA or RIA drug screens or may be used to determine cocaine blood level to assess a state of acute intoxication. Its sensitivity allows GCMS to pick up cocaine metabolites for up to 7 days after heavy usage (Ambre 1985).

In sum, clinical information and impressions should be checked by drug screens. EIA or RIA methods provide adequate screening techniques, with GCMS providing sensitive and fingerprint-certain confirmation. Finally, for drug testing to be reliable, the sample being tested must have a chain of accountability that is unbroken, beginning with the person responsible for collecting the specimen tested and ending with the person who runs and reports the test on that sample. Failure to have such a chain in the testing process allows for the possibility of misdiagnosis and significant adverse consequences for the person misdiagnosed.

PREVALENCE

Cocaine is a drug whose use has skyrocketed in the past 10 years. An estimated 30–60 tons of cocaine worth 55 billion dollars is imported into the United States yearly (Grabowski and Dworkin 1985). Twenty-five million Americans have tried cocaine during their lifetime, and 6 million use it regularly (National Institute on Drug Abuse 1985). Three thousand people try it for the first time each day (Gold 1984). In 1972, 1.5% of all adolescents, 9.1% of all young adults, and 1.6% of all adults had tried or were using cocaine regularly. By 1986, 6.9% of all adolescents, 28.7% of all young adults, and 8.7% of all adults had tried or were using cocaine regularly (Grabowski and Dworkin 1985). Unlike many other drugs, these data demonstrate that risk for initiation of cocaine use does not end with young adulthood. Between 1976 and 1981, there was a 300% increase in emergency room visits, a 400% increase in deaths, and a 450% increase in treatment program admissions for cocaine abuse (Adams and Durrell 1984). In one study, 5% of surveyed college students tried or used cocaine in 1969 (Walters et al. 1972); by 1977, 33% of the students had tried or were using cocaine (Pope et al. 1981). In another study, 18% of pregnant women were found to have used cocaine while pregnant (Zuckerman et al. 1989).

In 1987, cocaine use in teenagers first showed evidence of decreasing prevalence. Prevalence rates of current cocaine use had decreased from 6.2% to 4.3% of high school seniors in 1987 (Bowen 1988). However, data suggest that abuse of "crack" is spreading beyond metropolitan areas (Macdonald 1987).

Rates of cocaine abuse have been highest in the major metropolitan areas of the East Coast and West Coast and lower in southern and north central portions of the United States (O'Malley et al. 1985). Data from the 1-800-COCAINE hotline studies suggest that cocaine abuse is increasing among young people, women, and lower income groups (Washton and Gold 1987). The data from this hotline receive confirmation from other researchers who find cocaine being tried by women at rates greater than or equal to males (Anthony et al. 1985). Existing data also suggest that cocaine does not discriminate racially, with significant cocaine abuse problems in black populations (Adams and Durrell 1984). Cocaine use is also prevalent among opiate addicts (Kosten et al. 1985; Nurco et al. 1985; Strug et al. 1985).

Several predictors of cocaine abuse are suggested. The use of marijuana has consistently been a predictor of later cocaine use. Alcohol or tobacco use, truancy or declining school performance, and early onset of drug use may also be predictive of cocaine use (Kandel et al. 1985; O'Malley et al. 1985).

Cocaine is, in most studies, not used alone. Cocaine use is increasingly prevalent among opiate abusers or addicts. Conversely, most cocaine users also abuse other drugs (Abelson and Miller 1985; Clayton 1985; Kandel et al. 1985; O'Malley et al. 1985).

Thus the dramatic increases in cocaine use that began in the 1970s are not abating. We can expect to continue to see more patients with cocaine abuse problems in the coming years.

PHARMACOLOGY

Cocaine can be obtained or prepared in forms that will be absorbed from the lung, the bloodstream, or any mucosal surface of the body. Cocaine hydrochloride, the white crystalline powder, is most commonly insufflated but can also be absorbed by rectal or vaginal mucosae and is also absorbed by the gastrointestinal tract after oral ingestion. Cocaine hydrochloride is also water soluble and can be absorbed from the bloodstream by injection after dissolution in water. By dissolving cocaine hydrochloride in a strong base, subsequently extracting the cocaine free base in a solvent, and then separating out the free base from the solvent, a solid form of cocaine that melts at 98° C and subsequently volatizes at increasing temperatures is formed (Gold 1984). This is free-base cocaine or "crack," which may be smoked, with the cocaine-containing smoke being absorbed from the lungs.

Cocaine bioavailability is not the same for all forms or sites of entry; 20–40% of oral or intranasal cocaine is bioavailable, whereas 100% of iv cocaine is absorbed (Jones 1984; Mayersohn and Perrier 1978). Oral cocaine bioavailability is decreased by first-pass hepatic metabolism. Insufflated cocaine absorption is decreased by the intense nasal vasoconstriction produced by the drug (Wilkinson et al. 1980). Various peak plasma levels have been reported. In a study of Peruvian chewers of erythroxylon leaves, peak plasma levels of 95 ng/ml were found (Paly et al. 1980). A single administration of 1.5 mg/kg intranasal cocaine produced peak blood levels of 120–475 ng/ml (Jatlow et al. 1978). A single 32-mg bolus of iv cocaine produced peak plasma levels of 300 ng/ml (Javaid et al. 1983). A single bolus of ½ g of free-based cocaine gave peak blood levels of 975 ng/ml and blood levels of 800–900 ng/ml 3 hours after ingestion (Siegel 1982b).

By whatever route cocaine enters the body, peak blood concentration is dose-dependent, as is time to peak blood level (Wilkinson et al. 1980). However, there is no research clearly defining dose versus plasma concentration correlation curves. Because of interindividual variability in absorption and metabolism, such correlations are probably not possible.

It is probably the rate of change in cocaine blood levels (presumably reflecting changes in cocaine brain levels), the time after intake for change in blood levels to occur, and to some extent the maximal change occurring that produces the sought-after euphoria (Zahler et al. 1982). Thus an iv bolus of 0.6 mg/kg of cocaine given over 1 minute with peak blood levels of 300–400 ng/ml produces a euphoria equal to that from 3 mg/kg given over 1 hour with blood levels up to 1,100 ng/ml (Jones 1984). With insufflation, peak subjective high, occurring approximately 30 minutes after intake, precedes peak plasma levels, and the euphoria wears off while cocaine is still detectable in plasma (Van Dyke et al. 1976). Oral ingestion has been shown by at least one group to give a significantly greater high than an equivalent intranasal dose (Van Dyke et al. 1978). However, with oral use, the euphoria peaks at 75 minutes; the delay in comparison to intranasal use is due to time required for gastrointestinal transport and subsequent absorption. With iv use, the high occurs within 1 minute of intake (Resnick et al. 1977). With a single iv injection, the euphoria parallels the increase and decrease in cocaine blood levels (Javaid et al. 1978). With free-base use of cocaine, the euphoria begins even more rapidly than with iv use (with circulation time from lung to brain being about 8 seconds).

Whatever the route of intake, tolerance occurs clinically with repeated usage, and this tolerance is both acute and chronic. Acutely, Siegel (1982b) showed that cocaine smokers increase the size of their hits during a given run. With iv users, Fischman (1984) found that subjective effects decreased if doses were repeated every 6–10 minutes unless the dosage was increased over time. With chronic use, the baseline dose needed to produce euphoria increases, the total euphoric change decreases, and side effects increase. Thus users may begin with insufflation of portions of a gram, increase to several grams, and then change to iv or free-base use. There is no definitive research to explain this tolerance, but Dackis and Gold's (1985b) dopamine depletion hypothesis is perhaps the best explanation to date.

Simply stated, this theory suggests that dopamine-dependent pleasure centers of the brain are outstripped of their ability to replenish dopamine and require increased stimulation to release enough dopamine to produce euphoria.

Once in the body, cocaine is primarily metabolized in two ways: de-esterification and *N*-demethylation. A major de-esterification product of cocaine is benzoylecgonine. This inactive metabolite is formed by the spontaneous hydrolysis of cocaine at physiologic pH, with 30–45% of ingested cocaine being excreted as benzoylecgonine. (Johns et al. 1977; Stewart et al. 1979). Clinically, when assaying for cocaine in the bloodstream, this spontaneous metabolism must be prevented or assay performed promptly, or the cocaine plasma levels will be artificially decreased (Stewart et al. 1977). Another major metabolite of cocaine is ecgonine methyl ester, a de-esterfied metabolite formed by the action of liver and plasma cholinesterases. This is an inactive metabolite that has been variously reported to account for 25–60% of ingested cocaine (Ambre et al. 1984). If one is going to test for cocaine, care must be taken either to assay the sample promptly or to inactivate serum cholinesterases with an inhibitor such as fluoride or physostigmine (Jones 1984). One *N*-demethylation metabolic product is norcocaine, the only known active metabolite of cocaine to date (Hawks et al. 1975; Misra et al. 1975; Spealman et al. 1979). Norcocaine kinetics are believed to be similar to cocaine kinetics (Misra et al. 1975). Other metabolites of cocaine have been described but are presumed to be inactive minor metabolites (Lowry et al. 1979; D Smith et al. 1984).

The clinical importance of metabolites derives from their use as markers of cocaine use. Cocaine itself has a relatively brief half-life that has been variously found to range from 45 minutes to 2.5 hours (Chow et al. 1985; Fischman 1984; Jones 1984; Mayersohn and Perrier 1978; Van Dyke et al. 1976; Wilkinson et al. 1980). Therefore, one typically assays for longer-lived metabolites. Benzoylecgonine is the metabolite most commonly assayed and can be tested for by TLC, RIA, EMIT, GCMS, and reverse HPLC methods (Jatlow et al. 1978; Kogan et al. 1977; Tindal et al. 1978; Valanzi et al. 1973; Van Dyke et al. 1976). By EMIT, GCMS, or RIA methods, benzoylecgonine may be detectable in urine for up to 543 hours after use (Weiss and Gawin 1988); the most sensitive of these methods (GCMS and RIA) can detect less than 100 ng/ml of benzoylecgonine in urine (Lehrer and Gold 1987).

ETIOLOGY

Little is known about the etiology of cocaine abuse. It appears that
there are some users who can maintain circumscribed, nonaddictive
use of cocaine over time (O'Malley et al. 1985; Siegel 1984). This
suggests that not everyone is a potential cocaine abuser, and studies
that clarify who is susceptible to cocaine addiction might provide important insight for both prevention and treatment of cocaine abuse.

Data from the 1-800-COCAINE hotline suggest that cocaine
abuse is a familial illness, similar to alcoholism. Thus approximately
50% of cocaine abusers had a positive family history of addictive illness. Further, those with a positive family history of addiction and for
whom cocaine was the first drug of abuse were significantly younger
than those for whom cocaine was the first drug of abuse but who
lacked a family history of addictive illness (Roehrich and Gold 1988).

Several studies have suggested that affective illness may be important in progression from cocaine use to abuse (Khantzian and
Khantzian 1984; Smith 1986; Weiss and Mirin 1986). In these studies, cocaine use is valued for its euphoria in depressed patients and for
its enhancement of hypomania in bipolar patients. Follow-up studies
have failed to replicate the finding of an overrepresentation of affective illness in cocaine addicts (Gawin 1988). Several studies also suggest that attention-deficit disorder may be a predispositional risk factor for cocaine abuse. In these individuals, cocaine acts paradoxically
to increase attention span and concentration (Khantzian 1983; Weiss
et al. 1985).

Several researchers found narcissistic and borderline personality
disorders overrepresented among cocaine abusers (Weiss and Mirin
1986; Wurmser 1974). It has been assumed that individuals with
these personality disorders find illusory self-esteem, enhanced pres-
tige, and diminished depression through cocaine-induced euphoria.

Both human and animal research suggest that behavioral conditioning is important to the development and maintenance of addictive behavior with cocaine, as well as in fostering relapse (Childress et
al. 1986; Gold et al. 1986). This conditioning effect has been demonstrated for other substances of abuse as well.

Biologically, the euphoria induced by cocaine appears to be mediated by dopaminergic reward centers of the brain (Dackis and Gold
1985b; DeWit and Wise 1977; Mendelson et al. 1988; Scheel-Kruger
1971). The nucleus accumbens, mesolimbic and mesocortical dopa-

mine systems, and the prefrontal cortex appear to be critical areas for the development of cocaine dependence (Dworkin and Smith 1988; Goeders 1988). Positron-emission tomography scanning studies have correspondingly shown that significant increases in glucose utilization occur in the prefrontal cortex and nucleus accumbens in association with cocaine use (Porrino and Kornetsky 1988). Sensitization to cocaine occurs within 4–7 days of use in laboratory studies (Post and Weiss 1988). It has also been postulated that these systems may have pathologic alterations in addicted and potentially addicted individuals (Koob and Hubner 1988). The addictive potency of cocaine analogues has been shown to correlate with their ability to bind to the dopamine uptake receptors and thereby inhibit dopamine uptake in critical brain areas (Ritz et al. 1987). Blockade of neurotransmission in these centers blocks behavioral responsivity to cocaine in animals.

Although much additional research is needed, the data now available suggest the importance of recognizing families with addiction as targets for intervention. Careful attention to affective illness and screening for attention-deficit disorder are warranted. Identification and treatment of borderline or narcissistic personality disorders may be important for successful recovery from cocaine addiction. Attention to behaviorally conditioned cues is important. Further understanding of cocaine neurophysiology may allow for medicines capable of blockading cocaine's euphoria as an adjunct means of sobriety maintenance. Attention to alcohol, marijuana, and tobacco abuse may also be important in preventing cocaine abuse.

CLINICAL SIGNS OF INTOXICATION

While high on cocaine, the abuser is euphoric and has a global feeling of self-confidence, alertness, and well-being. The user is likely to be talkative, expressing self-confidence and perceived intelligence. While high, the abuser feels intense energy, and fatigue or need for sleep are diminished. While high, the abuser also may experience heightened sexual drive (Gold 1984; Horberg and Schnoll 1983). The duration of the high is practically determined by access to cocaine. With free access, the severely addicted individual may binge for several days, nonstop.

As the amount used and duration of use increases, the rewarding effects are increasingly replaced by side effects. Pleasure turns into agitation, anxiety, and at times panic attacks. The intoxicated individual may pace and have stereotyped movements and grinding of the teeth and jaws. Decreased need for sleep turns into insomnia. Sexual drive is lost. Concentration is lost as the individual is dominated by anxiety and craving for more cocaine. By this time, attention to personal hygiene is usually abandoned. Paranoia may be present, usually a delusion that cocaine use is known to law enforcement officials and that arrest is imminent. Visual or auditory hallucinations may also be present. Medically, pupils are dilated, and blood pressure is increased, as is the respiratory rate. As usage increases, the risk of seizure, cardiac arrhythmia, respiratory arrest, or other medical complications increase (Gold 1984, 1986).

After the "high" comes the "crash," which resembles an acute onset of agitated depression. The abuser is depressed, insomniac, anorexic, and agitated and has intense cravings for additional cocaine. If untreated, this phase may last for hours or days. Abusers will often self-medicate with a sedative-hypnotic drug as this point to "knock themselves out" and, on awakening, will be in a state resembling a retarded depression. They become hypersomnolent, hyperphagic, anhedonic, anergic, motorically slowed, depressed, irritable, and unmotivated. This phase may also last for a period of hours to days.

With chronic use, the euphoric and pleasurable effects are increasingly lost, and the side effects become increasingly prominent. Nonetheless, the abuser will continue to use because the crash persists. The addiction is now reinforced by avoidance of the crash.

MEDICAL COMPLICATIONS

The widespread use of cocaine may have been fostered by the myth that it is a medically safe drug (Gold 1986; Isner et al. 1986). Yet, between 1976 and 1981, while cocaine use was rising dramatically, there was a threefold increase in the rate of cocaine-related emergencies and a fourfold increase in the rate of cocaine-related deaths. There is no amount of cocaine or route of use that is medically safe. Further, at this time, cocaine's adverse medical effects remain largely unpredictable.

Cocaine's most serious adverse effect is death. Unpublished personal contacts suggest that cocaine-related fatalities are underreported in the medical literature. These fatalities result from both direct use of cocaine and from crimes committed to procure the drug. Death has been reported after intranasal, intravenous, free-base, or intravaginal use (Finkle and McCloskey 1977; Mittleman and Wetli 1984). Blood levels at time of autopsy have been as low as 110 ng/dl (DiMaio and Garriott 1978).

Individuals who are sensitive to succinylcholine may be particularly at risk (Jatlow et al. 1979). Succinylcholine sensitivity results from an abnormal cholinesterase, which is responsible for cocaine metabolism. Thus cocaine may accumulate to toxic levels in these individuals more rapidly.

Two rapidly fatal syndromes following cocaine use have been described. One presentation consists of headache, cold sweat, rapid pulse, tremor, and nausea followed by convulsions, loss of consciousness, and death within minutes of onset (DiMaio and Garriott 1978). In this syndrome, death is believed to result from respiratory paralysis. Direct effects on the heart may also be important. A second fatal syndrome is characterized by an excited, paranoid delirium with associated panic and violent behavior, fever as high as 106° F, mydriasis, tachypnea, and death (Catravas and Waters 1981; Wetli and Fishbain 1985). This syndrome has been postulated to be a variant of the neuroleptic malignant syndrome (Kosten and Kleber 1988). Further, another group has suggested that a D_1 dopamine receptor antagonist, given before cocaine use, may block cocaine's lethal effect (Witkin et al. 1989). In both of these syndromes, autopsy findings were nonspecific. Lidocaine may prevent ventricular ectopy in these patients (Gay 1982). If immediately available, diazepam may prevent seizures. Correction of acidosis may help, and cooling by any means must be undertaken (Jonsson et al. 1983; Siegel 1985). The importance of hyperthermia in cocaine-related fatalities has been confirmed by animal research (Catravas and Waters 1981). Jones (1984) reported that fatalities also occur in cocaine abusers who relapse and falsely presume they have retained the tolerance they had previously developed. Specific medical causes of death related to cocaine use include myocardial infarction (Isner et al. 1986), rupture of the ascending aorta (Barth et al. 1986), cardiac arrhythmia (Barth et al. 1986), seizures, central nervous system (CNS) infections from cocaine use (Wetli et al. 1984), intestinal infarction (Nalbandian et al. 1985), bacteremia (Alonso et al. 1986), renal infarction (Sharff 1984), suicide (Washton et al. 1984b), and respiratory failure (DiMaio and Garriott 1978). Additionally, pregnant cocaine abusers have increased rates of spontaneous abortion in comparison to abstinent women (Chasnoff et al. 1985). An animal study by Bozarth and Wise (1985) clearly demonstrated cocaine's toxic potential. After 30 days, rats given free access to cocaine lost an average of 47% of their body weight, and 90% succumbed.

Cardiovascular morbidity associated with cocaine use includes nonfatal myocardial infarction (Coleman et al. 1987; Cregler and Mark 1985; Howard et al. 1985; Kossowsky and Lyon 1984; Pasternack et al. 1985; Schachne et al. 1984; Simpson and Edwards 1986). While the majority of these people have demonstrable preexisting coronary artery disease, some have no history of heart disease or have normal coronary arteriograms, or both. By constricting coronary arteries, decreasing coronary blood flow, and increasing blood pressure and heart rate (thereby increasing cardiac oxygen needs), cocaine use presents an increased risk of angina or myocardial infarction (Lange et al. 1989). Cocaine may also cause thrombosis in individuals with normal coronary arteries. Deep vein thrombosis has been associated with cocaine use (Lisse and Davis 1989). Cocaine use has also been associated with vascular headaches (Satel and Gawin 1989a).

The use of cocaine has also been associated with cardiac arrhythmias, including asystole, ventricular fibrillation, sinus tachycardia, and ventricular tachycardia (Barth et al. 1986; Benchimol et al. 1978; Weiss 1986). The arrhythmias presumably occur due to relative hypoxemia induced by cocaine use, secondary to cocaine-induced seizures, via direct toxic effect on myocardial tissue, and due to elevated catecholamine levels associated with cocaine intoxication. In an unconfirmed animal study, amitriptyline given at least 24 hours before cocaine administration prevented sudden cardiac death (Antelman et al. 1981). More recently, an experimental calcium-channel blocker, nitrendipine, has been reported effective against cocaine-associated cardiac arrhythmia in an animal model (Nahas et al. 1985).

Cocaine has also been associated with sudden cardiac death (Nanji and Filipenko 1985), dilated cardiomyopathy (Wiener et al. 1986), myocarditis (Virmani et al. 1988), and pulmonary edema (Alfred and Ewer 1981).

Cocaine also causes hypertension in association with its use. Propranolol has been variously reported to worsen this hypertension or antagonize the hypertension (Ramoska and Sacchetti 1985; Rappolt et al. 1977). The group reporting successful amelioration of hypertension used higher doses safely, and this suggests that the unsuccessful report may represent inadequate dosing (Rappolt et al. 1977).

Obstetric-neonatal morbidity is also associated with cocaine use.

Several studies have demonstrated an increased rate of abruptio placentae in cocaine-abusing women (Acker et al. 1983; Chasnoff et al. 1985). Chasnoff et al. (1986) also described a case of an infant born with a cerebrovascular accident (CVA) in progress at the time of birth, in association with maternal cocaine abuse. Chasnoff et al. (1989) also reported that cocaine use in the first trimester resulted in abnormalities on the Brazelton Neonatal Exam. Cocaine use throughout pregnancy correlated with increased rates of preterm birth, low birth weight, intrauterine growth retardation, decreased length, and decreased head circumference (Chasnoff et al. 1989). Another group also presented evidence of cocaine's teratogenicity (Bingol et al. 1987). They found that cocaine-abusing women had increased stillbirth rates, accounted for by abruptio placentae. Only infants born to cocaine-abusers had skull defects and congenital heart defects. Another group confirmed the finding of increased congenital cardiac anomalies in infants born to cocaine-abusing mothers (Little et al. 1989). These findings coincide with demonstrated teratogenicity associated with cocaine use in animal models (Fantel and Macphail 1982; Mahalik et al. 1980; Mitchell et al. 1988). One pathophysiologic mechanism for fetal anomalies may be a dose-dependent decrease in uterine blood flow, with accompanying fetal hypoxemia, tachycardia, and hypertension with cocaine use (Bingol et al. 1987).

Following delivery, infants born to mothers who have used cocaine in pregnancy may be at increased risk of sudden infant death syndrome (Bouchner et al. 1988). Newborns have been brought to emergency rooms with cocaine intoxication and seizures from breastfeeding while their mothers were using cocaine (Chaney et al. 1988; Chasnoff et al. 1987). Intoxication leading to overdose death has also been reported in infants who are several weeks old (Cravey 1988). Fatal and nonfatal child abuse has also been linked to cocaine use (Chasnoff 1989; Press 1988). In infants whose mothers had been actively using cocaine during pregnancy, a lack of ability to bond to parents has been strongly suggested (Rodning et al. 1988).

There is a variety of CNS toxicity associated with cocaine abuse. CVAs have been reported in temporal association with cocaine abuse by several groups (Brust and Richter 1977; Golbe and Merkin 1986; Lichtenfeld et al. 1984; Schwartz and Cohen 1984; Tuchman et al. 1987). Headaches occurring during cocaine abuse may be a premonitory symptom of an impending CVA (Cregler and Mark 1986b). Aneurysms or arteriovenous malformations may predispose cocaine abusers to have a CVA (Schwartz and Cohen 1984). Elevation of blood pressure in association with cocaine abuse is the most frequently proffered pathophysiologic explanation, although one group has postulated an immune mechanism, and another group has suggested cerebral vasoconstriction as an etiologic mechanism for cocaine-related CVAs (Brust and Richter 1977; Caplan et al. 1982; Lichtenfeld et al. 1984).

Seizures have also been reported in association with cocaine abuse and appear to originate in the limbic system (Jonsson et al. 1983; Myers and Earnest 1984; Siegel 1982b). They may result from kindling-reverse tolerance, secondary to associated hyperpyrexia, secondary to anoxia resulting from cardiac arrhythmia, or from lowering of the seizure threshold (Cohen 1984; Post et al. 1976; Roberts et al. 1984). Unlike amphetamines, which produce seizures only after repeated use, cocaine may precipitate a seizure with first use (Van Dyke and Byck 1982). These seizures are reported to be resistant to most anticonvulsants, but do respond to iv diazepam (Jonsson et al. 1983).

One group has reported two cases of fatal CNS fungal infection associated with iv cocaine abuse and one case with severe neurologic sequelae (Wetli et al. 1984). They suggested that immune function may have been altered in these cases, but do not offer substantiating evidence. Botulism has also been reported as a complication of cocaine abuse (Kudrow et al. 1988). Other infections have also been reported in association with cocaine abuse. Staphylococcal septicemia resulting in death has been reported in intranasal cocaine abusers (Alonso et al. 1986; Sharff 1984; Silverman and Smith 1986; Wetli et al. 1984). In one case, the person was a known nasopharyngeal carrier of staphylococcus. Brain abscesses have also been associated with cocaine use (Rao 1988). The acquired immune deficiency syndrome (AIDS) has been and is likely to continue to be a complication of iv cocaine abuse (Chaisson et al. 1989). Cocaine might, in fact, have effects on the immune system that compromise immune system function and increase susceptibility to human immunodeficiency virus (HIV) infection (Guynn et al. 1986).

Pulmonary function, specifically CO_2 diffusing capacity, has been shown to be decreased in free-base cocaine abusers (Itkonen et al. 1984; Weiss et al. 1981). The postulated mechanism is damage to alveolar surface secondary to pulmonary vasoconstriction associated with cocaine use. At follow-up, one group reported lack of normalization of gas exchange in some subjects. Pneumomediastinum and pneumopericardium have also been reported with cocaine freebasing (Adrouny and Magnusson 1985; Aroesty et al. 1986; Bush et al. 1984). Both disorders resolved spontaneously in the reported cases and are presumed to result from the positive pressure ventilation used to inhale the cocaine smoke, resulting in localized alveolar rupture. Pulmonary edema has also been reported in cocaine abusers who "speedball" heroin and cocaine (Cregler and Mark 1986a). Pulmonary hemorrhage has also been reported with cocaine use (Goodwin et al. 1989).

Intestinal infarct and ischemia have also been reported in association with cocaine abuse (Fishel et al. 1985; Nalbandian et al. 1985). These conditions are believed to result from increased intestinal vasoconstriction secondary to cocaine-induced catecholamine release. Cocaine is also a hepatotoxin in several animal models (Chardoukian and Shuster 1985; Gottfried et al. 1986). However, it is less clear that cocaine is a human hepatotoxin. A single case of renal infarction associated with cocaine abuse has also been reported (Scharff 1984).

Several ear, nose, and throat complications of cocaine abuse have also been reported. These include loss of smell, nasal mucosal erosion, and nasal septal perforation (Estroff and Gold 1985; Schweitzer 1986; Vilensky 1982). Central retinal artery occlusion has also been associated with cocaine use (Derenyi et al. 1988). We have commonly encountered bacterial rhinitis and various types of sinusitis in cocaine abusers.

The majority of cocaine abusers also have untreated dental problems. A majority have been reported to have one or more vitamin deficiencies on admission to treatment (Gold 1984). Finally, skin and muscle infarction have been reported in association with free-base cocaine use (Zamora-Quezada et al. 1988).

PSYCHIATRIC COMPLICATIONS

Cocaine abuse may present with major psychiatric illness or its abuse may result in syndromes mimicking psychiatric illness. While actively using, cocaine abusers may present for treatment of depression, sexual dysfunction, or eating disorders (Estroff and Gold 1984, 1985; Jonas and Gold 1986; Post 1975; Siegel 1982a; R Smith et al. 1984; Washton and Gold 1984; Washton et al. 1984b). The depression may include neurovegetative features, and the cocaine abuser may be

contemplating or have already attempted suicide. However, more recent studies suggest that cocaine abusers have an incidence of affective disorder similar to that found in the general population (Gawin
1988). Therefore, it is critical that psychiatric diagnoses not be made
before adequate abstinence from cocaine (Pollack et al. 1989). The
sexual dysfunction may include impotence, anorgasmia, and spontaneous ejaculation (Washton and Gold 1987). Cocaine abusers also
have elevated rates of anorexia and bulimia. Cocaine has also been
reported to precipitate manic episodes (Dackis et al. 1985–86). Increased cocaine craving has been reported as a consequence of winter
depression in individuals with seasonal affective disorder (Satel and
Gawin 1989b). The paranoia that heavy cocaine abusers experience
may lead to violence and subsequent arrest, or it may first be noted at
presentation for treatment (Gawin and Kleber 1986a; Lehrer and
Gold 1987). Psychosis and violent behavior are believed to be dispro-
portionately increased among crack-cocaine users (Honer et al. 1987).

Cocaine-induced panic disorder has been proposed as a psychiatric entity. A group of panic disorder patients has been described for
whom anxiety attacks did not begin until after cocaine use was established. It has been suggested that this group of patients can be distinguished by electroencephalographic abnormalities and that they may
not respond well to typical antidepressant treatment or alprazolam
(Xanax). However, clonazepam (Klonopin) or carbamazepine (Tegre-
tol) appeared promising as treatments (Abraham 1989; Louie et al.
1989).

ABSTINENCE

Several groups of researchers have presented phenomenological and
biological evidence for a cocaine withdrawal syndrome and have pro-
posed etiologic theories and treatments (Baxter 1983; Dackis and
Gold 1985b; Dackis et al. 1985-86; Extein et al. 1987b; Gawin and
Kleber 1984, 1986a; Post 1975; Rowbotham et al. 1984; Tennant and
Sagherian 1987).

The abstinence syndromes proposed have features of both agitated and retarded depression accompanied by intense cocaine craving (Dackis and Gold 1985a, 1985c; Gawin and Kleber 1986b;
Tennant and Sagherian 1987). Table 5-1 presents a comparison of the
various withdrawal syndromes proposed. Clinically, the abstinence
syndrome is important because the associated dysfunction, combined

with craving for cocaine, is instrumental in leading to relapse. Thus a vicious cycle of discontinuation of cocaine, leading to abstinence symptoms, leading to relapse occurs.

Dopamine depletion, with resultant postsynaptic receptor super-sensitivity, has been proposed as the basis for cocaine withdrawal symptoms (Dackis and Gold 1985a, 1985b, 1985c; Dackis et al. 1985-86; Extein et al. 1987b). The dopamine depletion hypothesis states that while cocaine acutely causes an increase in dopaminergic neurotransmission, chronically it causes depletion of dopamine. This depletion causes a functional inhibition of central dopamine circuits, which results in craving. Depletion occurs because cocaine blocks do-pamine reuptake and decreases presynaptic vesicular binding (Scheel-Kruger 1971; Taylor and Ho 1978). Therefore dopamine turnover outstrips the brain's ability to synthesize it (DiGuilio et al. 1978; Memo et al. 1981; Patrick and Barchas 1977; Taylor et al. 1979). There are a variety of data to support this hypothesis. Persistently elevated prolactin levels have been found in cocaine abusers and presumably result from decreased dopaminergic inhibition due to decreased available dopamine (Dackis et al. 1984a; Mendelson et al. 1988). In animals exposed to cocaine, an increase in postsynaptic do-pamine receptors occurs, reflecting denervation hypersensitivity (Gawin and Kleber 1986b; Memo et al. 1981; Taylor and Ho 1977, 1979). Further, in animals exposed to cocaine, brain dopamine levels are decreased (Taylor and Ho 1977). Evidence for a persistent de-crease in dopamine metabolites in abstinent cocaine abusers has been reported and further serves to confirm the dopamine depletion hy-pothesis (Small and Purcell 1985). A variety of antidepressants, tyro-sine, carbamazepine (Halikas et al. 1989), amantadine, and bromocriptine have been used to augment CNS catecholamine func-tion, decrease postsynaptic receptor sensitivity, and relieve abstinence symptoms (Dackis and Gold 1985a, 1985b; Extein et al. 1987a; Gawin 1988; Gawin and Kleber 1984, 1986b; Gawin et al. 1989; Gold et al. 1983; Rowbotham et al. 1984; Taylor and Ho 1978) (see Table 5-2). However, only bromocriptine, amantadine, and desipramine have withstood the test of double-blind trials with demonstrated effi-cacy as of this writing (Gawin 1988; Tennant and Sagherian 1987). However, amantadine's efficacy has not been replicated by one group (Gawin et al. 1989). Bromocriptine was first tried at 0.625 mg and was found to relieve cocaine craving with the first dose (Dackis and Gold 1985a). An open clinical trial has replicated this rapid onset of

Table 5-1. A comparison of proposed cocaine withdrawal syndromes

Baxter (1983)	Dackis and Gold (1985b) Dackis et al. (1985-86)	Gawin and Kleber (1986a)	Gold et al. (1983)	Horberg and Schnoll (1983)	Rowbotham et al. (1984)	Small and Purcell (1985)	Tennant and Sagherian (1987)
Depression, hypersomnolence, ↑dreaming	Depression, hypersomnia	*Phase I* (9 hours to 4 days) Agitation, depression, craving ↓	Depression, sleep disturbed, craving, anergia	Depression, sleep disturbed	Depression, sleep disturbed	Depression	Depression, sleep disturbed, craving, anergia, irritable
No time sequence proposed	Craving anergia, hyperphagia, irritability, ↓libido, ↓concentration, motor retardation, amotivation	fatigue, depression, no craving, insomnia ↓ exhaustion, hypersomnolence, hyperphagia, no craving ↓	Irritable Amotivated	Irritable Gastrointestinal upset, headache	Time course not specified	Fatigue ↓Concentration Anhedonia	↓Concentration Anxiety

Time: Lasts 3–5 days

Phase II (1–10 weeks)
Normal sleep, euthymic, low craving, low anxiety
Anhedonia, anergia, anxiety, craving
Euthymic, episodic craving, normal hedonic, response

Time course not specified

Begins 24–48 hours after last use and lasts 7–10 days

No time course given

Anorexia, diarrhea, confusion, diaphoresis, myalgia, nausea

Table 5-2. A comparison of treatments for cocaine abstinence symptoms

Researcher	Treatment	Dosage	Treatment timing	Symptoms relieved	Study method
Baxter (1983)	Desipramine	75–200 mg/day	Relief within 24 hours, duration not specified	Hypersomnolence, anergia, dysphoria	Open study
Dackis et al. (1985-86)	Bromocriptine	(a) 1.25 mg challenge (b) 0.625 mg po (c) up to 2.5 mg po tid	(b) Relief within hours (c) 10-day treatment protocol	Cocaine craving	(a) Open study (b) Single-blind (c) Double-blind (in progress)
Gawin (1988)	Desipramine	Unknown		Significantly better than placebo for maintaining abstinence	Double-blind
Gawin (1988)	Desipramine	200 mg/day	Relief from craving in 2–3 weeks	Cocaine craving	Open clinical trial
Gold et al. (1983)	Tyrosine	100 mg/kg/po tid	2nd–14th day of hospitalization	Depression, irritability: effect seen on days 2,3,4,5	Open clinical trial

Study	Medication	Dosage	Duration	Results	Design
Small and Purcell (1985)	Trazodone	100 mg/po qhs increased to 200 mg po qhs after 1 week	Remains on medication at 11 months after initiation	Depression, hypersomnia, agitation, craving	Open clinical trial in one patient
Tennant and Rawson (1982)	Desipramine			Relieved craving, depression, sleep disturbance	Open trial
Tennant and Tarver (1984)	Desipramine	100–150 mg/ po/qd	Up to 42 days	No significant differences versus placebo	Double-blind
Tennant and Sagherian (1987)	(a) Bromocriptine[a] (b) Amantadine	(a) 2.5 mg po bid–tid (b) 100 mg po bid–tid	10-day study	Craving, anergia	(a) Double-blind (b) Double-blind

[a]Two patients were withdrawn from study because of side effects: headache, vertigo, and syncope.

effective anticraving action of bromocriptine (Extein et al. 1987a). Our current protocol utilizes doses of up to 2.5 mg, as seen in Table 5-3 (Dackis and Gold 1985a).

TREATMENT ISSUES

At the outset, we would recommend that all identified cocaine abusers be evaluated and treated by specialists in addictive illness and that any proposed treatment must have complete and permanent abstinence as its expectation. We also note that there are few empirical data regarding the treatment of cocaine abuse. The one study located comparing inpatient, outpatient, or no treatment found outpatient treatment associated with the highest abstinence rates (Rawson et al. 1985). Another study suggests those with urines positive for cocaine at admission to outpatient treatment are less likely to remain abstinent and may imply the utility of inpatient treatment for this group of patients (Tennant et al. 1986). Several studies suggest that length of treatment is a key variable and that 6 months may be the minimal time of treatment for a reasonable chance of continued abstinence (American Psychiatric Association 1980; WJ Annitto, personal communication 1986; Washton 1987; Washton et al. 1985). Finally, several studies suggest that desipramine may facilitate long-term ab-

Table 5-3. Suggested treatment regimen of oral bromocriptine in acute cocaine withdrawal

Day	Bromocriptine dose (mg)	Frequency
1	0.625	tid
2	0.625	tid
3	0.625	qid
4	1.25	bid
5	1.25	tid
6	1.25	tid
7	1.25	tid
8	2.5	tid
9	2.5	tid
10	2.5	tid

Note. Bromocriptine appears to be effective in very small doses, perhaps due to dopamine receptor supersensitivity with cocaine exposure. Titration of the dose is necessary, weighing anticraving and anticrashing effects against possible side effects.

stinence in cocaine abusers (Gawin 1988; Gawin and Kleber 1984, 1986a). Despite the lack of empirical data, assessment and treatment methods for cocaine abuse will be offered.

Once cocaine abuse has been identified, the next decision is whether to treat on an inpatient or outpatient basis. We suggest that inpatient treatment be recommended for 1) those abusing cocaine uncontrollably by iv or free-base routes; 2) those with serious associated medical or psychiatric problems; 3) those who have failed previous outpatient treatment; 4) those with no existing abstinent support systems; and 5) those who require detoxification from and treatment for another drug or drugs (Gold and Washton 1985).

Whatever the setting, the initial phase of treatment must include assessment of Axis I, Axis II, and Axis III problems (Dackis et al. 1989). Final assessment of Axis I and Axis II problems must be deferred until 2–3 weeks after completion of detoxification (Pollack et al. 1989). During this time, organic illness secondary to drug abuse will be resolving (Washton et al. 1987). The thyrotropin-releasing hormone test is generally unreliable as a diagnostic tool for affective illness in cocaine abusers, and the dexamethasone suppression test is best used 3–4 weeks after completion of detoxification (Dackis et al. 1984b; Kosten 1986). Concurrent treatment of major affective, anxiety, psychotic, or personality disorders is necessary to facilitate treatment of the addiction.

One group of researchers reported that cocaine addicts do not differ significantly from opiate addicts (Craig 1988). Other groups reported that cocaine addicts are more likely to have narcissistic or borderline personality styles than either psychiatric controls or the general population (Dougherty and Lesswig 1989; Yates et al. 1989). Research to date suggests that depression, bipolar illness, attention-deficit disorder, and borderline and narcissistic personality disorders may be associated with cocaine abuse (Jonas and Gold 1986; D Smith et al. 1984; Washton and Gold 1984; Washton et al. 1985; Weiss and Mirin 1986; RD Weiss et al. 1985). Antidepressants, lithium, pemoline (Cylert), bromocriptine, and individual psychotherapy, respectively, have been reported to have efficacy in treating these psychiatric disorders in cocaine abusers (Dackis and Gold 1985c; Gawin and Kleber 1984, 1986b; Khantzian 1983; Resnick and Resnick 1985; Rowbotham et al. 1984; Spotts and Shantz 1984; Treece and Khantzian 1986; RD Weiss et al. 1985; Woody et al. 1983).

However, desipramine may also cause agitation rather than relief. For individuals who develop an agitated response to desipramine, switching to maprotiline (Brotman et al. 1988), doxepin, or trazodone (Louie et al. 1989) may be useful. It must also be emphasized that identification and treatment of Axis I and Axis II psychiatric disorders do not constitute treatment of the addiction but are necessary to permit treatment of the addiction.

Finally, it must be noted that, even with treatment, relapse rates run 50–80% at 1 year posttreatment (Gawin and Ellinwood 1989). Testing for and acceptance of HIV status has not been shown to impair treatment in one research report (Weddington and Brown 1988). This is an important issue, because as discussed earlier in this chapter, iv cocaine users are at increased risk for contracting HIV infection.

The initial goal in the treatment of cocaine abusers is complete abstinence from all mind- or mood-altering drugs (Dackis et al. 1989; Gawin 1988; Resnick and Resnick 1985; Wolpe and Lazarus 1966). Patients must be assisted in identifying the progression of their addiction and the accompanying negative impacts on their life and must understand their inability to control their drug usage. The inability to control one's addiction and life also requires that the abuser be assisted in recognizing the need to relinquish control of major life decisions to treatment providers to prevent decisions that will foster relapse. The patient must also learn to identify drug cravings and how to work them through. The patient must understand the conditioned nature of many urges. Urges are often tied to stimuli-arousing affects that are difficult to modulate, and the patient must therefore develop the ability to identify the stimuli more effectively and to modulate these affects. Abusers need to evaluate carefully all important people, places (e.g., home, work, and social settings), and things (e.g., television programs, movies, and music) for stimuli that foster urges and learn how to manage the urges or make appropriate life-style changes (Schulman 1989). Behavioral desensitization to cocaine as a means to decrease cocaine craving may also be beneficial (O'Brien et al. 1988). Regular but random drug screens should be a part of the treatment program (Wesson and Smith 1985). Treatment will ideally utilize individual and group therapy, Twelve-Step work, family therapy, drug education, assertiveness training, and relaxation training (Jarbe 1978; Marlatt and Gordon 1985; Wesson and Smith 1985; Wolpe and Lazarus 1966).

The Twelve-Step programs of Alcoholics Anonymous (AA), Narcotics Anonymous (NA), and Cocaine Anonymous (CA) can help the patient understand the nature of his or her illness and provide an abstinent support network. Like the addict, family members become increasingly affected by the addiction and can benefit from a recovering process for themselves whether or not they remain with the addicted person. Many abusers have difficulty with self-assertion, alternating between passivity and aggression. Assertiveness training can be a powerful tool for helping the addicted individual to neutralize drug urges by learning how to assert his or her needs properly. Relaxation therapy may help the recovering addict to neutralize distressing affects associated with urges. This first stage of treatment also depends on helping the patient establish external controls and should conclude with a treatment contract that delineates the consequences of a relapse.

Although antipsychotic medications, which are dopamine-blocking agents, theoretically might attentuate cocaine-induced euphoria, they have not been found to do so (Sharer et al. 1989). One interesting report details the use of phenelzine for the treatment of cocaine addicts who had failed previous treatments (Golwyn 1988). The phenelzine was used to deter cocaine use in a fashion analogous to disulfiram (Antabuse) for alcoholics.

The next phase of treatment, lasting 6–12 months, will focus further on preventing relapse and on developing a new and drug-free lifestyle. These goals may be met by a combination of individual and group therapies. In the second phase of treatment, relapse prevention focuses on issues of euphoric recall of cocaine "highs"; how to modulate and manage painful emotional states; the strength of conditioned stimuli; the role of narcissistic pathology in heightening denial; the risk associated with stress; and the risk in "taking back control" too soon (Wallace 1989). Relapse must be reframed as a very high risk situation that can be contained and in which learning can occur rather than as a sign of complete and irreversible failure (Washton 1988).

The recovering individual must be assisted to recall the numerous negative impacts on his life associated with cocaine abuse. The recovering person will require assistance in discerning warning signs of impending relapse so that relapse may be avoided. The patient must be assisted not to take back control of major life decisions prematurely as it is likely to be followed by placing oneself in situations that risk relapses. Patients must be educated about the sense of defeat and failure that accompanies relapse and learn how to seek help immediately if a relapse occurs. Finally, the individual requires assistance in developing a satisfying, drug-free life-style. Recovering addicts need to be able to resolve interpersonal problems, find recreation, develop friendships, and have fun without drugs (Marlatt and Gordon 1985). Developing a peer support network in AA, NA, and CA fellowships is crucial to the process. Urine screening remains helpful and necessary during this second phase.

REFERENCES

Abelson HI, Miller JD: A decade of trends in cocaine use in the household population. Natl Inst Drug Abuse Res Monogr Ser 61:35–49, 1985

Abraham HD: Stimulants, panic and beam EEG abnormalities (letter). Am J Psychiatry 146:947, 1989

Acker D, Sachs BP, Tracey KJ, et al: Abruptio placentae associated with cocaine use. Am J Obstet Gynecol 146:220–221, 1983

Adams EH, Durrell J: Cocaine: a growing public health problem. Natl Inst Drug Abuse Res Monogr Ser 50:9–14, 1984

Adrouny A, Magnusson P: Pneumopericardium from cocaine inhalation. N Engl J Med 313:49–50, 1985

Alfred RJ, Ewer S: Fatal pulmonary edema following intravenous freebase cocaine use. Ann Emerg Med 10:441–442, 1981

Alonso K, Solomons ET, Dawson JB: Bacteremic death: sequel of persistent rhinitis precipitated by intranasal cocaine abuse. South Med J 79:1049, 1986

Ambre J: The urinary excretion of cocaine and metabolites in humans: a kinetic analysis of published data. J Anal Toxicol 9:241–245, 1985

Ambre J, Fischman M, Ruo TI: Urinary excretion of ecgonine methyl ester, a major metabolite of cocaine in humans. J Anal Toxicol 8:23–25, 1984

American Psychiatric Association: Diagnostic and Statistical Manual of Mental Disorders, 3rd Edition. Washington, DC, American Psychiatric Association, 1980

Antelman SM, Kocan D, Rowland N, et al: Amitriptyline provides long-lasting immunization against sudden cardiac death from cocaine. Eur J Pharmacol 69:119–120, 1981

Anthony JC, Ritter CJ, Vonkorff MR, et al: Descriptive epidemiology of adult cocaine use in four US communities. Natl Inst Drug Abuse Res Monogr Ser 67:283–289, 1985

Aroesty DJ, Stanley RB, Crockett DM: Pneumomediastrium and cervical emphysema from the inhalation of 'freebase' cocaine. Otolaryngol Head Neck Surg 94:372–374, 1986

Barth CW, Bray M, Roberts WC: Rupture of the ascending aorta during cocaine intoxication. Am J Cardiol 57:496, 1986

Baxter LR: Desipramine in the treatment of hypersomnolence following abrupt cessation of cocaine use. Am J Psychiatry 140:1525–1526, 1983

Benchimol A, Bartall H, Desser KB: Accelerated ventricular rhythm and cocaine abuse. Ann Intern Med 88:519–520, 1978

Bingol N, Fuchs M, Diaz V, et al: Teratogenicity of cocaine in humans. J Pediatr 110:93–96, 1987

Bouchner H, Zuckerman B, McClain M, et al: Risk of sudden infant death syndrome among infants with in utero exposure to cocaine. J Pediatr 113:831–834, 1988

Bowen OR: U.S. Department of Health and Human Services press release, Washington, DC, January 13, 1988

Bozarth MA, Wise RA: Toxicity associated with long-term intravenous heroin and cocaine self-administration in the rat. JAMA 254:81–83, 1985

Brotman AW, Wilkie SM, Gelenberg AJ: An open trial of maprotiline for the treatment of cocaine abuse: a pilot study. J Clin Psychopharmacol 8:125–127, 1988

Brust JC, Richter RW: Stroke associated with cocaine abuse. NY State J Med 77:1473–1475, 1977

Bush MN, Rubenstein R, Hoffman I, et al: Spontaneous pneumomediastinum as a consequence of cocaine use. NY State J Med 84:618–619, 1984

Caplan LR, Hier DB, Bans G: Current concepts of cerebrovascular disease-stroke: stroke and drug abuse. Stroke 13:869–872, 1982

Catravas JD, Waters IW: Acute cocaine intoxication in the conscious day: studies on the mechanism of lethality. J Pharmacol Exp Ther 217:350–356, 1981

Chaisson RE, Bacchetti P, Osmond D, et al: Cocaine use and HIV infection in intravenous drug users in San Francisco. JAMA 261:561–565, 1989

Chaney NE, Franke J, Waddington WB: Cocaine convulsions in a breast-feeding baby. J Pediatr 112:134–135, 1988

Chardoukian JC, Shuster L: Electrochemistry of norcocaine introxide and related compounds: implications for cocaine hepatotoxicity. Biochem Biophys Res Commun 130:1044–1051, 1985

Chasnoff IJ: A nation's health in jeopardy (letter). West J Med 150:456–457, 1989

Chasnoff IJ, Burns WJ, Schnoll SH, et al: Cocaine use in pregnancy. N Engl J Med 313:666–669, 1985

Chasnoff IJ, Bussey ME, Savich R: Perinatal cerebral infarction and maternal cocaine use. J Pediatr 108:456–459, 1986

Chasnoff IJ, Lewis DE, Squires L: Cocaine intoxication in a breast-fed infant. Pediatrics 6:836–838, 1987

Chasnoff IJ, Griffith DR, MacGregor S, et al: Temporal patterns of cocaine use in pregnancy. JAMA 261:1741–1744, 1989

Childress AR, McClellan AT, O'Brien CP: Role of conditioning factors in the development of drug dependence. Psychiatr Clin North Am 9:413–426, 1986

Chow MJ, Ambre JJ, Ruo TI, et al: Kinetics of cocaine distribution, elimination, and chromotropic effects. Clin Pharmacol Ther 38:318–324, 1985

Clayton RR: Cocaine in the United States: in a blizzard or just being snowed? Natl Inst Drug Abuse Res Monogr Ser 61:8–35, 1985

Cohen S: Cocaine: acute medical and psychiatric complications. Psychiatric Annals 14:747–749, 1984

Coleman DL, Ross TF, Naughton JL: Myocardial ischemia and infarction related to recreational cocaine use. West J Med 136:444–446, 1987

Cone EJ, Weddington WW: Prolonged occurrence of cocaine in human saliva and urine after chronic use. J Anal Toxicol 13:65–68, 1989

Cone EJ, Kumor K, Thompson LK, et al: Correlation of saliva cocaine levels with plasma levels and with pharmacologic effects after intravenous cocaine administration in human subjects. J Anal Toxicol 12:200–206, 1988

Cone EJ, Menchen SL, Paul BD, et al: Validity testing of commercial urine metabolite assays, I: assay detection times, individual excretion patterns and kinetics after cocaine administration to humans. J Forensic Sci 34:15–31, 1989

Craig RJ: Psychological functioning of cocaine freebasers derived from objective psychological tests. J Clin Psychol 44:599–606, 1988

Cravey RH: Cocaine deaths in infants. J Anal Toxicol 12:354–355, 1988

Cregler LL, Mark H: Relation of acute myocardial infarction to cocaine abuse. Am J Cardiol 56:794, 1985

Cregler LL, Mark H: Cardiovascular dangers of cocaine abuse. Am J Cardiol 57:1185–1186, 1986a

Cregler LL, Mark H: Medical complications of cocaine abuse. N Engl J Med 315:1495–1499, 1986b

Dackis CA, Gold MS: Bromocriptine as a treatment of cocaine abuse. Lancet 1:1151–1152, 1985a

Dackis CA, Gold MS: New concepts in cocaine addiction: the dopamine depletion hypothesis. Neurosci Biobehav Rev 9:469–477, 1985b

Dackis CA, Gold MS: Pharmacological approaches to cocaine addiction. J Subst Abuse Treat 2:139–145, 1985c

Dackis CA, Gold MS, Estroff TW, et al: Hyperprolactinemia in cocaine abuse. Neuroscience 10:1099, 1984a

Dackis CA, Estroff TW, Pottash ALC, et al: Thyrotropin-releasing hormone testing of cocaine abusers. Paper presented at the annual meeting of the American Psychiatric Association, Los Angeles, CA, May 1984b

Dackis CA, Gold MS, Davies RK, et al: Bromocriptine treatment for cocaine abuse: the dopamine depletion hypothesis. Int J Psychiatry Med 15:125–135, 1985-86

Dackis CA, Gold MS, Estroff TW: Inpatient treatment of addiction, in Treatment of Psychiatric Disorders, Vol. 2. Edited by Karasu TB. Washington, DC, American Psychiatric Press, 1989, pp 1359–1379

Derenyi P, Schneiderman JF, Derenyi RG, et al: Cocaine-induced central retinal artery occlusion. Can Med Assoc J 138:129–130, 1988

DeWit H, Wise RA: A blockade of cocaine reinforcement in rats with the dopamine receptor blockade pimozide but not with the noradrenergic blockers phentolamine or phenoxybenzamine. Can J Psychol 31:195–203, 1977

DiGuilio AM, Groppetti A, Cattabeni F, et al: Significance of dopamine metabolites in the evaluation of drugs acting on dopaminergic neurons. Eur J Pharmacol 52:201–207, 1978

DiMaio VJ, Garriott JC: Four deaths due to intravenous injection of cocaine. Forensic Sci Int 12:119–125, 1978

Dougherty RJ, Lesswig NJ: Inpatient cocaine abusers: an analysis of psychological and demographic variables. J Subst Abuse Treat 6:45–47, 1989

Dworkin SI, Smith JG: Neurobehavioral pharmacology of cocaine. Natl Inst Drug Abuse Res Monogr Ser 88:185–197, 1988

Estroff TW, Gold MS: Psychiatric misdiagnosis, in Advances in Psychopharmacology: Predicting and Improving Treatment Response. Edited by Gold MS, Lydiard RB, Carman JS. Boca Raton, FL, CRC Press, 1984, pp 34–66

Estroff TW, Gold MS: Medical and psychiatric complications of cocaine abuse with possible points of pharmacological treatment. Adv Alcohol Subst Abuse 5:61–76, 1985

Extein IL, Gold MS, Gross DA: Dopamine agonists in treating stimulant abuse. Paper presented at the annual meeting of the American Psychiatric Association, Chicago, IL, May 1987a

Extein IL, Potter WZ, Gold MS, et al: Persistent neurochemical deficit in cocaine abuse. Paper presented at the annual meeting of the American Psychiatric Association, Chicago, IL, May 1987b

Fantel AG, Macphail BJ: The teratogenicity of cocaine. Teratology 26:17–19, 1982

Finkle BS, McCloskey KL: The forensic toxicology of cocaine. Natl Inst Drug Abuse Res Monogr Ser 13:153–193, 1977

Fischman MW: The behavioral pharmacology of cocaine in humans. Natl Inst Drug Abuse Res Monogr Ser 50:72–91, 1984

Fishel R, Hamamoto G, Barbul A, et al: Cocaine colitis. Dis Colon Rectum 28:264–266, 1985

Gawin FH: Chronic neuropharmacology of cocaine: progress in pharmacotherapy. J Clin Psychiatry 49:511–516, 1988

Gawin F, Ellinwood E: Cocaine and other stimulants: action, abuse and treatment. N Engl J Med 318:1173–1182, 1989

Gawin FH, Kleber HD: Abstinence symptomatology and psychiatric diagnosis in cocaine abusers. Arch Gen Psychiatry 43:107–113, 1986a

Gawin F, Kleber H: Pharmacologic treatments of cocaine abuse. Psychiatr Clin North Am 9:573–583, 1986b

Gawin FH, Morgan C, Kosten TR: Double-blind evaluation of the effect of acute amantadine on cocaine craving. Psychopharmacology 97:402–403, 1989

Gay GR: Clinical management of acute and chronic cocaine poisoning. Ann Emerg Med 11:562–572, 1982

Goeders NE: Intracranial cocaine self-administration. Natl Inst Drug Abuse Res Monogr Ser 88:199–215, 1988

Golbe LI, Merkin MD: Cerebral infarction in a user of freebase cocaine ("crack"). Neurology 36:1602–1604, 1986

Gold MS: 800-COCAINE. New York, Bantam Books, 1984

Gold MS: The Facts About Drugs and Alcohol. New York, Bantam Books, 1986

Gold MS, Washton AM: Cocaine abuse: neurochemistry, phenomenology, and treatment. Natl Inst Drug Abuse Res Monogr Ser 61:130–150, 1985

Gold MS, Pottash ALC, Annitto WJ, et al: Cocaine withdrawal: efficacy of tyrosine. Neuroscience 9:157, 1983

Gold MS, Byron JP, Dackis CA, et al: Paraphernalia-induced cocaine craving. Neuroscience 12:936, 1986

Goldwyn DH: Cocaine abuse treated with phenelzine. Int J Addict 23:897–905, 1988

Goodwin JE, Harley RA, Miller KS: Cocaine pulmonary hemorrhage and hemoptysis. Ann Intern Med 110:843, 1989

Gottfried MR, Kloss MW, Graham D, et al: Ultrastructure of experimental cocaine hepatotoxicity. Hepatology 6:299–304, 1986

Grabowski J, Dworkin SI: Cocaine: an overview of current issues. Int J Addict 20:1065–1088, 1985

Guynn RW, Biehl K, Merrill DK, et al: Urinary neoplerin in cocaine-abusing individuals, in Chemistry and Biology of Pteridines. Edited by Cooper BA, Whitehead VM. Berlin, Walter de Gruyter, 1986, pp 257–262

Halikas J, Kemp K, Kuhn K: Carbamazepine for cocaine addiction. Lancet 1:623–624, 1989

Hansen JH, Caudill SP, Boone DJ: Crisis in drug testing: results of CDC blind study. JAMA 25:2382–2387, 1985

Hawks RL, Kopin IJ, Colburn RW, et al: Norcocaine: a pharmacologically active metabolite of cocaine found in brain. Life Sci 15:2189–2195, 1975

Honer WG, Gewirtz G, Turey M: Psychosis and violence in cocaine smokers. Lancet 2:451, 1987

Horberg LK, Schnoll SH: Treatment of cocaine abuse. Current Psychiatric Therapeutics 22:177–187, 1983

Howard RE, Hueter DC, Davis GJ: Acute myocardial infarction following cocaine abuse in a young woman with normal coronary arteries. JAMA 254:95–96, 1985

Isner M, Estes NA, Thompson PD, et al: Acute cardiac events temporally related to cocaine abuse. N Engl J Med 315:1438–1443, 1986

Itkonen J, Schnoll S, Glassroth J: Pulmonary dysfunction in "freebase" cocaine users. Arch Intern Med 144:2195–2197, 1984

Jarbe TUC: Cocaine as a discriminative cue in rats: interactions with neuroleptics and other drugs. Psychopharmacology 59:183–187, 1978

Jatlow PI, Van Dyke C, Barash P, et al: Measurement of benzoylecgonine and cocaine in urine, separation of various cocaine metabolites during reversed phase high performance liquid chromatography. J Chromatogr 152:115–121, 1978

Jatlow P, Barash PG, Van Dyke C, et al: Cocaine and succinylcholine sensitivity: a new caution. Anesth Analg 58:235–238, 1979

Javaid JE, Fischman MW, Schuster CR, et al: Cocaine plasma concentration: relation to physiological and subjective effects in humans. Science 202:227–228, 1978

Javaid JI, Musa MN, Fischman MW, et al: Kinetics of cocaine in humans after intravenous and intranasal administration. Biopharm Drug Dispos 4:9–18, 1983

Johns ME, Berman AR, Price JC, et al: Metabolism of intranasally applied cocaine. Annals of Otology 86:342–347, 1977

Jonas JM, Gold MS: Cocaine abuse and eating disorders. Lancet 1:390–391, 1986

Jones RT: The pharmacology of cocaine. Natl Inst Drug Abuse Res Monogr Ser 50:34–52, 1984

Jonsson S, O'Meara M, Young JB: Acute cocaine poisoning: importance of treating seizures and acidosis. Am J Med 75:1061–1064, 1983

Kandel DB, Murphy D, Kraus D: Cocaine use in young adulthood: patterns of use and psychosocial correlates. Natl Inst Drug Abuse Res Monogr Ser 61:76–110, 1985

Khantzian EJ: An extreme case of cocaine dependence and marked improvement with methylphenidate treatment. Am J Psychiatry 140:784–785, 1983

Khantzian EJ, Khantzian NJ: Cocaine addiction: is there a psychological predisposition? Psychiatric Annals 14:753–759, 1984

Kogan MJ, Verebey K, DePace AC, et al: Quantitative determination of benzoylecgonine and cocaine in human biofluids by gas liquid chromatography. Anal Chem 49:1965–1969, 1977

Koob GF, Hubner CB: Reinforcement pathways for cocaine. Natl Inst Drug Abuse Res Monogr Ser 88:137–159, 1988

Kossowsky WA, Lyon AF: Cocaine and acute myocardial infarction: a probable connection. Chest 86:729–731, 1984

Kosten TR: Diagnosing depression with the DST and TRH in cocaine and opioid abusers. J Subst Abuse Treat 3:47–49, 1986

Kosten TR, Kleber HD: Rapid death during cocaine abuse: a variant of the neuroleptic malignant syndrome. Am J Drug Alcohol Abuse 14:335–346, 1988

Kosten TR, Gawin FH, Rounsaville BJ, et al: Abuse of cocaine with opioids: psychological aspects of treatment. Natl Inst Drug Abuse Res Monogr Ser 67:278–282, 1985

Kudrow DB, Henry DA, Haake DA, et al: Botulism associated with clostordium botulinum sinusitis after intranasal cocaine abuse. Ann Intern Med 109:984–985, 1988

Lange RA, Cigarroa RG, Yancy CW, et al: Cocaine-induced coronary-artery vasoconstriction. N Engl J Med 321:1557–1562, 1989

Lehrer M, Gold MS: Laboratory diagnosis of cocaine: intoxication and withdrawal. Adv Alcohol Subst Abuse 6:123–141, 1987

Lichtenfeld PJ, Rubin DB, Feldman RS: Subarachnoid hemorrhage precipitated by cocaine snorting. Arch Neurol 41:223–224, 1984

Lisse JR, Davis CP: Deep venous thrombosis of the upper extremity associated with IV cocaine use. Ann Intern Med 110:571, 1989

Little BB, Snell LM, Klein VM, et al: Cocaine abuse during pregnancy: maternal and fatal outcomes. Obstet Gynecol 73:157–160, 1989

Louie AK, Lannon RA, Ketter TA: Treatment of cocaine-induced panic disorder. Am J Psychiatry 146:40–44, 1989

Lowry WT, Lomonte JN, Hatchette D, et al: Identification of two novel cocaine metabolites in bile by gas chromatography and gas chromatography/mass spectrometry in a case of acute intravenous cocaine overdose. J Anal Toxicol 3:91–95, 1979

Macdonald DI: High school senior drug use declines. JAMA 257:2699, 1987

Mahalik MP, Gantiere RF, Mann DE: Teratogenetic potential of cocaine hydrochloride in CF-1 mice. J Pharm Sci 69:703–706, 1980

Marlatt GA, Gordon JR: Relapse Prevention. New York, Guilford, 1985

Mayersohn M, Perrier D: Kinetics of pharmacologic response to cocaine. Res Commun Chem Pathol Pharmacol 22:465–474, 1978

Memo M, Pradhan S, Hanbauer I: Cocaine-induced supersensitivity of striatal dopamine receptors: role of endogenous calmodulin. Neuropharmacology 20:1145–1150, 1981

Mendelson JH, Teoh SK, Lange U, et al: Hyperprolactinemia during cocaine withdrawal. Natl Inst Drug Abuse Res Monogr Ser 81:67–73, 1988

Misra AL, Nayark PK, Block R, et al: Estimation and disposition of [3H] benzoylecgonine and pharmacological activity of some cocaine metabolites. Journal of Brain Pharmacology 27:784–786, 1975

Mitchell M, Sabbagha R, Keith L, et al: Ultrasonic growth parameters in fetuses of mothers with primary addiction to cocaine. Am J Obstet Gynecol 159:1104–1109, 1988

Mittleman RE, Wetli CV: Death caused by recreational cocaine use. JAMA 252:1889–1893, 1984

Mule SJ, Jukofsky D, Kogan M, et al: Evaluation of the radioimmunoassay for benzoylecgonine in human serum. Clin Chem 23:796–801, 1977

Myers JA, Earnest MP: Generalized seizures and cocaine abuse. Neurology 34:675–676, 1984

Nahas G, Trouve R, Demus JF: A calcium channel blocker as antidote to the cardiac effects of cocaine intoxication. N Engl J Med 313:519–520, 1985

Nalbandian H, Sheth N, Dietrich R, et al: Intestinal ischemia caused by cocaine ingestion. Surgery 97:374–376, 1985

Nanji A, Filipenko JD: Asystole and ventricular fibrillation associated with cocaine intoxication. Chest 85:132–133, 1985

National Institute on Drug Abuse: National Household Survey on Drug Abuse: Main Findings. Rockville, MD, National Institute on Drug Abuse, 1985

Nurco DN, Asin IH, Ball JC: Use of nonnarcotic drugs by narcotic addicts. Natl Inst Drug Abuse Res Monogr Ser 67:295–299, 1985

O'Brien CP, Childress AR, Arndt IO, et al: Pharmacological and behavioral treatments of cocaine dependence: controlled studies. J Clin Psychiatry 49(suppl):17–22, 1988

O'Malley PM, Johnston LD, Bachman JG: Cocaine use among American adolescents and young adults. Natl Inst Drug Abuse Res Monogr Ser 61:50–75, 1985

Paly D, Jatlow P, Van Dyke C, et al: Plasma levels of cocaine in native Peruvian coca chewers, in Cocaine, 1980s. Edited by Jeri FR. Lima, Pacific Press, 1980, pp 86–89

Pasternack PF, Colvin SB, Baumann FG: Cocaine-induced angina pectoris and myocardial infarction in patients younger than 40 years. Am J Cardiol 55:847, 1985

Patrick RL, Barchas JD: Potentiation by cocaine of the stimulus-induced increase in dopamine synthesis in rat brain striatal synaptosomes. Neuropharmacology 16:327, 1977

Pollack MH, Brotman AW, Rosenbaum JF: Cocaine abuse and treatment. Compr Psychiatry 30:31–44, 1989

Pope HG, Ionescu-Pioggia M, Cole JO: Drug use and life-style among college undergraduates: nine years later. Arch Gen Psychiatry 38:588–591, 1981

Porrino LJ, Kornetsky C: The effects of cocaine on local cerebral metabolic activity. Natl Inst Drug Abuse Res Monogr Ser 88:92–106, 1988

Post RM: Cocaine psychoses: a continuum model. Am J Psychiatry 132:225–231, 1975

Post RM, Weiss SB: Psychomotor stimulant vs local anesthetic effects of cocaine: role of behavioral sensitization and kindling. Natl Inst Drug Abuse Res Monogr Ser 88:217–238, 1988

Post RM, Kopanda RT, Black KE: Progressive effects of cocaine on behavior and central amine metabolism in rhesus monkeys: relationship to kindling and psychosis. Biol Psychiatry 11:403–419, 1976

Press S: Crack and fatal child abuse. JAMA 260:3132, 1988

Ramoska E, Sacchetti AD: Propranolol-induced hypertension in treatment of cocaine intoxication. Ann Emerg Med 14:1112–1113, 1985

Rao AN: Brain abscess: a complication of cocaine inhalation. NY State J Med 89:548–550, 1988

Rappolt RT, Gay GR, Inaba DS: Propranolol: a specific antagonist to cocaine. Clin Toxicol 10:265–271, 1977

Rawson RA, Obert JL, McCann MD: Cocaine treatment outcome: cocaine use following inpatient, outpatient and no treatment. Natl Inst Drug Abuse Res Monogr Ser 67:271–277, 1985

Resnick RB, Resnick E: Psychological issues in the treatment of cocaine abuse. Natl Inst Drug Abuse Res Monogr Ser 67:290–294, 1985

Resnick RB, Kestenbaum RS, Schwartz LK: Acute systemic effects of cocaine in man: a controlled study by intranasal and intravenous routes. Science 195:696–699, 1977

Ritz MC, Lamb RJ, Goldberg SR, et al: Cocaine receptors on dopamine transporters are related to self-administration of cocaine. Science 237:1219–1223, 1987

Roberts JR, Quattrocchi E, Howland MA: Severe hyperthermia secondary to intravenous drug abuse. Am J Emerg Med 2:373, 1984

Rodning C, Beckwith L, Howard J: Presentation at New York Academy of Sciences Conference on Prenatal Abuse of Licit and Illicit Drugs. Bethesda, MD, September 7–9, 1988

Roehrich H, Gold MS: 800-COCAINE: origin, significance and findings. Yale J Biol Med 61:149–155, 1988

Rowbotham MC, Jones RT, Benowitz NL: Trazodone-oral cocaine interactions. Arch Gen Psychiatry 41:895–899, 1984

Satel S, Gawin F: Migraine-like headaches and cocaine use. JAMA 261:2995–2996, 1989a

Satel SL, Gawin FH: Seasonal cocaine abuse. Am J Psychiatry 146:534–535, 1989b

Schachne JS, Roberts BH, Thompson PD: Coronary-artery spasm and myocardial infarction associated with cocaine abuse. N Engl J Med 310:1665–1666, 1984

Scheel-Kruger J: Comparative studies of various amphetamine analogues demonstrating different interactions with the metabolism of catecholamine in the brain. Eur J Pharmacol 14:45–59, 1971

Schulman GD: Experience with the cocaine trigger inventory. Adv Alcohol Subst Abuse 8:71–85, 1989

Schwartz KA, Cohen JA: Subarachnoid hemorrhage precipitated by cocaine snorting. Arch Neurol 41:705, 1984

Schweitzer VG: Osteolytic sinusitis and pneumomediastinum: deceptive otolaryngologic complications of cocaine abuse. Laryngoscope 96:206–210, 1986

Sharer MA, Kumor K, Jaffe JH: Effects of intravenous cocaine are partially attenuated by haloperidol. Psychiatry Res 27:117–125, 1989

Sharff JA: Renal infarction associated with intravenous cocaine use. Ann Emerg Med 13:1145–1147, 1984

Siegel R: Cocaine and sexual dysfunction: the curse of mama coca. J Psychoactive Drugs 14:71–74, 1982a

Siegel RK: Cocaine smoking. J Psychoactive Drugs 14:271–359, 1982b

Siegel RK: Changing patterns of cocaine use: longitudinal observations, consequences, and treatment. Natl Inst Drug Abuse Res Monogr Ser 50:92–110, 1984

Siegel R: Treatment of acute cocaine intoxication. J Psychoactive Drugs 17:1–9, 1985

Silverman HS, Smith AL: Staphylococcal sepsis precipitated by cocaine sniffing. N Engl J Med 314:1706, 1986

Simpson RW, Edwards WD: Pathogenesis of cocaine-induced ischemic heart disease. Arch Pathol Lab Med 110:479–484, 1986

Small GW, Purcell JJ: Trazodone and cocaine abuse. Arch Gen Psychiatry 42:524, 1985

Smith DE: Cocaine-alcohol abuse: epidemiological, diagnostic, and treatment considerations. J Psychoactive Drugs 18:117–129, 1986

Smith DE, Wesson DR, Apter-Marsh M: Cocaine and alcohol induced sexual dysfunction in patients with addictive diseases. J Psychoactive Drugs 18:359–361, 1984

Smith DE, Schwartz RH, Martin DM: Heavy cocaine use by adolescents. Pediatrics 83:539–542, 1989

Smith RM, Poquette MA, Smith PJ: Hydroxy methoxy benzoyl-methylecgonines: new metabolites of cocaine from human urine. J Anal Toxicol 8:29–34, 1984

Spealman RD, Goldberg SR, Kelleher RT: Effects of norcocaine and some norcocaine derivatives on schedule-controlled behavior of pigeons and squirrel monkeys. J Pharmacol Exp Ther 210:196–205, 1979

Spotts JV, Shantz FC: Drug-induced ego states, I: cocaine: phenomenology and implications. Int J Addict 19:119–151, 1984

Stewart DJ, Inaba T, Tang BK, et al: Hydrolysis of cocaine in human plasma by cholinesterase. Life Sci 20:1557–1564, 1977

Stewart DJ, Inaba T, Lucassen M, et al: Cocaine metabolism: cocaine and norcocaine hydrolysin by liver and serum esterases. Clin Pharmacol 25:464–468, 1979

Strug DL, Hunt DE, Lipton DS, et al: Patterns of cocaine use among methadone clients. Int J. Addict 20:1163–1175, 1985

Taylor D, Ho BT: Neurochemical effects of cocaine following acute and repeated injection. J Neurosci Res 3:95–101, 1977

Taylor D, Ho BT: Comparison of inhibition of monoamine uptake by cocaine, methylphenidate, and amphetamines. Res Commun Chem Pathol Pharmacol 21:67–75, 1978

Taylor D, Ho BT, Fagen JD: Increased dopamine receptor binding in rat brain by repeated cocaine injections. Community Psychopharmacology 3:137–142, 1979

Tennant FS, Rawson RA: Cocaine and amphetamine dependence treated with desipramine. Natl Inst Drug Abuse Res Monogr Ser 43: 351–355, 1982

Tennant FS, Sagherian AA: Double-blind comparison of amantadine and bromocriptine for ambulatory withdrawal from cocaine dependence. Arch Intern Med 147:109–112, 1987

Tennant FS, Tarver AL: Double-blind comparison of desipramine and placebo in withdrawal from cocaine dependence. Natl Inst Drug Abuse Res Monogr Ser 55:159–163, 1984

Tennant FS, Tarver A, Seecof R: Cocaine plasma concentrations in persons admitted to outpatient treatment: relationship to treatment outcome. J Subst Abuse Treat 3:27–32, 1986

Tindal S, Lutz T, Vestergaard P: Mass spectrometric determination of cocaine and its biologically active metabolite, norcocaine, in human urine. Biomedical Mass Spectrometry 5:658–663, 1978

Treece C, Khantzian EJ: Psychodynamic factors in the development of drug dependence. Psychiatr Clin North Am 9:399–412, 1986

Tuchman AJ, Daras M, Zalzal P: Intracranial hemorrhage after cocaine abuse. JAMA 257:1175, 1987

Valanzi NN, Baden MM, Valanzi SN, et al: Detection of biotransformed cocaine in urine from drug abusers. J Chromatogr 81:1701–1773, 1973

Van Dyke C, Byck R: Cocaine. Sci Am 246:128–141, 1982

Van Dyke C, Barash PG, Jatlow P, et al: Cocaine: plasma concentrations after intranasal applications in man. Science 191:859–861, 1976

Van Dyke C, Byck R, Barash P, et al: Urinary excretion of immunologically reactive metabolites after intranasal administration of cocaine followed by enzyme immunoassay. Clin Chem 23:241–244, 1977

Van Dyke C, Jatlow P, Ungerer J, et al: Oral cocaine: plasma concentrations and central effects. Science 200:211–213, 1978

Vilensky W: Illicit and licit drugs causing perforation of the nasal septum. J Forensic Sci 27:958–962, 1982

Virmani R, Robinowitz M, Smialek JE, et al: Cardiovascular effects of cocaine: an autopsy study of 40 patients. Am Heart J 115:1068–1076, 1988

Wallace BC: Psychological and environmental determinants of relapse in crack cocaine smokers. J Subst Abuse Treat 6:95–106, 1989

Walters PA, Goethals GW, Pope HG: Drug use and life-style among 500 college undergraduates. Arch Gen Psychiatry 26:92–96, 1972

Washton AM: Nonpharmacologic treatment of cocaine abuse. Psychiatr Clin North Am 9:563–571, 1987

Washton AM: Preventing relapse to cocaine. J Clin Psychiatry 49:34–38, 1988

Washton AM, Gold MS: Chronic cocaine abuse: evidence for adverse effects on health and functioning. Psychiatric Annals 14:733–743, 1984

Washton AM, Gold MS: Recent trends in cocaine abuse: a view from the national hotline, 800-COCAINE. Adv Alcohol Subst Abuse 6:31–47, 1987

Washton AM, Gold MS, Pottash AC, et al: Adolescent cocaine abusers. Lancet 2:746, 1984a

Washton AM, Gold MS, Pottash AC: Upper-income cocaine abusers. Adv Alcohol Subst Abuse 4:51–57, 1984b

Washton AM, Gold MS, Pottash AC: Treatment outcome in cocaine abusers. Natl Inst Drug Abuse Res Monogr Ser 67:381–384, 1985

Washton AM, Gold MS, Pottash ALC: Cocaine abuse: techniques of assessment, diagnosis and treatment. Psychiatr Med 3:185–195, 1987

Weddington W, Brown BS: Acceptance of HIV antibody testing by persons seeking outpatient treatment for cocaine abuse. J Subst Abuse Treat 5:131–137, 1988

Weiss RD: Recurrent myocardial infarction caused by cocaine abuse. Am Heart J 111:793, 1986

Weiss RD, Gawin FH: Protracted elimination of cocaine metabolites in long-term, high dose cocaine abusers. Am J Med 85:879–880, 1988

Weiss RD, Mirin SM: Subtypes of cocaine abusers. Psychiatr Clin North Am 9:491–503, 1986

Weiss RD, Goldenheim PD, Mirin SM, et al: Pulmonary dysfunction in cocaine smokers. Am J Psychiatry 138:1110–1112, 1981

Weiss RD, Pope HG, Mirin SM: Treatment of chronic cocaine abuse and attention-deficit disorder, residual type, with magnesium pemoline. Drug Alcohol Depend 15:69–72, 1985

Wesson DR, Smith DE: Cocaine: treatment perspectives. Natl Inst Drug Abuse Res Monogr Ser 61:193–203, 1985

Wetli CV, Fishbain DA: Cocaine-induced psychosis and sudden death in recreational cocaine users. J Forensic Sci 30:873–880, 1985

Wetli CV, Weiss SD, Cleary TJ, et al: Fungal cerebritis from intravenous drug abuse. J Forensic Sci 29:260–268, 1984

Wiener RS, Lockhart JT, Schwartz RG: Dilated cardiomyopathy and cocaine abuse. Am J Med 81:699–701, 1986

Wilkinson P, Van Dyke C, Jatlow P, et al: Intranasal and oral cocaine kinetics. Clin Pharmacol Ther 27:386–393, 1980

Witkin JM, Goldberg SR, Katz JL: Lethal effects of cocaine are reduced by the dopamine-1 receptor antagonist but not by haloperidol. Life Sci 44:1285–1291, 1989

Wolpe J, Lazarus AA: Behavior Therapy Techniques. London, Pergamon, 1966

Woody GE, Luborsky L, McClellan AT: Psychotherapy for opiate addicts. Arch Gen Psychiatry 40:639–645, 1983

Wurmser L: Psychoanalytic consideration of the etiology of compulsive drug usc. J Am Psychoanal Assoc 22:820–843, 1974

Yates WY, Fulton AI, Gabel JE, et al: Personality risk factors for cocaine abuse. Am J Public Health 79:891–892, 1989

Zahler R, Wachtel P, Jatlow P, et al: Kinetics of drug effect by distributed lay analysis: an application to cocaine. Clin Pharmacol Ther 31:775–782, 1982

Zamora-Quezada JC, Diverman H, Stadecker MJ, et al: Muscle and skin infarction after freebasing cocaine. Ann Intern Med 108:564–566, 1988

Zuckerman B, Frank DA, Hingson R, et al: Effects of maternal marijuana and cocaine use on fetal growth. N Engl J Med 320:762–768, 1989

Chapter 6

Stimulants

Donald C. Goff, M.D.
Domenic A. Ciraulo, M.D.

The study of stimulant abuse is complicated by the existence of many different patterns of stimulant use, as well as the availability of a wide variety of centrally active stimulants. In this chapter, we will focus on the amphetamines, since they are the most commonly abused of the major stimulants and the best studied. Cocaine will not be discussed in this chapter, but is specifically covered by Roehrich and Gold (Chapter 5, this volume).

Stimulants are valuable therapeutic agents, prescribed for a number of medical indications, including narcolepsy and attention deficit disorder (see Tables 6-1 and 6-2). Stimulants are also commonly used to enhance performance by combating fatigue or by improving concentration, although, with the exception of caffeine, such use is not advised. A wide variety of stimulants are used as appetite suppressants for weight control, some with considerable abuse potential and others with minimal risk. Some users take stimulants episodically to elevate their mood and for increased energy. When this form of use becomes chronic, it can lead to escalating doses and a withdrawal syndrome consisting of sleep and mood disturbances when the drug is stopped. Intravenous use is practiced by the "speed freaks" and is characterized by runs during which extremely high cumulative

Table 6-1. Major stimulants: trade and street names

Chemical name	Trade names	Street names	Schedule
D, L-amphetamine	Benzedrine[a]	Bennies, beans, whites	II
D, L-amphetamine plus dextroam- phetamine	Biphetamine Obetrol Delcobese	Black beauties	II
Dextroamphetamine	Dexedrine Dexampex Ferndex Oxydess	Dexies, brownies	II
Methamphetamine	Desoxyn Methedrine Methampex	Meth, speed, crystal	II
Dextroamphetamine plus amobarbital	Dexamyl[a]	Greenies	II
Dextroamphetamine plus prochlorper- azine	Eskatrol[a]		II
Methylphenidate	Ritalin		II
Phenmetrazine	Preludin		II
Pemoline	Cylert		IV

[a]No longer commercially available.

Table 6-2. Major stimulants: half-life and dose range

Chemical name	Half-life (hours)	Therapeutic dose range (mg/day)
Amphetamine	10–30	10–40
Dextroamphetamine	10–30	10–40
Methamphetamine	10–30	10–40
Methylphenidate	4–5	10–40
Phenmetrazine	10–20	37.5–75
Pemoline	10–15	56.25–112.5

levels of stimulant are attained, often leading to exhaustion and psychosis. Finally, a smokable form of methamphetamine, known as "ice," has appeared in some areas and threatens to supplant cocaine as a major drug of abuse.

HISTORY

The synthetic stimulants have a long history of controversy, during which they have posed considerable problems for many societies (Iversen et al. 1978). Amphetamine, the prototypic major stimulant, was first synthesized in Germany in 1887 (Edeleano 1887), but its effects on humans were not discovered until Alles (1928) experimented with it 30 years later as a possible substitute for ephedrine in treating asthma. Methamphetamine was synthesized in Japan in 1888 and introduced to Western medicine in 1929 (Ellinwood 1979). Amphetamine became available to the American public in 1932 in the form of the Benzedrine inhaler, which contained a wick of paper saturated with 250 mg of amphetamine. Four years later Benzedrine tablets were marketed and, like the Benzedrine inhaler, were available without a prescription.

Initially, narcolepsy was the only identified disorder responsive to amphetamine. However, clinicians soon tried it in a wide range of conditions, and many enthusiastic claims of efficacy soon followed (Reifenstein and Davidoff 1939). A review by Bett in 1946 cited 158 references describing amphetamine use in 39 disorders, including depression, migraine, hypotension, seasickness, nasal congestion, nausea of pregnancy, and Parkinson's disease. In addition, amphetamine was widely recognized and prescribed as an "energizer" and mood elevator in people without defined psychiatric illness. The psychological effects of amphetamine were studied at the University of Minnesota in 1937, and accounts of amphetamine's ability to alleviate fatigue and of its euphoriant effect spread to other college campuses, where amphetamine became popular as a study aid and as a recreational drug (Iversen et al. 1978). It was not until 1939 that amphetamine became a prescription drug; the inhaler remained available over the counter despite widespread abuse until 1959 (Morgan 1981).

Additional experience with amphetamine's effects was accumulated as a result of heavy use during World War II (Iversen et al. 1978). Approximately two million amphetamine tablets were dispensed to British and American troops to counteract battle fatigue. In Japan, methamphetamine was also given to civilians working in defense-related industries to increase productivity. After the war, large wartime stocks of amphetamines, including intravenous methamphetamine, were dumped on the open market in Japan and advertised to the demoralized population as a drug to restore low spirits (Masaki 1956). An epidemic of amphetamine addiction subsequently developed, peaking in 1954 with an estimated 500,000 to one million users in a population of 83 million people (Nagahama 1968). Enforcement of strict antiabuse laws is credited with an almost complete disappearance of methamphetamine abuse in Japan by 1957 (Hemmi 1969). However, methamphetamine abuse has reemerged as a major problem in Japan (Sato 1986).

In the United States, nonmedical use of amphetamines steadily increased through the 1960s, particularly among students and truck drivers. A major factor in the proliferation of amphetamine use allegedly was a considerable laxity in screening of distributors by the pharmaceutical companies (Grinspoon and Hedblom 1975). It has been estimated that 50% of commercially produced amphetamine was diverted into illicit channels, of which 90% was distributed from truck stops, restaurants, and gas stations (Sadusk 1966). In the 1960s, amphetamines were a common choice among the drug culture and often used in combination with sedatives and narcotics (Grinspoon and Hedblom 1975). Intravenous amphetamine abuse, as practiced by the speed freaks, followed a distinct pattern of episodic "runs" lasting a few days, with escalating doses usually leading to a period of exhaustion and abstinence before the cycle was repeated (Kramer 1969; Kramer et al. 1967). Amphetamine psychosis frequently resulted from this pattern of use.

Beginning in 1987, a new smokable form of methamphetamine, known as ice, began appearing in Hawaii and has gradually spread to a number of West Coast communities. This drug originated in Asia, but increasingly is produced in small laboratories in the United States. Ice threatens to become a major and very serious drug of abuse in this country for a number of reasons. First, it is synthesized by a relatively simple and inexpensive process; if efforts to reduce importation of cocaine are successful, ice may serve as a readily available substitute. Second, ice produces a sustained euphoria, often lasting up to 48 hours compared to 15 minutes for crack cocaine. Finally, ice is associated with a high rate of psychosis, aggressive behavior, and withdrawal depression. The psychological adverse effects and violence resulting from this form of methamphetamine abuse may exceed those of cocaine.

PREVALENCE

Amphetamine abuse appears to have increased slightly in prevalence since the early 1970s (Morgan 1981; National Institute on Drug Abuse 1985). Surveys conducted in the mid-1970s found amphetamine use to be generally very light, with only about 10% of users taking it daily (Abelson and Fishburne 1976; Blackford 1977). Intravenous abuse was believed to be rare. Amphetamine was used most commonly by college-educated urban white males and was predominately obtained from nonmedical sources. The 1985 National Household Survey on Drug Abuse (National Institute on Drug Abuse 1985) interviewed 8,038 randomly selected subjects and reported the following rates of stimulant use within the previous year: 4.4% among 12–17 year olds, 10.4% among 18–25 year olds, and 2.7% among those older than 26 years. These rates have all remained relatively stable over the past decade, with an increasing trend that has been greatest in the age group above 25 years of age. Data are not available on the relative severity of stimulant use or on the prevalence of intravenous use.

Following the tighter regulations controlling the production and prescription of amphetamines in 1972, the quality of illicit amphetamines dramatically declined. Morgan and Kagan (1979) reported that whereas samples of street drugs submitted in 1971–1972 contained amphetamine or methamphetamine 65% of the time, by 1976 this had dropped to 10%. The most common substance misrepresented as amphetamine is caffeine, followed by ephedrine and phenylpropanolamine. Of patients reporting amphetamine use to the Drug Abuse Warning Network (DAWN) System emergency room survey (Food and Drug Administration 1977), approximately 25% obtained the drug by prescription and the remaining 75% either bought illicit drug or stole it.

Another important development in the history of stimulant abuse has been the recent popularity of the so-called designer drugs, methylenedioxyamphetamine (MDA) and 3,4-methylenedioxymethamphetamine (MDMA or "ecstasy") (Climko et al. 1987; Nichols 1986; Reidlinger 1985; Shulgin 1986). These drugs appear to have similar properties: a combination of amphetamine-like stimulant effects and mescaline-like hallucinogenic effects. Both drugs were first synthesized in the early 1900s, but were only recently rediscovered.

MDA has been widely abused in the United States since 1960, although its classification in 1973 as a schedule I controlled substance reduced its production to a few illicit laboratories. MDMA has more recently emerged as a drug of abuse and was emergently classified as schedule I in July 1985. MDMA is infrequently detected by forensic laboratories; one laboratory reported that only 27% of samples identified as MDMA actually contained the drug (Climko et al. 1987). Additional attention has also been focused on MDA and MDMA over the past few years following a number of reports claiming efficacy for these drugs as enhancers of psychotherapy (Riedlinger et al. 1985; Shulgin 1986). Although much has been written about this potential role for these drugs, controlled studies have not been performed.

Another stimulant that is receiving attention as a drug of abuse is propylhexedrine, which is the active ingredient in Benzedrex nasal decongestant inhalers (Wesson 1986). Propylhexedrine was substituted for amphetamine in Benzedrex inhalers in 1949 to prevent abuse. Increasingly common among stimulant abusers is the practice of heating the contents of the nasal inhaler with hydrochloric acid and dissolving the resulting crystals in water for injection. This preparation is known as "stovetop speed." Although inhalation and oral ingestion of propylhexedrine are associated with only mild abuse patterns, significant abuse and toxicity occur with intravenous use. Cases of brain, heart, and lung injury from vasoconstriction have been reported, in addition to chronic pulmonary hypertension.

PHARMACOLOGY

Amphetamine

Amphetamine exists as two isomers, dextroamphetamine and levamphetamine. The racemic amphetamine mixture and the dextro-isomer are commercially available, whereas the levo-isomer, which has less central activating effects and greater peripheral side effects (Smith and Davis 1977), is not commercially available. Methamphetamine, an amphetamine analogue, is equivalent to dextroamphetamine in potency (Martin et al. 1971) and is frequently the choice of intravenous abusers. Although the amphetamines are quite similar in action, the range of drug effects is diverse, depending in part on whether the drug is taken orally or intravenously and in low or high dosage.

When taken orally, amphetamine's onset of action occurs in about 30 minutes, and peak blood levels occur after 2–3 hours. Duration of action is quite long, between 10 and 30 hours, depending on the rate of urinary excretion. Although metabolized by deamination and hydroxylation in the liver, as much as 80% can be excreted unchanged in the urine (Caldwell and Sever 1974). Urinary excretion is determined by urinary pH; excretion increases with acidification of urine. For example, acidification of the urine to a pH of 5.6 can reduce amphetamine's half-life to 8 hours. Methamphetamine has a much shorter half-life of 4–5 hours and is also less influenced by urinary pH.

The amphetamines produce their complex stimulant effects primarily by increasing dopaminergic and noradrenergic activity (Groves and Tepper 1983). Dopamine is released from a newly synthesized, reserpine-resistant pool. Catecholamine reuptake is blocked, and degradation by the monoamine oxidase enzyme is inhibited (Kuczenski 1983).

Amphetamine has been extensively investigated in animals, where distinct behavioral patterns have been used for models of human response. At low doses, amphetamine produces an increase in locomotor activity, which is believed to correspond to the energizing or activating effect in humans. This motoric response is believed to be mediated by norepinephrine and by mesolimbic dopamine pathways (Solanto 1984). Higher doses produce stereotyped behaviors that are species-specific and, in humans, commonly take the form of disassembling or reassembling mechanical objects, protracted sexual activity, or psychosis. The stereotypy in animals has been linked to activation of nigrostriatal dopamine pathways (Solanto 1984).

In humans, subjective and behavioral responses to amphetamine are very complex and depend on many variables, including: 1) dose; 2) route of administration; 3) previous experience with stimulants; 4) the environment in which the drug is taken; and 5) the unique response pattern of the individual user, which may in part be genetically determined. In most subjects, low doses administered orally produce a sense of relaxation, well-being, diminished fatigue, self-confidence, and mental alertness (Martin et al. 1971). Increasing doses result in greater activation, anxiety, insomnia, and anorexia. The mood response can vary from elation to extreme dysphoria; an antidepressant effect is seen in some depressed patients (Silberman et al. 1981). Intravenous administration produces an intensely pleasurable response, which users commonly liken to sexual climax (Smith and Fischer 1970).

A large body of literature has examined the effects of amphetamine on athletic and cognitive performances (Weiss and Laties 1962). Although some of the data conflict, most studies indicate that stimulants improve performance when fatigue, boredom, or apathy interfere with concentration. Surprisingly, amphetamine is also reported to improve athletic performance significantly in such areas as the shot put and discus throw (Smith and Beecher 1959), activities that do not seem to involve endurance and sustained attention.

Side effects are numerous and are discussed later. Briefly, they include hypertension, tachycardia and tachyarrhythmias, urinary sphincter contraction, hyperthermia, anorexia, insomnia, and delayed gastric emptying. Amphetamine has a mild analgesic effect (Forrest et al. 1977), but lacks the anesthetic and seizure-inducing properties of cocaine.

Tolerance develops to the anorectic and hyperthermic responses and to the acute euphoric effect (Schuster 1981). Patients treated for narcolepsy or apathetic states find that the stimulant properties usually persist without development of tolerance. Evidence is accumulating that sensitization occurs for some effects, most notably amphetamine-induced psychosis. In animal studies, repeated administration of amphetamine produces dopaminergic hypersensitivity that correlates with stereotyped behaviors (Klawans and Margolin 1975; Schuster 1981; Segal and Mandell 1974). Sensitization is demonstrated in humans by the production of psychosis with progressively lower doses and shorter periods of consumption of amphetamine following repeated use over time (Sato 1986). Sensitization for amphetamine-induced psychosis may persist despite long periods of abstinence.

Methylphenidate

Methylphenidate is very similar to amphetamine in its clinical effects but differs in certain pharmacologic properties (Shaywitz et al. 1982; Smith and Davis 1977). Peak levels are achieved in 2 hours after oral administration. Methylphenidate is metabolized in the liver; its primary metabolite, ritalinic acid, does not have significant stimulant activity. Although methylphenidate's half-life has been calculated to be as short as 1–2 hours, methylphenidate's clinical duration of action is considerably longer (6–9 hours). Methylphenidate inhibits hepatic enzymes, thereby elevating blood levels of many drugs, including phenytoin, phenobarbital, warfarin (Coumadin), and tricyclic antidepressants. By avoiding first-pass hepatic metabolism, intravenous administration produces blood levels approximately 10 times higher than are produced by oral administration. Methylphenidate is roughly two-thirds as potent a stimulant as dextroamphetamine. Although methylphenidate produces a range of symptoms very similar to amphetamine, some evidence suggests that individual subjects may have quite different mood responses to methylphenidate than to amphetamine (Smith and Davis 1977). Methylphenidate has relatively less noradrenergic activity than amphetamine. Like amphetamine, methylphenidate acts on dopamine pathways, but the mechanism of dopaminergic activation differs between the two drugs (Solanto 1984). The dopamine released by methylphenidate is from a reserpine-sensitive storage pool. Whereas dextroamphetamine increases dopamine and phenylethylamine synthesis, methylphenidate administration decreases dopamine synthesis and does not affect urinary phenylethylamine (Zametkin et al. 1985). It was originally believed that methylphenidate did not produce psychosis or abuse. Increasing experience suggests that both of these adverse effects occur (Rioux 1960). In fact, drug-abusing subjects equally prefer methylphenidate and dextroamphetamine to placebo when given under double-blind conditions (Martin et al. 1971).

Anorectics

A variety of stimulant drugs are used primarily for their appetite-suppressant effects and are commonly referred to as "diet pills" (Table 6-3). The amphetamines were widely prescribed as diet pills until physicians recognized the risk of abuse. The drugs listed in Table 6-3 as anorectics represent a wide range of central nervous system (CNS) stimulant activity and of addiction potential (Ellinwood et al. 1973; Griffith 1977). Like amphetamine and the other major stimulants, tolerance generally develops for the appetite suppressant effect after 6–12 weeks; discontinuation can result in fatigue, sleep disorders, and depression. The anorectics produce less CNS stimulation than amphetamine and vary considerably in their peripheral side effects (Bartholomew and Marley 1959). Most cause insomnia, anxiety, and restlessness, which can limit their use.

Table 6-3.   Anorectics

Chemical name	Brand names	Schedule
Phenmetrazine	Preludin	II
Benzphetamine	Didrex	III
Phendimetrazine	Statobex, Wehless, Adipost, Bontril, Dyrexan, Hyrex, Trimcaps, Obezine, Trimstat, Weightrol, Trimtabs, Phenazine, Unicelles, Prelu-2, Timecelles, Bacarate, Melfiat, Metra, Obalan, Plegine	III
Diethylpropion	Tenuate, Tepanil, Ten-tab	IV
Fenfluramine	Pondimin	IV
Mazindol	Mazanor, Sanorex	IV
Phentermine	Ionamin, Fastin, Obephen, Obermine, Obestin, Parmine, Phentride, Unifast, Wilpower, Adipex-p, Dapex, Phentrol	IV
Phenylpropanolamine	Prolamine, Dexatrim, Westrim, Dex-A-Diet, Rhindecon, Didax, Propagest, Acutrim, Help, Ornex, Deconex, Diatrim	Over the counter

Phenmetrazine is the anorectic most similar to amphetamine and is one-fourth to one-third as potent (Martin et al. 1971). Abuse and psychosis are both reported with its use (Rylander 1969). Diethylpropion is also similar to amphetamine and can be abused; unlike amphetamine, however, it is reported to cause minimal cardiovascular stimulation (Caplan 1963; Clein and Benady 1962; Jonsson 1969). Fenfluramine, a serotonin agonist, is unique among the phenylethylamines in being a CNS depressant and has minimal potential for self-administration in animal studies (Bartholomew and Marley 1959). Mazindol resembles the tricyclic antidepressants in mechanism of action and can potentiate tricyclic antidepressant effects while producing weak CNS stimulation. Lastly, phenylpropanolamine is the most commonly used anorectic and is available without prescription. It is similar to ephedrine and produces mild central and peripheral stimulation along with blood pressure elevation. Phenylpropanolamine is not recognized as an amphetamine by human subjects and does not produce self-administration behavior in animals.

Pemoline

Pemoline is structurally dissimilar to amphetamine and methylphenidate and produces mild CNS stimulation (Garattini and Samanin 1981). It is believed to present less abuse potential because of its gradual onset of action and its lack of a euphoric mood response. Pemoline is used as an alternative to the major stimulants in attention-deficit disorder and is prescribed occasionally for atypical depressive disorders. Clinical improvement in conditions such as attention-deficit disorder can require 3–4 weeks, in contrast to the rapid response seen following amphetamine or methylphenidate treatment. Rare cases of abuse, psychosis, and precipitation of mania have been reported with pemoline (Polchert and Morse 1985; Sternbach 1981). In addition, elevation of liver enzymes representing possible hepatotoxicity has been reported (Nehra et al. 1990).

Pemoline's central activating effects were previously believed to result from augmentation of dopaminergic activity, although more recent work has not supported this view (Molina and Orsingher 1981). While pemoline does not appear to increase levels of brain catecholamines, it may decrease their turnover.

MDA and MDMA

MDA resembles amphetamine in producing central and peripheral stimulation, anorexia, and hyperthermia. In addition, MDA has hallucinogenic properties similar to mescaline and lysergic acid diethylamide (LSD) (Climko et al. 1987; Nichols 1986; Riedlinger 1985; Shulgin 1986). The stimulant effects are believed to result from amphetamine-like release and reuptake blockade of norepinephrine and by activation of dopamine. MDA is also a potent releaser of serotonin; the hallucinogenic effect is believed to be mediated by 5-hydroxytryptamine (5-HT) receptors (Nichols 1986). At oral doses of 100–200 mg, MDA is reported to produce a sense of well-being, diminished anxiety, and increased desire for interpersonal contact and is described as enhancing access to emotions and memories in psychotherapy. Hallucinogenic effects occur at higher doses. MDA causes self-infusion behavior in monkeys. Less is known about the pharmacology of MDMA, which appears to be similar to MDA, although with less hallucinogenic effect. MDMA can also produce self-infusion behaviors in animals, but of less intensity than produced by cocaine (Shulgin 1986).

MDMA, administered twice daily in subcutaneous doses of 2.5, 3.75, and 5.0 mg/kg, produced dose-dependent depletion of serotonin and 5-hydroxyindoleacetic acid (5-HIAA) in macaque monkeys (Ricaurte et al. 1988). Serotonergic cell bodies of the dorsal, but not medial, raphe nucleus developed intracytoplasmic inclusions accompanied by a loss of serotonin-immunoreactive nerve fibers in the cerebral cortex. Depletion of serotonin was seen in the cortex, caudate, putamen, hippocampus, hypothalamus, and thalamus. Although the applicability to humans is not entirely clear, it raises the possibility that MDMA may cause structural damage to serotonergic neurons. The doses in this study were somewhat higher than the typical human dose of a single 1.7–2.7 mg/kg oral dose separated by several days or weeks.

Caffeine

Caffeine, a methylxanthine, produces significant central stimulation that is dose-related. A typical cup of brewed coffee contains 100–150 mg of caffeine; instant coffee contains 85–100 mg of caffeine; and brewed tea contains 60–75 mg of caffeine. Cola drinks also contain caffeine, usually about 40–75 mg per 12 ounces (Table 6-4). Caffeine is believed to exert its CNS-stimulating action by inhibition of phosphodiesterase, which increases levels of cyclic adenosine monophosphate. In addition, caffeine competitively blocks adenosine receptors (Katims et al. 1983). Caffeine causes cardiac stimulation, dilatation of coronary and peripheral blood vessels, constriction of cerebral blood vessels, increased gastric acid secretion, diuresis, and stimulation of skeletal muscle. Like amphetamine, caffeine has been demonstrated to improve performance on many tasks that require sustained concentration (Weiss and Laties 1962). When more than 1 g is ingested, caffeine can produce insomnia, dyspnea, delirium, muscle twitching, and arrhythmias. Doses above 5 g can be lethal. The half-life is 3–7 hours; it is much longer in infants and in pregnant women, both of whom can become toxic at relatively low doses.

Caffeinism is a syndrome of excessive consumption of caffeine and is characterized by symptoms of anxiety, dysphoria, sleep disturbance, diarrhea, palpitations, and tremulousness (Greden 1979). Although tolerance develops to most of these symptoms, caffeine con-

Table 6-4. Common sources of caffeine

	Caffeine (mg)
Coffee (1 cup)	
Brewed	100–150
Instant	85–100
Tea (1 cup)	60–75
Cola drinks (12 ounces)	40–75
Cocoa (1 cup)	50
Bittersweet chocolate (1 ounce)	25
OTC cold preparations (1 tablet)	15–60
OTC stimulants	100–200

Note. OTC = over the counter.

sumption greater than 500–700 mg/day probably produces symptoms of caffeine toxicity in most people. The typical patient with caffeinism consumes about 1 g/day, or the equivalent of 6–10 cups of brewed coffee. Gilbert (1976) estimated that as many as 10% of Americans may suffer from caffeinism.

Like the other CNS stimulants, caffeine also produces a withdrawal syndrome. Caffeine withdrawal generally appears within 18–24 hours and is characterized by headache, malaise, irritability, and dysphoria (Greden 1979). Relief of symptoms, particularly headache, often occurs soon after ingesting additional caffeine, a response that tends to promote patterns of caffeine abuse.

ETIOLOGIC THEORIES OF STIMULANT ABUSE

Rats (Pickens 1968), cats (Balster et al. 1976), and monkeys (Balster and Schuster 1973) all self-administer amphetamine in cyclic patterns resembling human stimulant abuse. When given unlimited amphetamines availability, animals will become emaciated, will self-mutilate, and often die of exhaustion and hyperthermia (Pickens and Harris 1968; Thompson and Pickens 1970). The mechanism responsible for amphetamine's reinforcing property is not clearly identified, but is believed to involve activation of catecholamine systems, particularly dopaminergic pathways. Dopamine antagonists, such as pimozide, block self-administration of amphetamine, as does ablatement of dopamine neurons in the nucleus accumbens (Fouriezos and Wise 1976). Like morphine, amphetamine decreases the amount of electrical stimulation necessary to activate brain reward centers. This decrease in the threshold for intracranial self-stimulation may correspond with the subjective experience of stimulation-seeking, which abusers report. Following withdrawal from long-term amphetamine administration, the rate of intracranial self-stimulation is significantly decreased (Cassens et al. 1981; Leith and Barret 1980), possibly representing a model for the anhedonia reported by human subjects. This decrease of intracranial self-stimulation following amphetamine withdrawal is reversed by tricyclic anti-depressants (Kokkinidis et al. 1980).

Social and psychological factors contributing to amphetamine abuse in humans are diverse and not well understood. Many low-dose users seem to take amphetamine for enhancement of performance in athletic pursuits, for repetitious cognitive tasks, or for occupational activities requiring prolonged concentration and alertness. These users are often able to discontinue use without significant difficulty. Users who rely on amphetamines for weight loss or to elevate their mood or energy level often develop a pattern of escalating the dose as tolerance occurs. These users may develop withdrawal syndromes, consisting of fatigue, depression, and irritability when they attempt to stop the drug. Another group of stimulant abusers may be self-medicating major psychiatric disorders, such as depression and attention deficit disorder (Khantzian 1985; McLellan et al. 1979; Pope 1979; Tennant and Swenseid 1985). Finally, the so-called speed freak or high-dose intravenous user appears to be driven by the reinforcing effect of the acute rush following intravenous administration (Smith 1969). As tolerance to the euphoric rush develops, such users steadily increase the dose, injecting subsequent doses before the previous dose has been cleared. Very high cumulative drug levels can thus be reached in a short period of time, with some users injecting as much as 10 g in a 24-hour period.

In one study, normal subjects given low-dose amphetamine (5 mg) or placebo under blind conditions preferred amphetamine to placebo approximately 80% of the time (Johanson and Uhlenhuth 1981). Although subjects reported increases in vigor, friendliness, elation, arousal, and positive mood following amphetamine administration, these effects did not correlate with drug preference. In addition, when the trial was repeated three times during a 1-week period, preference for amphetamine dropped to 42% despite continuation of positive subjective effects. This study suggests that the positive subjective effects of low-dose, oral amphetamine may not account directly for repetitive patterns of use in normal subjects.

ACUTE INTOXICATION

As previously described, many patterns of stimulant use occur. Oral amphetamine abuse typically follows a pattern of gradually increasing doses as tolerance to the euphoric effect develops over weeks or months. Alcohol or other sedatives are commonly used in combination, particularly for sleep at night. The intravenous abuse pattern usually occurs in cycles of 4–6 days during which increasing doses may reach as high as 1–2 g every 2–3 hours until the run ends due to exhaustion, psychotic disorganization, or simply running out of the drug (Kramer et al. 1967). A prolonged sleep follows, lasting 12–24 hours, followed by a period of fatigue, hunger, and depression. Most intravenous users do not tolerate this stage for long before starting another cycle of stimulant injection.

The most striking characteristic of high-dose stimulant abuse is the development of psychosis. The amphetamines, methylphenidate, and phenmetrazine all produce psychosis (Ellinwood et al. 1973; Iversen et al. 1978; Lucas and Weiss 1971; McCormick and McNeil 1962). Although some schizophrenic patients are particularly sensitive to exacerbation of psychosis from stimulants (Janowsky et al. 1973), paranoid delusions can probably be produced in most people if given an adequate dose of stimulant (Griffith et al. 1968). The dose required to produce psychosis varies greatly among individuals (Bell 1973). In one study of normal volunteers, 100 mg of amphetamine was sufficient in one subject, whereas another subject required 955 mg (Angrist and Gershon 1970). Prior to the onset of overt psychosis, most users begin to exhibit suspiciousness and a fascination with details of objects in their environment and often will begin to perform repetitive behaviors, such as picking at their skin, disassembling mechanical objects, and prolonged masturbation or coitus (Connell 1958). With higher doses or continued administration, users begin to experience paranoid delusions; ideas of reference; visual, auditory, or olfactory hallucinations; and agitation (Ellinwood 1967). Unlike most toxic psychoses, disorientation does not typically occur. Violence, including homicide, is reported as a consequence of this activated, para-noid state (Ellinwood 1967; Kramer 1969). The clinical presentation of stimulant psychosis has frequently been described as being indis-tinguishable from paranoid schizophrenia (Angrist and Gershon 1970; Ellinwood 1971). However, agitation, hypersexuality, affective lability, and grandiosity also frequently occur, thus leading to confu-sion with mania. In addition, many symptoms are suggestive of tem-poral lobe epilepsy, such as olfactory hallucinations, déjà vu, philo-sophical preoccupation, and the very atypical course of the illness (Ellinwood 1968). Stimulant psychosis generally clears within a few days of discontinuation of the drug (Beamish and Kiloh 1960), al-though prolonged psychoses are associated with stimulant abuse (Iversen et al. 1978).

CHRONIC USE

The effects of chronic stimulant use vary widely and are largely de-termined by the dosage and pattern of use. Low-dose users can main-tain effects of behavioral activation and mood elevation for long peri-ods, while developing tolerance to anoretic and euphoric effects. Sleep often normalizes in such users, as do signs of autonomic arousal. Chronic low to moderate use can thus be clinically undetect-able unless the user increases the dose to produce intoxication or abruptly stops it and exhibits withdrawal. Those who develop a pat-tern of escalating dose generally exhibit obvious dysfunction within a few months. In addition to symptoms of stimulant intoxication, gen-eral deterioration in work and social interactions is usually apparent. Sexual dysfunction, including perversions and hypersexuality or hyposexuality, is common in chronic users; however, evidence of sex-ual maladaptation as well as personality disorders is usually apparent prior to the onset of stimulant abuse (Bell and Trethowan 1961a, 1961b). Preoccupation with the drug often occurs, and users may be-come paranoid, withdrawn, and isolated within the drug culture. The course of chronic stimulant abuse is further complicated by concomi-tant abuse of sedatives and alcohol, particularly for nighttime sleep.

It has been estimated that 50% of people who abuse amphet-amine 30–100 mg/day for 3 months will develop psychotic symptoms (Sato 1986). Amphetamine psychosis can become chronic; in addi-tion, as sensitization to psychosis occurs, small doses of stimulant can trigger psychotic episodes despite long periods of abstinence (Sato 1986).

Withdrawal symptoms are an important characteristic of high-dose, chronic stimulant abuse. Discontinuation is associated with an initial period of hypersomnia and rebound of rapid-eye-movement sleep (Oswald and Thacore 1963). Depression usually peaks at 48–72 hours, but can persist for months (Watson et al. 1972). During the first few days, dysphoria can be intense, with suicidality and an overwhelming desire to relieve the depression by restarting the drug. The depression is associated with a significant decrease in excretion of urinary 3-methoxy-4-hydroxyphenylglycol (MHPG) excretion, which gradually increases over days and weeks (Watson et al. 1972).

Animal studies suggest that some neurotransmitter effects of stimulant abuse may be long lasting. In monkeys treated with methamphetamine for 3–6 months, brain norepinephrine and serotonin levels are significantly decreased. When monkeys were studied 6 months after discontinuing methamphetamine, dopamine levels in the caudate were decreased by 70%, and norepinephrine levels were reduced 33% in the midbrain and 52% in the frontal cortex (Seiden et al. 1975). Whether such animal work has implications for human stimulant abusers is unclear.

MEDICAL AND PSYCHOLOGICAL CONSEQUENCES

Adverse effects of stimulant consumption are numerous. Following a single, low to moderate oral dose, some individuals will experience dysphoria, agitation, anxiety, headache, or palpitations. Mania can be triggered in bipolar patients, and exacerbation of psychosis can occur in schizophrenic patients (Janowsky et al. 1973; O'Flannagan and Taylor 1950). High doses can produce delirium, hypertension, arrhythmias, hyperthermia, seizures, coma, and death (Oswald and Thacore 1963). Consequences of high-dose intravenous use include psychosis, dehydration, malnutrition, and the hazards of shared needle use. Intravenous users can lose 6–7% of total body weight during a run (Anggard et al. 1970). One common manifestation of chronic malnutrition is the impaired healing of excoriations inflicted during runs (Ellinwood 1967). Chronic use can also produce permanent damage to cerebral blood vessels. Cerebral vasculitis, necrotizing angitis, and cerebral hemorrhage have been attributed to chronic amphetamine use (Bostwick 1981; Citron et al. 1970; Salanova 1984). A characteristic "beading" pattern is found on angiography. Animal studies suggest that vascular segments of low flow, petechial hemorrhages, and cerebral edema result from amphetamine-induced hypertension and vasoconstriction (Rumbaugh et al. 1971). Finally, a variety of movement disorders are associated with stimulant abuse, including choreoathetoid movements, tics, bruxism, and orofacial dyskinesias (Goetz and Klawans 1983; Iversen et al. 1978).

Overdose

Amphetamine overdose is characterized by signs of adrenergic stimulation: dilated pupils, diaphoresis, tachycardia, hypertension, and hyperreflexia. Hyperpyrexia and acidosis may also occur. Patients often display mental status changes, most commonly anxiety, paranoid psychoses, or delirium. Massive overdoses may result in seizures, severe hyperthermia, and cardiovascular collapse. Cooling measures and intravenous diazepam should be administered promptly in such cases. Gastric lavage is generally helpful, since amphetamine can reduce gastric motility. Acidification of the urine with ascorbic acid or ammonium chloride will substantially increase urinary excretion of the drug. Hypertension may require treatment with nitroprusside or the alpha-adrenergic antagonist, phentolamine. Psychiatric management is focused on preventing self-injury and reducing agitation. Patients should be kept in a quiet environment with minimal external stimulation. Limb restraints may be necessary to prevent injury or elopement. Benzodiazepines are often effective in treating agitation, although treatment with high-potency neuroleptics, such as haloperidol, will rapidly reduce psychotic symptomatology and can usually be stopped within a few days (Angrist et al. 1974). Chlorpromazine probably should not be used because of its cardiovascular side effects and since it may slow the metabolism of amphetamine (Lemberger et al. 1970).

TREATMENT

Throughout the 1960s and early 1970s, treatment of stimulant abuse remained largely unsuccessful (Tennant 1979, 1983). Anderson et al. (1972) reported that of a series of 18 amphetamine abusers seen in an outpatient clinic, none followed the recommendation for continued care. As for all substance abuse disorders, treatment outcome for stimulant abuse is strongly influenced by the duration of treatment, whether inpatient or outpatient. In one study, only after 90 days of treatment was outcome superior for amphetamine abusers compared with those who did not receive treatment (Simpson 1981). After completing 90 days of treatment, prognosis correlated with length of continued treatment. McLellan et al. (1982) reported a 50% reduction in stimulant use and dramatic improvement in social functioning among substance abusers who completed a 60-day program of individual and group psychotherapy, educational and vocational counseling, and participation in a structured therapeutic community. Abusers who received a favorable discharge after less than 15 days of treatment did not display significant improvement. Data are not available on the relative efficacy of different treatment approaches or on individual components of treatment programs.

Within the past few years, attention has begun to focus on the possible use of pharmacologic interventions as an additional component of stimulant abuse treatment. Tennant and colleagues (Tennant and Rawson 1983; Tennant et al. 1986) have reported an open study and one small double-blind study ($N = 4$) in which desipramine appeared to improve outcome in amphetamine abusers. Patients receiving desipramine remained in treatment longer and reported less drug craving, depression, and sleep disorder than did patients receiving placebo. This work remains preliminary due to the very small number of subjects studied as of this writing; however, impressive early results in cocaine abusers further support the likelihood that desipramine may play an important role in the treatment of stimulant abuse (Gawin and Kleber 1984). Two other drug strategies may also decrease amphetamine use, but have not been studied yet in abusers. Lithium is known to attenuate the euphoric effect of amphetamines and so may decrease the psychological reinforcement of its use (Van Kammen and Murphy 1975). Serotonergic agonists may also be of value; fluoxetine (5-HT reuptake blocker), L-tryptophan (5-HT precursor), and quipazine (5-HT receptor agonist) all significantly reduce amphetamine self-administration in rats (Leccese and Lyness 1984; Yu et al. 1986).

REFERENCES

Abelson H, Fishburne P: National survey—main findings 1976: nonmedical use of psychoactive substances (NTIS PB 268-144). Springfield, VA, National Technical Information Service, 1976

Alles GA: The comparative physiological action of phenylethanolamine. J Pharmacol Exp Ther 32:121, 1928

Anderson WH, O'Malley JE, Lazare A: Failure of outpatient treatment of drug abuse, II: amphetamines, barbiturates, hallucinogens. Am J Psychiatry 128:1572–1576, 1972

Anggard E, Gunne LM, Jonsson LE, et al: Pharmacokinetic and clinical studies on amphetamine dependent subjects. Eur J Clin Pharmacol 3: 3–11, 1970

Angrist B, Gershon S: The phenomenology of experimentally induced amphetamine psychosis: preliminary observations. Biol Psychiatry 2:95–107, 1970

Angrist B, Lee HK, Gershon S: The antagonism of amphetamine-induced symptomatology by a neuroleptic. Am J Psychiatry 131:817–819, 1974

Balster RL, Schuster CR: A comparison of d-amphetamine, l-amphetamine, and methamphetamine self-administration in rhesus monkeys. Pharmacol Biochem Behav 1:67, 1973

Balster RL, Kilbey MM, Ellinwood EH: Methamphetamine self-administration in the cat. Psychopharmacologia (Berlin) 46:222, 1976

Bartholomew AA, Marley E: Toxic response to 2-phenyl-3-methyl-tetrahydro-1,4-oxazine hydrochloride "Preludin" in humans. Psychopharmacologia (Berlin) 1:124–139, 1959

Beamish P, Kiloh LG: Psychosis due to amphetamine consumption. Journal of Mental Science 106:337–343, 1960

Bell DS: The experimental reproduction of amphetamine psychosis. Arch Gen Psychiatry 29:35–40, 1973

Bell DS, Trethowan WH: Amphetamine addiction. J Nerv Ment Dis 133: 489–496, 1961a

Bell DS, Trethowan WH: Amphetamine addiction and disturbed sexuality. Arch Gen Psychiatry 4:74–78, 1961b

Bett WR: Benzedrine sulfate in clinical medicine: a survey of the literature. Postgrad Med J 22:205–218, 1946

Blackford L: Summary report: surveys of student drug use: San Mateo County, CA. San Mateo County, CA, Research and Statistics Section, Department of Health and Welfare, 1977

Bostwick DG: Amphetamine induced cerebral vasculitis. Hum Pathol 1: 1031–1033, 1981

Caldwell J, Sever PA: The biochemical pharmacology of abused drugs, I: amphetamines, cocaine and LSD. Clin Pharmacol Ther 16:625–638, 1974

Caplan J: Habituation to diethylpropion (Tenuate). Can Med Assoc J 88: 943–944, 1963

Cassens G, Acton C, Kling M, et al: Amphetamine withdrawal: effects on threshold of intracranial reinforcement. Psychopharmacology (Berlin) 73:318–322, 1981

Citron BP, Halpern M, McCarron M, et al: Necrotizing angiitis associated with drug abuse. N Engl J Med 283:1003–1011, 1970

Clein LJ, Benady DR: Case of diethylpropion addiction. Br Med J 2:456, 1962

Climko RP, Roehrich H, Sweeney DR, et al: Ecstacy: a review of MDMA and MDA. Int J Psychiatry Med 16:359–372, 1987

Connell PH: Amphetamine Psychosis (Maudsley Monographs No 5). London, Oxford University Press, 1958

Edeleano L: Uber einige derivate der phenylmethocrylsure wid der Phenyl-
   isobu ttersaure. Berichte Deutsche Chemische Gesellschaft (Berlin)
   20:616, 1887
Ellinwood EH Jr: Amphetamine psychosis, I: description of the individuals
   and process. J Nerv Ment Dis 144:273–283, 1967
Ellinwood EH Jr: Amphetamine psychosis, II: theoretical implications.
   J Neuropsychiatry 4:45–54, 1968
Ellinwood EH Jr: Assault and homicide associated with amphetamine
   abuse. Am J Psychiatry 127:1170–1175, 1971
Ellinwood EH Jr: Amphetamines/anorectants, in Handbook on Drug
   Abuse. Edited by Dupont RI, Godstein A, O'Donnell J, et al. Rock-
   ville, MD, National Institute on Drug Abuse, 1979, pp. 221–232
Ellinwood EH Jr, Sudilovsky A, Nelson L: Evolving behavior in the clinical
   and experimental amphetamine (model) psychosis. Am J Psychiatry
   130:1088–1093, 1973
Food and Drug Administration: Amphetamines. Federal Register 42:
   55374–55379, 1977
Forrest WH, Brown BW, Brown CR, et al: Dextroamphetamine with morphine for the treatment of postoperative pain. N Engl J Med 296:712,
   1977
Fouriezos G, Wise RA: Pimozide-induced extinction of intracranial self-
   stimulation: response patterns rule out motor or performance deficits.
   Brain Res 103:377–380, 1976
Garattini S, Samanin R: The pharmacological profile of some psychomotor
   stimulant drugs including chemical, neurophysiological, biochemical,
   and toxicological aspects, in Psychotropic Agents, Part II. Edited by
   Hoffmeister F, Stille G. New York, Springer-Verlag, 1981, pp 545–
   585
Gawin FH, Kleber HD: Cocaine abuse treatment: open pilot trial with desi-
   pramine and lithium carbonate. Arch Gen Psychiatry 41:903, 1984
Gilbert RM: Caffeine as a drug of abuse, in Research Addresses in Alcohol
   and Drug Problems, Vol 3. Edited by Gibbin RG, Hiklart YI, Pophom
   RE, et al. New York, John Wiley, 1976
Goetz CG, Klawans HL: Stimulant-induced chorea: clinical studies and an-
   imal models, in Stimulants: Neurochemical, Behavioral and Clinical
   Perspectives. Edited by Creese I. New York, Raven, 1983, pp 227–235
Greden JF: Caffeinism and caffeine withdrawal, in Handbook on Drug
   Abuse. Edited by Dupont RI, Godstein A, O'Donnell J, et al. Rock-
   ville, MD, National Institute on Drug Abuse, 1979
Griffith JD: Structure-activity relationships of several amphetamine drugs
   in man, in Cocaine and Other Stimulants. Edited by Ellinwood EH Jr,
   Kilbey MM. New York, Plenum, 1977
Griffith J, Oates JA, Cavanaugh JH: Paranoid episodes induced by drug.
   JAMA 205:39, 1968
Grinspoon L, Hedblom P: The Speed Culture. Cambridge, MA, Harvard
   University Press, 1975
Groves PM, Tepper JM: Neuronal mechanisms of action of amphetamine,
   in Stimulants: Neurochemical, Behavioral, and Clinical Perspectives.
   Edited by Creese I. New York, Raven, 1983

Hemmi T: How we handled the problem of drug abuse in Japan, in Abuse of Central Stimulants. Edited by Sjoqvist F, Tottie M. Stockholm, Almqvist & Wiksell, 1969, pp 147–153

Iversen LL, Iversen SD, Snyder SH: Stimulants: Handbook of Psychopharmacology, Vol 11. New York, Plenum, 1978

Janowsky DS, El-Yousef MK, Davis JM, et al: Provocation of schizophrenic symptoms by intravenous administration of methylphenidate. Arch Gen Psychiatry 28:185–191, 1973

Johanson CE, Uhlenhuth EH: Drug preference and mood in humans: repeated assessment of d-amphetamine. Pharmacol Biochem Behav 14:159–163, 1981

Jonsson CO: Behavioral studies of diethylpropion in man, in Abuse of Central Stimulants. Edited by Sjoqvist F, Tottie M. Stockholm, Almqvist & Wiksell, 1969

Katims JJ, Murphy MM, Snyder SH: Xanthine stimulants and adenosine, in Stimulants: Neurochemical, Behavioral and Clinical Perspectives. Edited by Creese I. New York, Raven, 1983, pp 63–79

Khantzian EJ: Self-medication hypothesis of addictive disorders. Am J Psychiatry 142:1259–1264, 1985

Klawans HL, Margolin DI: Amphetamine induced dopaminergic hypersensitivity in guinea pigs. Arch Gen Psychiatry 32:723–732, 1975

Kokkinidis L, Azcharko RM, Predy PA: Post-amphetamine depression of self-stimulation responding from the substantia nigra: reversal with tricyclic antidepressants. Pharmacol Biochem Behav 13:379–383, 1980

Kramer JC: Introduction to amphetamine abuse. Journal of Psychedelic Drugs 2:1, 1969

Kramer JC, Fischman VS, Littlefield DC: Amphetamine abuse: pattern and effects of high doses taken intravenously. JAMA 201:305–309, 1967

Kuczenski R: Biochemical actions of amphetamine and other stimulants, in Stimulants: Neurochemical, Behavioral, and Clinical Perspectives. Edited by Creese I. New York, Raven, 1983

Leccese AP, Lyness WH: The effects of putative 5-hydroxytryptamine receptor active agents on d-amphetamine self-administration in controls and rats with 5,7 dihydroxytryptamine median forebrain bundle lesions. Brain Res 303:153–162, 1984

Leith NJ, Barret RJ: Effects of chronic amphetamine or reserpine on self stimulation responding: animal model of depression? Psychopharmacology (Berlin) 72:9–15, 1980

Lemberger L, Witt EI, Davis JM, et al: The effects of haloperidol and chlorpromazine on amphetamine metabolism and amphetamine stereotype behavior in the rat. J Pharmacol Exp Ther 174:428–433, 1970

Lucas AR, Weiss M: Methylphenidate hallucinosis. JAMA 217:1079–1081, 1971

Martin WR, Sloan JW, Sapira JD, et al: Physiologic, subjective and behavioral effects of amphetamine, methamphetamine, ephedrine, phenmetrazine and methylphenidate in man. Clin Pharmacol Ther 12:245–258, 1971

Masaki T: The amphetamine problem in Japan. WHO Tech Rep Ser 102: 14–21, 1956

McCormick TC Jr, McNeil TW: Acute psychosis and Ritalin abuse. Texas State Journal of Medicine 59:99–100, 1962

McLellan AT, Woody GE, O'Brien CP: Development of psychiatric illness in drug abusers. N Engl J Med 301:1310–1314, 1979

McLellan AT, Luborsky L, O'Brien CP, et al: Is treatment for substance abuse effective? JAMA 247:1423–1428, 1982

Molina VA, Orsingher OA: Effects of Mg-pemoline on the central catecholaminergic system. Arch Int Pharmacodyn Ther 251:66–79, 1981

Morgan JP: Amphetamine, in Substance Abuse: Clinical Perspectives and Problems. Edited by Lowinson JH, Ruiz P. Baltimore, MD, Williams & Wilkins, 1981, pp 167–184

Morgan JP, Kagan D: Street amphetamine quality and the controlled substances act of 1970, in Amphetamine Use, Misuse, and Abuse. Edited by Smith DE, Boston, MA, GK Hall, 1979

Nagahama M: A review of drug abuse and counter measures in Japan since World War II. UN Bulletin on Narcotics 20:19, 1968

National Institute on Drug Abuse: National household survey on drug abuse: main findings. Rockville, MD, National Institute on Drug Abuse, 1985

Nehra A, Mullick F, Ishak KG, et al: Pemoline-associated hepatic injury. Gastroenterology 99:1517–1519, 1990

Nichols DE: Differences between the mechanism of action of MDMA, MBDB, and the classic hallucinogens: identification of a new therapeutic class: entactogens. J Psychoactive Drugs 18:305–313, 1986

O'Flannagan PM, Taylor RB: A case of recurrent psychosis associated with amphetamine addiction. Journal of Mental Science 76:1033–1036, 1950

Oswald I, Thacore VR: Amphetamine and phenmetrazine addiction. Br Med J 427–431, 1963

Pickens R: Self administration of stimulants by rats. Int J Addict 3:215, 1968

Pickens R, Harris WC: Self administration of d-amphetamine by rats. Psychopharmacologia (Berlin) 12:158–163, 1968

Polchert SE, Morse RM: Pemoline abuse. JAMA 254:946–947, 1985

Pope HG: Drug abuse and psychopathology. N Engl J Med 301:1341–1342, 1979

Reifenstein EC Jr, Davidoff E: Benzedrine sulfate therapy, the present status. NY State J Med 42–57, 1939

Ricaurte GA, Forno LS, Wilson MA, et al: (±) 3,4-Methylenedioxymethamphetamine selectively damages central serotonergic neurons in nonhuman primates. JAMA 260:51–55, 1988

Riedlinger JE: The scheduling of MDMA: a pharmacists' perspective. J Psychoactive Drugs 17:167–171, 1985

Rioux B: Is Ritalin an addiction producing drug? Diseases of the Nervous System 21:346–349, 1960

Rumbaugh CL, Bergeron RT, Fang HXH, et al: Cerebrovascular changes secondary to amphetamine abuse in the experimental animal. Neuro-radiology 101:345–351, 1971

Rylander G: Clinical and medica-criminological aspects of addiction to central stimulating drugs, in Abuse of Central Stimulants. Edited by Sjoqvist F, Tottie M. Stockholm, Almqvist & Wiksell, 1969, pp 251–273

Sadusk JR: Non-narcotic addiction, size and extent of the problem. JAMA 196:707–709, 1966

Salanova V: Intracerebral haemorrhage and vasculitis secondary to amphetamine use. Postgrad Med J 60:429–430, 1984

Sato M: Psychotoxic manifestations in amphetamine abuse. Psychopharmacol Bull 22:751–756, 1986

Schuster CR: The behavioral pharmacology of psychomotor stimulant drugs, in Psychotropic Agents, Part II. Edited by Hoffmeister F, Stille G. New York, Springer-Verlag, 1981, pp 587–605

Segal DA, Mandell AJ: Long-term administration of d-amphetamine: progressive augmentation of motor activity and stereotypy. Pharmacol Biochem Behav 2:249–255, 1974

Seiden LS, Fischman MW, Schuster CR: Long-term methamphetamine induced changes in brain catecholamines in tolerant rhesus monkeys. Drug Alcohol Depend 1:215–219, 1975

Shaywitz SE, Hunt RD, Jatlow P, et al: Psychopharmacology of attention deficit disorder: pharmacokinetic, neuroendocrine and behavioral measures following acute and chronic treatment with methylphenidate. Pediatrics 69:688–694, 1982

Shulgin AT: The background and chemistry of MDMA. J Psychoactive Drugs 18:291–304, 1986

Silberman EK, Reus VI, Jimerson DC, et al: Heterogeneity of amphetamine response in depressed patients. Am J Psychiatry 138:1302–1307, 1981

Simpson DD: Treatment for drug abuse. Arch Gen Psychiatry 38:875–880, 1981

Smith DE: Analysis of variables in high dose methamphetamine dependence. Journal of Psychedelic Drugs 2:132–137, 1969

Smith DE, Fischer CM: An analysis of 310 cases of acute high-dose methamphetamine toxicity in Haight Ashbury. Clinical Toxicology 3:117–124, 1970

Smith GM, Beecher HK: Amphetamine sulfate and athletic performance. JAMA 170:542–557, 1959

Smith RC, Davis JM: Comparative effects of d-amphetamine, l-amphetamine and methylphenidate on mood in man. Psychopharmacology (Berlin) 53:1–12, 1977

Solanto MV: Neuropharmacological basis of stimulant drug action in attention deficit disorder with hyperactivity: a review and synthesis. Psychol Bull 94:387–409, 1984

Sternbach H: Pemoline-induced mania. Biol Psychiatry 16:987–989, 1981

Tennant FS Jr: Outpatient treatment and outcome of prescription drug abuse. Arch Intern Med 139:154–156, 1979

Tennant FS Jr: Treatment of dependence upon stimulants and hallucinogens. Drug Alcohol Depend 11:111–114, 1983

Tennant FS Jr, Rawson RA: Cocaine and amphetamine dependence treated with desipramine. Natl Inst Drug Abuse Res Monogr Ser 43:351–355, 1983

Tennant FS Jr, Swendseid ME: Alterations in catecholamine metabolism partially corrected during amphetamine-dependence. Drug Alcohol Depend 15:57–60, 1985

Tennant FS Jr, Tarver A, Pumphrey E: Double-blind comparison of desipramine and placebo for treatment of phencyclidine or amphetamine dependence. Natl Inst Drug Abuse Res Monogr Ser 67:310–317, 1986

Thompson T, Pickens T: Stimulant self-administration by animals: some comparisons with opiate self-administration. Federal Process 29:6–12, 1970

Van Kammen DP, Murphy DL: Attenuation of the euphoriant and activating effects of *d*- and *l*-amphetamine by lithium carbonate treatment. Psychopharmacologia (Berlin) 44:215–224, 1975

Watson R, Hartmann E, Schildkraut JJ: Amphetamine withdrawal: affective state, sleep patterns and MHPG excretion. Am J Psychiatry 129:263–269, 1972

Weiss B, Laties VG: Enhancement of human performance by caffeine and the amphetamines. Pharmacol Rev 14:1–36, 1962

Wesson DR: Propylhexedrine. Drug Alcohol Depend 17:273–278, 1986

Yu DSL, Smith FL, Smith DG, et al: Fluoxetine-induced attenuation of amphetamine self-administration in rats. Life Sci 39:1383–1388, 1986

Zametkin AJ, Karoum F, Linnoila M, et al: Stimulants, urinary catecholamines and indoleamines in hyperactivity: a comparison of methylphenidate and dextroamphetamine. Arch Gen Psychiatry 42:251–255, 1985

Chapter 7

Hallucinogens

Ulrich Tacke, M.D.
Michael H. Ebert, M.D.

The term *hallucinogens* refers to a chemically and pharmacologically heterogenous group of substances that have in common the potency to cause in the user a distortion of perception (hallucinations) and a mental state resembling psychosis. The term *hallucinogenic* emphasizes the perceptual effects. The term *psychotomimetic*, which is alternatively used to describe these drugs, emphasizes the similarity between their effect on affect, cognition, and perception and the symptoms of naturally occurring psychosis. The term *psychedelic* (mind-manifesting) is more vague but less restrictive and is also frequently used. Aside from naturally occurring plant-derived drugs (e.g., mescaline and psilocybin), these psychotomimetic substances also include semisynthetic (e.g., lysergic acid diethylamide [LSD]) and synthetic compounds (e.g., methylenedioxyamphetamine [MDA]). Frequently included in this group but discussed elsewhere are cannabis (Mendelson and Mello, Chapter 4, this volume) and phencyclidine (PCP) (Domino, Chapter 8, this volume). For practical purposes, the hallucinogens described here can be divided into tryptamine-related compounds, phenylalkylamines, and anticholinergics (Table 7-1).

Table 7-1.   Major groups of hallucinogens

Tryptamine-related compounds
  LSD (lysergic acid diethylamide)
  LSD derivatives contained in plants
    Morning glory seeds
  Dialkyltryptamines
    Psilocybin and psilocin
    DMT (*N,N*-dimethyltryptamine)
    DET (*N,N*-diethyltryptamine)
Phenylalkylamines
  Mescaline
  Synthetic amphetamine derivatives
    DOM (2,5-dimethoxy-4-methylamphetamine)
    MDA (3,4-methylenedioxyamphetamine)
    MDMA (3,4-methylenedioxymethamphetamine)
Anticholinergics
  Herbal anticholinergics
    Deadly nightshade (*Solanum dulcamara*)
    Atropa belladonna
    Jimsonweed (*Datura stramonium*)
  Prescription and nonprescription anticholinergics
    Antiparkinson drugs
      Trihexyphenidyl (Artane)
      Benztropine (Cogentin)
    Anticholinergics used in gastrointestinal disorders
    Over-the-counter antiasthma drugs

Note.   Phencyclidine (PCP) and cannabis not included here.

TRYPTAMINE-RELATED HALLUCINOGENS (INDOLEALKYLAMINES)

Tryptamine-related hallucinogens are naturally occurring plant alkaloids or their chemically synthesized derivatives. Some of them are related to substances (ergot alkaloids) produced by a rye-plant-inhabiting fungus (*Claviceps purpurea*).

Tryptamine itself is found in all major centers of the brain. Its physiologic role in central nervous system (CNS) function, however, remains unclear. 5-Hydroxytryptamine (5-HT, serotonin) is an important neurotransmitter in the CNS. The structural similarity of the tryptamine-related hallucinogens with 5-HT presumably forms the neurochemical basis for their action within the CNS.

History and Prevalence of
Abuse of Tryptamine-related Hallucinogens

The hallucinogenic and psychotomimetic effects of LSD were serendipitously discovered in 1943 by A. Hofmann, a chemist with a major Swiss pharmaceutical company who accidently ingested a minute quantity of the substance while working on ergot derivatives. His detailed report of his hallucinatory experience prompted intense research on this class of substances. It was believed that their experimental administration to normal volunteers could give new insights into the biochemical basis of psychosis. In the 1950s and 1960s, LSD was used by some psychiatrists in a variety of psychiatric patient populations, with the intention of accelerating the psychotherapeutic process by increasing insight and resurrecting repressed material. However, results from this "LSD-assisted psychotherapy" were not proven to be useful, and the therapeutic use of this substance was abandoned (Hollister 1986). In the mid-1960s, with the increasing public interest in the recreational use of mind-altering drugs, LSD found its way into American and European university campuses and countercultures. LSD was outlawed in the United States in 1968. Its abuse, however, increased during the 1970s and started to decline by 1980. Today, abuse is of a low-dose recreational type, and its level has been stable since 1985 (Robinson et al. 1987). Increased knowledge among users about dealing with "bad trips" (see below) has had an effect on the incidence of LSD-induced acute hallucinogenic crisis seen in the emergency room. However, other drugs (e.g., PCP and MDA), deceptively sold as LSD, or adulterants in street preparations (e.g., strychnine) continue to cause acute problems. The fact that LSD can be manufactured easily without profound knowledge in chemistry has helped make it a popular and profitable drug of abuse. Most of the different street names (Table 7-2) for LSD allude to the various forms in which the drug is offered to the consumer: as tablets (microdot), as capsules (blue devils or Mr. Natural), in gelatinous form (window pane), soaked on paper (blotter), or in Mickey Mouse decals (mickeys) (Giannini et al. 1986). Besides its oral use, LSD is also occasionally mixed with tobacco and smoked, or injected intravenously or subcutaneously. Morning glory seeds have been used in past cultures for religious ceremonies (Lewin et al. 1986). The small, black, round-shaped seeds of the flower *Ipomoea purpurea* and related varieties can be purchased from seed companies. Seeds are

Table 7-2. Street names of hallucinogens

LSD	Acid, blotter, blue devils, California sunshine, haze, microdot(s), mickeys, Mr. Natural, paper acid, purple haze, sunshine, wedges, window pane(s)
Morning glory seeds	Flying saucers, licorice drops, heavenly gates, pearly gates
Psilocybin	Magic mushroom, mushroom
DMT, DET	Businessman's lunch, snuff
Peyote/mescaline	Button(s), cactus, mesc, mescal, mescal buttons, moon, peyote
DOM	Golden eagle, STP, psychodrine, tile
MDA	Love drug
MDMA	Adam, ecstasy, MDM, XTC
MDEA	Eve

Note. LSD = lysergic acid diethylamide. DMT = *N,N*-dimethyltryptamine. DET = *N,N*-diethyltryptamine. DOM = 2,5-dimethoxy-4-methylamphetamine. MDA = methylenedioxyamphetamine. MDMA = methylenedioxymethamphetamine. MDEA = 3,4-methylenedioxyethamphetamine.

sometimes sprayed with paraquat to discourage inappropriate usage. However, dipping the seeds in ether effectively dissolves the herbicide (Giannini et al. 1986). Ingestion of the seeds produces an hallucinatory state that is due to the LSD-related compounds lysergol, D-lysergic acid amide, and D-isolysergic acid amide. Street names refer to the appearance of the seeds, or to the commercial names by which the seeds are marketed by seed companies (Table 7-2).

Psilocybin and psilocin were isolated and identified from the hallucinogenic mushroom *Psilocybe mexicana* in 1958 by Hoffman (Nichols 1986). "Magic" or "sacred" mushrooms have been used by American Indians for religious purposes since pre-Columbian times. Many of the psilocybin-containing mushrooms are found in different parts of the United States. Most of them belong to the genus *Psilocybe*, which includes about 100 species; however, not all of them contain psilocybin (Lincoff and Mitchel 1977). The outstanding feature of the psychotropic *Psilocybe* species is the color change to blue or blue-green on the cap or stalk from handling or age. *Psilocybe caerulipes* (blue foot) grows on debris under trees or rotting logs; *Psilocybe cubensis* can be found on rich pastures where it grows on dung (Lincoff and Mitchel 1977).

Psilocybin intoxication is seen either as accidental poisoning from ingestion of mushrooms falsely regarded as eatable, or from intentional seeking of a hallucinogenic "high." Although United States law prohibits shipping of mushrooms across state lines, the purchase of *Psilocybe cubensis* spores as mail-order kits for domestic cultivation has become part of the drug culture (Kulberg 1986; Kulberg et al. 1986). Sporadic cases of intravenous use of hallucinogenic mushrooms have been reported in the United States (Curry and Rose 1985) and in Australia (Sivyer and Dorrington 1984).

DMT (N,N-dimethyltryptamine) and DET (N_2N-diethyltryptamine) are constituents of snuff (cohoba) prepared from seeds and pods of *Piptademia peregrina*, a plant native to the West Indies and to Central and South America. Similar snuffs from other South American plants (Epena and Yopo snuffs) have been found to contain DMT 5-methoxy-DMT and bufotenine (5-hydroxy-DMT), a hallucinogenic substance originally isolated from the secretion of the skin glands of the poisonous toad *Bufo vulgaris*. DMT- and DET-containing *Piptademia* preparations can also be smoked, and the synthetic form of DMT is sometimes used by intravenous or intramuscular injection. DMT is known as snuff, or the businessman's lunch, the latter name referring to the high incidence of abuse in this particular population and the short duration of action (about 30 minutes).

Pharmacology of Tryptamine-related Hallucinogens

Pharmacokinetics. All drugs of this class are well absorbed from the gastrointestinal tract. LSD is the most potent hallucinogen known, with oral doses as low as 20–25 μg being sufficient for a marked sympathomimetic effect (Strassman 1984). Twice that amount ingested by a 160-pound man can produce an hallucinatory state lasting up to 12 hours. All of the structural modifications made to the LSD molecule have yielded less potent compounds. Also plant preparations containing LSD-like substances cause psychotomimetic symptoms at relatively low doses; for example, five morning glory seeds may be sufficient for a high of 12 hours or longer (Giannini et al. 1986). LSD is longer acting (8–12 hours) and more potent than psilocybin or psilocin (average duration of action, 4–12 hours). One or two mushrooms of the *Psilocybe* family (equivalent to about 20–70 mg of active substance) can produce hallucinosis for 4–12 hours. When inhaled, smoked, or used parenterally, DMT and DET show a short duration of action, limiting the psychotomimetic experience to not more than 30 minutes.

The impairment of cognitive functioning in healthy volunteers receiving LSD intravenously has been shown to correlate positively with the plasma concentration of the drug. Tryptamine-related compounds are mainly cleared by the liver; LSD concentrations in the urine are extremely low. Since the complete, intact structure of the LSD molecule is crucial for its biological activity, there are no active metabolites. Most LSD metabolites are excreted in the feces (Strassman 1984). Psilocybin is hydrolyzed in vivo to generate psilocin, which represents the active hallucinogen (Nichols 1986). DMT and DET undergo extensive first-pass oxidation, which makes these drugs ineffective after oral ingestion (Nichols 1986).

Mechanism of action. Although the exact mechanisms of action of LSD and other tryptamine-related compounds are still incompletely understood (Freedman 1986), there is convincing evidence relating the psychotomimetic effects of these substances to serotonergic transmission in the brain (Davis 1987; Freedman 1986; McCall 1986). An antagonism of 5-HT and LSD can be appreciated from the fact that a 15% depletion of 5-HT in the rat brain is sufficient to cause a decrease in the threshold dose of LSD by fourfold (Appel and Freedman 1964). Receptor binding studies have shown that ^{3}H-LSD labels $5-HT_2$ receptors in neuronal tissue (Peroutka 1987). LSD also binds with high affinity to a subtype of the $5-HT_1$ receptor ($5-HT_{1c}$), a site that also displays a high affinity for 5-HT (Glennon et al. 1986; Peroutka 1987).

The action of 5-HT on brain neuronal systems is complex; depending on the neurons involved, it can induce inhibition or excitation. Experiments with iontophoretic application of LSD to neurons have shown that 5-HT-induced excitation is invariably blocked by LSD, whereas LSD mimics inhibition at sites where 5-HT exerts an inhibiting effect (Aghajanian et al. 1987; Martin and Sloane 1986). Tryptamine itself is found in all major regions of the brain and produces pharmacologic effects that are similar to those seen with LSD, psilocybin, DMT, and the hallucinogens of the phenylalkylamine-group (mescaline and 2, 5,-dimethoxy-4-methylamphetamine [DOM]) (Martin and Sloane 1986). Inhibitory serotonergic input to the raphe nuclei, the cortex, and the limbic system is regarded as essential for the filtering of extracerebral (perception) and intracerebral (feeling and cognition) stimuli (Strassman 1984). It has been hypothesized that an inhibition of these serotonergic functions, which normally process physical and mental events as they arise, may lead to the experience of common stimuli as novel or "psychedelic." The dense innervation of the limbic and visual systems by 5-HT axons could make them a major target for this hallucinogenic disinhibition, leading to the major clinical drug effects: alteration of affect and visual hallucinations. LSD and other tryptamine-related compounds (psilocin and DMT) have been shown to produce a complete but reversible inhibition of the serotonin-mediated neuronal discharges in the raphe nucleus (McCall 1986). The relationship of this phenomenon to the hallucinogenic action of these compounds is stressed by the finding that brom-LSD, a nonhallucinogenic analogue of LSD, does not influence 5-HT neuronal discharge.

However, simple disinhibition of 5-HT neurons originating in the raphe cannot explain the following findings. First, lisuride, which is devoid of hallucinogenic properties, is 5–10 times more potent than LSD in blocking neuronal firing in the raphe. Second, the psychotomimetic effect of LSD lasts considerably longer than its inhibitory effect on raphe neuron firing. Third, while tolerance develops to the behavioral effects of LSD, no such tolerance can be seen for its neurophysiologic action. It has been proposed that a mechanism of 5-HT receptor sensitization may account for the psychedelic action of the hallucinogens (McCall 1986). This mechanism of action is similar to the 5-HT$_2$ agonist effect of the phenylalkylamines (Davis 1987; Hollister 1986), which may actually be the neurochemical substrate of hallucinogenic action in general (Lyon et al. 1988).

Acute and Chronic Effects of Tryptamine-related Hallucinogens

Clinical symptoms of LSD intoxication. Since the minimal lethal or toxic dose of LSD is not very well established in the literature, assessment of severity of intoxication should always be made on clinical grounds. The DSM-III-R (American Psychiatric Association 1987) criteria for hallucinogenic hallucinosis are presented in Table 7-3. The normally used quantity of LSD ingested ranges from 30 to 400 µg, but doses as low as 20 µg may cause clinically detectable symptoms (Strassman 1984). However, tolerance to the effect of LSD develops relatively quickly, so that chronic users will increase their dose over time.

Because of the rapid absorption from the gastrointestinal tract, symptoms start to occur within 30 minutes. Drug effects are at a

Table 7-3. DSM-III-R diagnostic criteria for hallucinogen hallucinosis

A. Recent use of a hallucinogen.
B. Maladaptive behavioral changes, e.g., marked anxiety or depression, ideas of reference, fear of losing one's mind, paranoid ideation, impaired judgment, impaired social or occupational functioning.
C. Perceptual changes occurring in a state of full wakefulness and alertness, e.g., subjective intensification of perceptions, depersonalization, derealization, illusions, hallucinations, synesthesias.
D. At least two of the following signs:
    (1) pupillary dilation
    (2) tachycardia
    (3) sweating
    (4) palpitations
    (5) blurring of vision
    (6) tremors
    (7) incoordination
E. Not due to any physical or other mental disorder.

Source.   Reprinted with permission from American Psychiatric Association (1987).

maximum at 1–4 hours after ingestion of the drug, with the symptoms subsiding during the following 8–16 hours. The predominant effects with small doses are autonomic nervous system changes and alterations of mood; higher doses cause the typical perceptional distortions and subjective changes in body image. Vegetative symptoms are mostly sympathomimetic (tachycardia, rise in blood pressure, mydriasis, and hyperthermia). However, a central parasympathomimetic component (diaphoresis, vomiting, and diarrhea) may complicate the clinical picture. Extreme agitation and marked muscular rigidity, causing lactic acidosis in combination with hyperthermia, should raise suspicion of adulteration of the ingested LSD by strychnine (Kulberg 1986).

The subjective experience under LSD is dependent on the personality of the user, his or her expectations, and the setting in which the drug is taken. While some subjects experience a state of excitement and activity, others become quiet and passive and withdraw from their surroundings. Changes of mood range from anxiety to ecstasy. Feelings of euphoria with symptoms of excitation are the most constant mood changes encountered during an LSD high. Episodes of depression and panic ("bad trip") may follow, or alternate with, the elevated state of affect (Strassman 1984).

The effect of LSD on perception is sometimes referred to as

"illusiogenic," since, rather than creating a perception of a nonexisting stimulus, LSD produces a distortion of the real sensory input from the environment (Kulberg 1986). Visual symptoms are most frequently experienced; for example, vision may be blurred, and the perception of distance and depth may be changed. Objects in the surroundings may be perceived as unusually intense in color, shape, and/or size. With the eyes closed, geometric and kaleidoscopic patterns are perceived. Synesthesia, by which a sensory stimulus of one modality is transformed into a perception from another sense, is a type of a perceptual distortion typically experienced under the influence of LSD; for example, smells and tactile stimuli seem to be visible, and colors become audible (Kulberg 1986). "Out-of-body" experiences, loss of ego boundaries causing the perception of being one with objects or others, and depersonalization are typical LSD-induced distortions of body image. Delusions of supernatural capabilities (e.g., the ability to fly) may lead to injury or death; suicidal impulses may also emerge during or after the acute state of intoxication. Tactile, gustatory, and olfactory hallucinations are frequently reported; auditory hallucinations are only rarely experienced. Insight into the drug-induced nature of these experiences is usually retained. Following the euphoric state with intense and vivid perceptions, reality is frequently experienced as dull and uninteresting after the acute toxic symptoms have subsided.

"Bad trip" describes a state of frightening illusions and panic that may be experienced instead of the heightened emotions and enjoyable hallucinations described above. This is frequently accompanied by the fear of insanity (Frosch et al. 1965; Kulberg 1986). Flashbacks in LSD users are reported to occur with an incidence of 15–77%. These spontaneous recurrences of symptoms may range from mild confusion to repeated intrusions into awareness of images from a previous LSD state. Flashbacks are most frequent during the first months following drug use and may be precipitated by periods of stress and anxiety. If the drug is not taken again, the frequency of flashbacks gradually decreases with time (Kulberg 1986).

Prolonged adverse reactions after the use of LSD (such as psychosis, paranoid states, or depression) have been reported (Cohen and Ditman 1962; Frosch et al. 1965; Hatrick and Dewhurst 1970; Strassman 1984). However, many of the reported cases have been in chronic schizophrenic patients and in subjects with personality disorders. Whether normal subjects are at risk for psychosis as a late adverse reaction after the use of LSD is not known.

High doses of LSD may cause chromosome damage in experimental animals (Dishotsky et al. 1971). In humans, chromosomal aberrations have been found to be related to drug abuse in general. Pharmacologically pure LSD, however, has not been demonstrated to cause a detectable increase in chromosome damage.

Treatment of LSD intoxication.   Patients with LSD-induced disorders come to the attention of medical care providers because of an acute overdose, because of a panic reaction during acute intoxication (bad trip), or because of episodes of flashbacks (Kulberg 1986; Slaby et al. 1981; Strassman 1984). LSD concentrations in body fluids are extremely low because of its high potency and its extensive metabolism, which poses a difficult analytical problem. Radioimmunoassay, high-pressure liquid chromatography, and gas chromatograph-mass spectrometry methods for LSD have been developed, but are rarely available for analysis in clinical settings. A routine urine drug screen does not reveal LSD. It helps, however, to rule out other intoxicants.

If the patient has ingested a substantial amount ($> 200 \ \mu g/kg$) of the drug fairly recently (ideally within 30 minutes) and is not obtunded, comatose, or convulsing, gastric lavage is most efficient in removing yet unabsorbed drug from the stomach. If this is not possible, emesis may be induced using ipecac syrup (children 1–12 years old, 15 ml; older children and adults, 30 ml). If emesis does not occur after the first dose, ipecac may be repeated once after 30 minutes. In most patients seen in the emergency room for symptoms from LSD intoxication, nearly complete absorption of the drug is most likely to have already occurred.

Convulsions are treated with diazepam given slowly intravenously (children, 0.1–0.3 mg/kg; adults, 10 mg; may be repeated if necessary). Acute anxiety can be managed with oral diazepam (adults, 5–20 mg). In the treatment of hallucinosis or acute delusions, neuroleptics should be used with great caution because they may induce or worsen hypotension and may cause convulsions through their effect of lowering the seizure threshold. Reassuring the patient that the alterations in his or her perception are due to the ingested drug ("talking down") is helpful in cases of acute anxiety. Placing the patient in a dimly lighted, quiet room and giving cues for orientation to place and time will assist in calming the patient. If hospitalization does not seem necessary, an outpatient clinic appointment should be made. Steps should be taken to ensure that a reliable person can look after the patient until symptoms have subsided completely.

Patients seen for flashbacks are treated with oral diazepam (adults, 15–30 mg) if symptoms of anxiety are severe (Rumack 1987). Neuroleptics, especially haloperidol, have been implicated in causing a transient increase in visual flashbacks and are not recommended (Moskowitz 1971; Strassman 1984). The patient needs assurance of the self-limiting nature of the phenomenon and its decreasing frequency of reoccurrence with time. The patient has to understand that any future use of hallucinogens or marijuana may precipitate similar symptoms (Strassman 1984). In those cases in which hospitalization is not necessary, arrangements for outpatient follow-up should be made.

Symptoms and treatment of intoxication with other tryptamine-related compounds (morning glory seeds, psilocybin, DMT, and DET). Clinical symptoms after ingestion of these substances are quite similar to LSD toxicity, including restlessness, nausea, and autonomic hyperactivity. Intoxication from mushrooms of the *Psilocybe* variety cause ataxia, hyperkinesis, and anticholinergic effects and chromatopsia (in which colorless objects are perceived to be in color) (Giannini et al. 1986). Clinical symptoms start 15–30 minutes after ingestion of the poisonous mushrooms. Psilocybin or morning glory seed intoxications are rarely fatal. DET and DMT may cause LSD-like clinical symptoms that are, however, much shorter lasting.

Therapeutic measures for the treatment of intoxication from psilocybin or morning glory seeds are the same as described above for LSD—that is, gastric lavage or induction of emesis with ipecac, treatment of anxiety with diazepam, and reassurance and psychological support (Rumack 1987). Acute treatment of DET or DMT intoxication in an emergency room setting is rarely necessary. Antipsychotics should be used with great caution, since the patient may have been exposed to PCP or DOM, which are frequently found as adulterants of street drugs. If these drugs are responsible for the clinical condition of the patient, antipsychotics may make symptoms worse.

PHENYLALKYLAMINE HALLUCINOGENS

The hallucinogenic substances of this group show a close structural resemblance to the catecholamines: noradrenaline and dopamine. The prototype structure is given by mescaline, a naturally occurring substance. Modification of the mescaline molecule has led to synthetic amphetamine derivatives with hallucinogenic action.

History and Prevalence of Abuse of Mescaline (Peyote)

Mescaline (3, 4, 5-trimethoxyphenylethylamine) is the hallucinogenic substance found in the peyote cactus (*Lophophora williamsii*), which is characterized by its red or pink flowers and soft spikes. One dried flower top of the cactus (mescal button) contains 6–45 mg of the active substance (Kulberg 1986), which represents up to 6% of its mass. Mescaline was isolated from peyote in 1896 and was synthesized in 1918. For centuries, peyote has played an important role in the religious ceremonies of the Indians of northern Mexico and southwestern United States. A "peyote cult" was established in the United States in the late 19th century, leading to the foundation of the Native American Church in 1918. In this congregation, the use of peyote as a religious sacrament during church services is legal under United States law.

   Peyote is ingested fresh (as whole dried buttons) or as powder (loose in capsules or pressed into tablets). Mescaline sold on the street (see Table 7-2) is generally not what it is claimed to be, but is most likely one of the following: DOM, PCP, LSD, caffeine, or amphetamine-related stimulants (Kulberg 1986). Only when the cactus buttons are found with the patient can there be certainty that the drug in question is peyote (mescaline) (Giannini et al. 1986).

History and Prevalence of Abuse of Hallucinogenic Phenylalkylamine Derivatives

The substituted phenethylamines, consisting of approximately 50 substances, form the largest chemical group of hallucinogenic substances known. The almost unlimited possibilities for modification of the amphetamine molecule encourages the development of "designer drugs," which are illegally synthesized in underground laboratories to supply the drug market with novel, yet unscheduled compounds, thus keeping the drug scene one step ahead of the law (Baum 1985). All hallucinogenic amphetamine-derivatives have structural similarities with mescaline as well as amphetamine; their clinical effects more or less mimic LSD.

DOM was found to be the active compound of the street drug "STP." The origin of this abbreviation remains obscure (one suggested explanation: *s*erenity, *t*ranquility, *p*eace). DOM or STP appeared on the North American drug scene in the late 1960s, but it lost importance during the last decade. The 4-bromo homolog of DOM has been sold in some cities as MDA or LSD.

MDMA (3,4-methylenedioxymethamphetamine) was synthesized in 1914 as an appetite suppressant but was never marketed (Dowling et al. 1987). In the early 1970s, it appeared on the United States drug scene under various street names (Table 7-2), the most popular being "ecstasy." It has also been used by some psychiatrists as an adjunct to psychotherapy (Dowling et al. 1987); the claims for a possible therapeutic benefit were basically the same as for the use of LSD 30 years ago (Hollister 1986).

Since 1983, MDMA has become very popular among American college students. It is sold as 100-mg "hits" in gelatin capsules or as loose powder that is sometimes mixed with juice. In 1985, MDMA was placed under an emergency Schedule I classification, mainly because of its rapidly increasing popularity and its similarity to MDA (see below). Although still available on the illicit drug market, it has been largely replaced by the nonscheduled, chemically related 3,4-methylenedioxyethamphetamine (MDEA) (Dowling et al. 1987).

MDA, the *N*-methylated derivative of MDMA, is a potent stimulant that was originally investigated by the U.S. Army as an incapacitating agent (Simpson and Rumack 1981). In the 1960s it became a popular drug of abuse. Its reputation as a safe recreational drug ("love drug"), providing the user with a "tranquil psychedelic experience," suffered from reports of several fatal intoxications (Climko et al. 1987). Some of the "ecstasy" sold to the user as MDMA is in reality MDA. Reports from clinical studies done several decades ago do not support the hallucinogenic nature of MDA, but instead indicated its closer relationship with the amphetamine stimulants.

Pharmacology of Hallucinogenic Phenylalkylamines

Pharmacokinetics of mescaline. This drug is considerably less potent than LSD; equipotent amounts are 5 mg and 1 μg, respectively. Peyote is readily absorbed from the gastrointestinal tract. Mescaline is mainly concentrated in the liver, spleen, and kidney. Up to 60% is excreted unchanged in the urine; mescaline metabolites are devoid of any psychoactive effect.

Clinical symptoms are similar to those seen in LSD intoxication. Nausea and vomiting occur 30 minutes to 2 hours after ingestion. Other symptoms are mydriasis, diaphoresis, hypertension, dizziness, and chills (Mack 1986). The hallucinogenic effects peak at 5–6 hours after ingestion of the drug (Kulberg 1986). Vivid colors, kaleidoscopic visions, and synesthesias similar to those experienced after LSD have been reported. The user may hallucinate that he or she is followed by marching geometric shapes; this symptom has been claimed to be pathognomonic for mescaline intoxication. After about 14 hours, when the effects of the drug have vanished, excellent recall of the experience is maintained. Since this is different from the state after PCP intoxication, it can have some practical significance for the differential diagnosis; on the street, PCP is frequently sold as mescaline (Giannini et al. 1986).

The lethal dose of mescaline varies because of the development of tolerance to the action of the drug. After a massive overdose, hypotension, bradycardia, CNS depression, and respiratory failure may be life threatening. Although fatal intoxications from mescaline are rare, they are usually attributed to traumatic fatalities resulting from altered perceptions.

Clinical toxicology of hallucinogenic amphetamine derivatives. Effective doses range from 1 to 5 mg for DOM and from 50 to 150 mg for MDMA. MDMA is well absorbed after ingestion, and its peak effect is experienced at about 1–5 hours. Three phases of action are frequently described by MDMA users. First there is an initial phase of disorientation. This is followed by a "rush," during which tingling and jerking movements in the extremities are experienced. The paresthesias and myoclonus subside within 1–4 hours and are followed by a short period (30–60 minutes) of "happy sociability" (Dowling et al. 1987). Death after the use of MDMA or MDEA is rare, but may occur due to induction of cardiac arrhythmias or as a consequence of risk-taking behavior. After the acute effects of MDMA, symptoms like anxiety, depression, and confusion may follow and, in some cases, continue for several weeks (Dowling et al. 1987). Due to its strong peripheral serotonin agonist effect, DOM may cause severe vasospasm (Bowen et al. 1983).

Mechanism of action. Behavioral effects of mescaline apparently result from an agonist action at the $5-HT_2$ receptors (Aghajanian and Haigler 1975). This hypothesis is supported by findings showing that $5-HT_2$ receptor antagonists are able to block selectively the increased reactivity of locus coeruleus neurons produced by these substances and that the potency of various phenylethylamine hallucinogens in producing this effect correlates well with their order of potency in binding to the $5-HT_2$ receptor (Aghajanian et al. 1987). In fact, since the agonist action at the $5-HT_2$ receptor is the one characteristic that the hallucinogenic indolealkylamines and phenylethylamines have in common, it has been proposed that this could be the ultimate neurochemical substrate for their behavioral and psychological effects (Aghajanian and Haigler 1975).

The mode of action of the amphetamine derivatives MDA and MDMA seems to be dissimilar, with MDMA possessing mescaline-like psychoactive properties. MDMA demonstrates greater serotonergic effects than does the more amphetamine-like MDA.

Treatment of Mescaline Intoxication

Active drug and metabolites can be detected from the urine by thin-layer chromatography, gas-liquid chromatography, or gas chromatography-mass spectrometry. However, assays are available only at specialized centers. Treatment of acute intoxication is virtually identical to the treatment outlines given for LSD intoxication. DOM-induced vasospasm responds well to intra-arterial tolazoline or sodium nitroprusside. Major life-threatening complications of hallucinogenic amphetamine derivatives include hyperthermia, hypertension, convulsions, cardiovascular collapse, and self-inflicted trauma.

ANTICHOLINERGICS

Anticholinergic Plants and Synthetic Anticholinergic Agents

Atropine and its ether analog scopolamine (hyoscine) are potent alkaloids that are found as active compounds in a large number of plants around the world (belladonna alkaloids).

The "deadly nightshades" ("European bittersweet," *Solanum dulcamara* or "belladonna," *Atropa belladonna*) were used in the Middle Ages as witches' brew. Intoxication from both plants mainly occurs in children who ingest the fruits or flowers because of their attractive appearance.

Jimsonweed (*Datura stramonium*, thorn apple, or "locoweed"), another member of the Solanaceae family, is found throughout the United States. The plant has large, jagged, bitter-tasting leaves, and large white or purple trumpet-like flowers. In the fall, the plant bears fruit in the form of thorny capsules, which contain brown or black seeds. All parts of the plant are poisonous; the seeds contain about 4% of anticholinergic alkaloids (scopolamine, hyoscyamine, and atropine). While accidental childhood poisonings with jimsonweed have been seen in the past, during the last 20 years there has been an increased incidence of inadvertent overdose in persons experimenting with mind-altering drugs (Goldfrank 1986). Leaves of the plant can be eaten raw, prepared as a tea, or smoked. There is even a preparation of *Datura stramonium* available in health food stores where it is sold as an asthma drug (Goldfrank 1986). Alkaloid contents of plants of the Solanaceae family vary between seasons and from year to year, which makes it difficult to make clinical inferences from the amount ingested; as little as 4–5 g of crude leaf from jimsonweed may be lethal for a child. Adolescents and young adults are known to smoke the dried leaves or consume the dried seeds to induce a state of toxic delirium.

Trihexyphenidyl (Artane), and benztropine (Cogentin) are prescription drugs used in the treatment both of Parkinson's disease and of extrapyramidal side effects from neuroleptic medication. They are occasionally abused for their mind-altering properties at toxic doses (Perry et al. 1978). Abusers often try to obtain these drugs by false representation of extrapyramidal symptoms, which are claimed to result from the use of phenothiazines or other neuroleptics (Rubinstein 1978).

Certain antiasthma drugs available in health food stores contain preparations from belladonna or stramonium leaves (Goldfrank 1986). Gastrointestinal anticholinergics containing atropine sulfate are used as adjunctive therapy for peptic ulcers and in other gastrointestinal conditions (e.g., functional diarrhea). Scopolamine has been introduced for the treatment of motion sickness. Over-the-counter sleeping pills containing scopolamine are also occasionally abused for their effect on the CNS.

Clinical Findings in Anticholinergic Intoxication

The clinical picture of anticholinergic intoxication is governed by the muscarinic effects of the drug (Table 7–4). Mydriasis is a consistent finding. Dry mouth, decreased gastrointestinal motility, urinary retention, tachycardia with dysrhythmias, and hyperpyrexia with a dry, flushed skin are also typically seen. These symptoms are markedly different from the sympathomimetic effects seen after the majority of the hallucinogens discussed above. Lilliputian hallucinations are frequently reported as a symptom of anticholinergic intoxication (Goldfrank 1986). Insight into the drug-induced nature of the sensory distortions and recall of the vivid illusions are typically lost (Shulgin 1981). In patients with narrow-angle glaucoma, anticholinergics may precipitate an acute attack.

Treatment of Anticholinergic Intoxication

Prevention of absorption. If the ingestion of the anticholinergic has been recent, and the patient is not obtunded or convulsing, gastric lavage or emesis with ipecac is indicated. Since absorption of the drug is slow due to the reduced motility of the gut, oral administration of activated charcoal and a cathartic enhances the probability of removing substantial amounts of unabsorbed drug.

Antidote treatment. In case of severe hallucinations, myoclonic seizures, hypertension, or arrhythmias, the anticholinesterase physostigmine is the drug of choice (Goldfrank 1986); it also can help to confirm the diagnosis in unclear cases. The effective dose of physo-

---

Table 7-4. Symptoms of anticholinergic intoxication

Peripheral signs
　　Mydriasis, tachycardia, hyperthermia, decreased salivation, dryness of skin and mucous membranes, facial flushing, difficulty urinating
Central symptoms
　　Visual hallucinations, drowsiness, distortion of body image, amnesia, heatstroke (from hyperthermia at high environmental temperatures)

stigmine is 0.5 mg in children and 1–2 mg (0.01–0.03 mg/kg) in adults, given im or iv over 2–5 minutes. Slow administration is essential because physostigmine may cause seizures if administered too rapidly. This dose may be repeated in 20–30 minutes if toxic effects persist and no cholinergic effect is produced. Since signs of cholinergic excess (bradycardia, heart block, and excessive secretions) may develop rapidly, use of physostigmine should be reserved for the intensive care setting. Neostigmine and pyridostigmine, which are quaternary amines, do not cross the blood-brain barrier and hence lack effect on the CNS. Relative contraindications to use of anticholinesterase treatment include a history of cardiovascular disease, asthma, glaucoma, and gastrointestinal or genitourinary obstruction. Symptomatic treatment of tachyarrhythmias with propranolol may be considered; beta-blockers, however, are less effective than physostigmine.

REFERENCES

Aghajanian GK, Haigler HJ: Hallucinogenic indoleamines: preferential action upon presynaptic serotonin receptors. Psychopharmacol Commun 1:619–629, 1975

Aghajanian GK, Sprouse JS, Rasmussen K: Physiology of the midbrain serotonin system, in Psychopharmacology: The Third Generation of Progress. Edited by Meltzer HY. New York, Raven, 1987, pp 141–149

American Psychiatric Association: Diagnostic and Statistical Manual of Mental Disorders, 3rd Edition, Revised. Washington, DC, American Psychiatric Association, 1987

Appel JB, Freedman DX: Chemically-induced alterations in the behavioral effects of LSD-25. Biochem Pharmacol 13:861–869, 1964

Baum RM: New variety of street drugs poses growing problem. Chemical Engineering News 63:7–16, 1985

Bowen JS, Davis GB, Kearney TE, et al: Diffuse vascular spasm associated with 4-bromo-2,5-dimethoxyamphetamine ingestion. JAMA 249:1477–1479, 1983

Climko RP, Roehrich H, Sweeney DR, et al: Ecstacy: a review of MDMA and MDA. Int J Psychiatry Med 16:359–369, 1987

Cohen S, Ditman K: Complications associated with lysergic acid diethylamide (LSD-25). JAMA 181:161–162, 1962

Curry SC, Rose MC: Intravenous mushroom poisoning. Ann Emerg Med 14:900–902, 1985

Davis M: Mescaline: excitatory effects on acoustic startle are blocked by serotonin 2 antagonists. Psychopharmacology (Berlin) 93:286–291, 1987

Dishotsky NI, Lougham WD, Mogar RE, et al: LSD and genetic damage. Science 172:431–440, 1971

Dowling GP, Mcdonough ET, Bost RO: 'Eve' and 'ecstasy': a report of five deaths associated with the use of MDEA and MDMA. JAMA 257: 1615–1617, 1987

Freedman DX. Hallucinogenic drug research: if so, so what? symposium summary and commentary. Pharmacol Biochem Behav 24:407–415, 1986

Frosch W, Robbins E, Stern M: Untoward reactions to lysergic acid diethylamide (LSD) resulting in hospitalization. N Engl J Med 273:1235–1239, 1965

Giannini AJ, Price WA, Giannini MC: Contemporary drugs of abuse. Am Fam Physician 33:207–216, 1986

Glennon RA, Titeler M, Young R: Structure-activity relationships and mechanism of action or hallucinogenic agents based on drug discrimination and radioligand binding studies. Psychopharmacol Bull 22:953–958, 1986

Goldfrank LR: Anticholinergic plant poisoning: jimson weed, in Goldfrank's Toxicologic Emergencies. Edited by Goldfrank LR, et al. Norwalk, CT, Appleton-Century-Crofts, 1986, pp 602–608

Hatrick JK, Dewhurst K: Delayed psychosis due to LSD. Lancet 2:742–744, 1970

Hollister L: Clinical aspects of abuse of phenylalkylamine and indolealkylamine hallucinogens. Psychopharmacol Bull 22:977–979, 1986

Kulberg A: Substance abuse: clinical identification and management. Pediatr Clin North Am 33:325–361, 1986

Kulberg AG, Goldfrank LR, Bresnitz EA: Mushrooms: toxic and hallucinogenic, in Goldfrank's Toxicologic Emergencies. Edited by Goldfrank LR, et al. Norwalk, CT, Appleton-Century-Crofts, 1986, pp 545–557

Lewin NA, Howland MA, Goldfrank LR, et al: Herbal preparations, in Goldfrank's Toxicologic Emergencies. Edited by Goldfrank LR, et al. Norwalk, CT, Appleton-Century-Crofts, 1986, pp 560–577

Lincoff GH, Mitchel DH: Toxic and Hallucinogenic Mushroom Poisoning: A Handbook for Physicians and Mushroom Hunters. Edited by Williams WK. New York, Van Nostrand Reinhold, 1977

Lyon RA, Titeler M, Seggel MR, et al: Indolealkylamines analogs share 5-HT2 binding characteristics with phenylalkylamine hallucinogens. Eur J Pharmacol 145:291–297, 1988

Mack RB: Marching to a different cactus: peyote (mescaline) intoxication. N Engl J Med 47:137–138, 1986

Martin WR, Sloan JW: Relationship of CNS tryptaminergic processes and the action of LSD-like hallucinogens. Pharmacol Biochem Behav 24: 393–399, 1986

McCall R: Effects of hallucinogenic drugs on serotoninergic neuronal systems. Pharmacol Biochem Behav 24:359:363, 1986

Moskowitz D: Use of haloperidol to reduce LSD flashbacks. Milit Med 136:754–757, 1971

Nichols DE: Studies of the relationship between molecular structure and hallucinogenic activity. Pharmacol Biochem Behav 24:335–340, 1986

Peroutka SJ: Serotonin receptors, in Psychopharmacology: The Third Generation of Progress. Edited by Meltzer HY. New York, Raven, 1987, pp 303–311

Perry PJ, Wilding OC, Juhl RP: Anticholinergic psychosis. Am J Hosp Pharm 35:725, 1978

Robinson TN, Killen JD, Taylor CB, et al: Perspectives on adolescent substance use: a defined population study. JAMA 258:2072–2076, 1987

Rubinstein JS: Abuse of antiparkinson drugs: feigning of extrapyramidal symptoms to obtain trihexyphenidyl. JAMA 239:2365, 1978

Rumack BH (ed): LSD, in Poisindex, Vol 54. Denver, CO, Micromedex, 1987

Schmidt CJ. Neurotoxicity of the psychodelic amphetamine, methylenedioxymethamphetamine. J Pharmacol Exp Ther 240:1–7, 1987

Shulgin AT: Hallucinogens, in Burger's Medicinal Chemistry, 4th Edition, part 3. Edited by Wolff ME. New York, John Wiley, 1981, pp 1109–1137

Simpson DL, Rumack BH: Methylenedioxyamphetamine: clinical description of overdose, death, and review of pharmacology. Arch Intern Med 141:1507–1509, 1981

Sivyer G, Dorrington L: Intravenous injection of mushrooms (letter). Med J Aust 140:182, 1984

Slaby AE, Lieb J, Trancredi LR: Handbook of Psychiatric Emergencies, 2nd Edition. Garden City, NY, Medical Examination Publishing, 1981

Strassman R: Adverse reactions to psychedelic drugs: a review of the literature. J Nerv Ment Dis 172:577–595, 1984

Chapter 8

Phencyclidine

Edward F. Domino, M.D.

HISTORICAL PERSPECTIVE

The history of the synthesis, early pharmacology, and clinical use of phencyclidine has been summarized by Maddox (1981), Chen (1981), McCarthy (1981), and Luby (1981) in a volume edited by Domino (1981). Briefly, phencyclidine was developed as a general anesthetic. Its early clinical trials were both encouraging and disappointing because of a rather high incidence (about 33%) of emergence delirium. Phencyclidine was given intravenously in surgical patients in doses of 0.25 mg/kg over a 15-minute period to achieve surgical anesthesia. Anesthetic induction occurred with doses of approximately 10 mg total. For various operative procedures, doses of 25–125 mg total were used. Large single doses of 0.5–1.0 mg/kg also produced convulsions in some subjects. The duration of anesthesia lasted 1–3 hours, depending on dose and whether a continuous infusion was used. Following recovery from anesthesia for the next 24 hours or longer, about 16% of patients showed hyperactivity and emergence delirium sufficient to be restrained. Because of these very undesirable and relatively long-lasting effects, it seemed that a shorter-acting compound that had less of a tendency to produce seizures and less emergence

279

delirium would be clinically more suitable. This led to the development of ketamine. Phencyclidine was abandoned as an unsuitable general anesthetic for humans. The unique state produced by this class of compounds led to the clinical description of dissociative anesthesia because the patients seemed disconnected from their environment. Ketamine still remains a useful, but seldom used, general anesthetic for humans in the United States (Domino 1990). However, ketamine is widely used as a general anesthetic for subhuman primates because of its wide margin of safety.

The history of the development of phencyclidine provides all of us with a number of surprises. Who would have predicted, in their wildest imagination, that a dissociative anesthetic, which produced a high incidence of anesthetic emergence phenomena and was a drug that mimicked the primary symptoms of schizophrenia by distorting body image, would become a drug of abuse in the United States? Yet that is what the drug culture has accomplished with phencyclidine. Surely a psychotomimetic drug in low dosage, an anesthetic, and a convulsant in large doses would not seem to be reinforcing—yet it is to many people. It is called by many different names, as listed in Table 8-1. People who abuse phencyclidine have been named parsley monsters when the drug is applied to parsley and smoked. Those who are "high" on phencyclidine are said to be crystallized. The drug is taken by inhalation, orally, intranasally (snorted), and intravenously.

PREVALENCE OF ABUSE

The prevalence of phencyclidine abuse varies markedly through the world. It appears that the major problem with phencyclidine is in the United States, especially in some of the larger cities such as Los Angeles and Washington, D.C. This fact may be related to the easy

Table 8-1. Street names for phencyclidine

PCP, synthetic THC, angel dust, dust, hog, crystal, animal tranquilizer, horse tranquilizer, peace pill, peaCe pill, crystal joint, CJ, KJ, sheet, rocket fuel, peace, peace weed, supergrass, super kools, superweed, elephant tranquilizer, seams, surfer, snorts, scuffle, cadillac, mist, goon, amoeba, cyclones, DOA (dead on arrival), killer weed, synthetic marijuana, lovely, lovely high chemical synthesis of phencyclidine so that it is available as a relatively cheap substitute for a large variety of street drugs. Phencyclidine used to be widely abused by college students in the 1970s but is no longer a major problem on college campuses. However, as long as phencyclidine is readily available on the illicit market, it will be abused, because the drug is highly reinforcing despite what one who does not use drugs would think. Apparently, some human beings enjoy a "body trip" that is more related to a schizophrenic-like state than any other known drug of abuse except chronic amphetamine and cocaine, which are drug models of paranoid schizophrenia.

DIAGNOSIS

Phencyclidine-induced behaviors vary widely, depending on dosage. Therefore, phencyclidine can mimic the actions of many other drugs of abuse. The only certain way of diagnosing phencyclidine use is by chemical assay involving plasma or serum and urine. In this regard, clinical laboratories vary widely in their sophistication of analytic methods used—from thin-layer chromatography to gas chromatography-mass spectroscopy. It is incumbent on the physician to know precisely what the clinical analytical laboratory is using and the specificity and sensitivity of their methods. The reason for this is that some chemical assays such as gas-liquid chromatography vary widely in sensitivity, depending on the detector used. Although this is technically a complex issue, the bottom line is sensitivity and specificity of the method used. One must demand this information from the analytical laboratory for each test they use. Lindgren and Holmstedt (1983) provided a technical guide to the analysis of phencyclidine and its metabolites in biological material.

Burns and Lerner (1981) provided information on the blood levels and clinical correlates of phencyclidine intoxication in humans (Table 8-2).

PHARMACOLOGY

Depending on the dose and personality of the patient, phencyclidine is an excitant or a cataleptoid anesthetic. While it is a general anesthetic, small doses (even less than 5 mg) can cause a rather remarkable psychotomimetic syndrome. Emergence delirium is seen often. Phencyclidine and related compounds have been called cataleptoid or

Table 8-2. Clinical spectrum of acute phencyclidine intoxication

Psychosis, confusion, or delirium	Coma	Coma plus seizure
Dose (mg)		
5–10	20+	70+
Plasma level		
25–50 ng/ml	100–200 ng/ml	200–500 ng/ml
Behavioral state		
Confusion, blank stare	Unresponsive, immobile	Prolonged coma
Vertical or horizontal nystagmus	Spontaneous vertical or horizontal nystagmus	
Increased blood pressure	Increased blood pressure	Sustained increase in blood pressure
Gait ataxia	Increased deep-tendon muscle rigidity	Muscle rigidity
		Decerebrate posturing
		Seizure activity
Excited, aggressive, or bizarre behavior	Theta slowing	Theta and delta slowing, periodic slow-wave complexes
		Hypoventilation, apnea
Body temperature		
Elevated if excited	Slightly lower	Decreased

sympathomimetic anesthetics. During induction, the patient often feels dissociated from his or her environment with analgesia and some amnesia. As described above, a related congener of phencyclidine is ketamine. Its anesthetic properties in humans were described as representing a new class of "dissociative" anesthetics because of its unique pharmacologic actions. During general anesthesia, the patient may keep his or her eyes open and appears "disconnected" from the environment. It seems as if higher associational functions of the brain are markedly depressed, a clinical impression for which there are some human and animal data. During emergence from dissociative anesthesia, the patient may go through a phase of vivid dreaming with or without psychomotor activity, manifested by confusion and irrational behavior. Chemically, phencyclidine, ketamine, and related compounds are arylcyclohexylamines. Although they have similar pharmacologic actions, they also have important differences both quantitatively and qualitatively. The major pharmacologic properties of these agents concerning the central nervous system can be summarized as follows:

- Small doses produce a "drunken" state with numbness of the extremities; some persons are excited.
- Moderate doses are analgesic and anesthetic.
- The psychic state crudely resembles sensory isolation; however, sensory impulses, if tested electrophysiologically, reach the neocortex, and neuronal signals are grossly distorted.
- Cataleptoid motor phenomena are seen.
- Large doses may produce convulsions, even through the person is anesthetized.
- Marked individual differences are present.

Effects of these agents on the autonomic and cardiovascular systems include sympathomimetic effects, tachycardia, hypertension, and potentiation of catecholamines through a cocainelike action.

To date, at least six cyclohexylamines have been either given to or taken by humans in the context of drug abuse. Their chemical structures are shown in Figure 8-1.

By far phencyclidine is the most abused and ketamine the least. PCC (1-piperidinocyclohexane-carbonitrile) is a contaminant of crude batches of phencyclidine. It does not possess the same pharmacologic properties as the other phencyclidine derivatives. However, its ingestion and biotransformation in the body leads to liberation of cyanide, and therefore the toxicity of the crude mixture is of great concern.

The neurochemical aspects of phencyclidine and related compounds have been summarized in the symposium volume by Domino and Kamenka (1988). Castellani and Bupp (1988) summarized the possible biochemical and behavioral mechanisms underlying phencyclidine psychosis, as shown in Table 8-3 with slight modifications.

It is apparent that phencyclidine alters a large variety of brain neurotransmitter functions, including dopamine, acetylcholine, serotonin, and the ion channel associated with the *N*-methyl-D-aspartate (NMDA) receptor of glutamic acid, as well as other membrane ion channels. These widespread neurochemical actions reflect the complexity of phencyclidine pharmacology and why a specific antagonist may be very difficult to discover. Especially intriguing is evidence that endogenous phencyclidine receptors and peptides exist in mam-

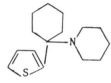

Phencyclidine (PCP)
1-(phenylcyclohexyl)
piperidine (CI-395)

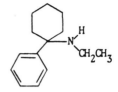

(Cyclohexamine (PCE)
N-ethyl-1-phenylcyclohexylamine
(CI-400)

1-(1-2-thienylcyclohexyl)
piperidine

1-(1-phenylcyclohexyl)
pyrrolidine

PCC
1-piperidinocyclohexane-
carbonitrile

Ketamine
2-(o-chlorophenyl)-2-methyl-
amine cyclohexanone (CI-581)

3057

Figure 8-1. Some abused phencyclidine derivatives.

malian brain (Di Maggio et al. 1988; Zukin and Zukin 1988). An important distinction between sigma and phencyclidine receptors has been made to avoid confusion in the literature (Quirion et al. 1988). Briefly, the term *opioid* in sigma opioid has been dropped. There are now two categories of receptors called sigma and PCP. The abbreviation PCP should be used only when discussing phencyclidine receptors. When the drug is referred to, the generic name phencyclidine should be spelled out. The reason for this is that the abbreviation PCP is also used in the literature on acquired immune difficiency syndrome (AIDS) and stands for *Pneumocystic carinii* pneumonia. The

Table 8-3. Possible biochemical and behavioral mechanisms underlying phencyclidine psychosis

Biochemical effect of phencyclidine	Animal model	Human model	Treatment
Enhanced dopamine	Stereotyped behaviors	Dopamine hypothesis; stimulation or psychosis	Neuroleptic drugs (selective D_2 antagonists)
Anticholinergic	Stereotyped behaviors	Anticholinergic psychosis; physostigmine treatment of mania	Cholinergic drugs (physostigmine)
Serotonin chronic, decreased acute, increased	Hallucinogen and chronic stimulant behaviors; serotonin syndrome	Hallucinogen; stimulation or psychosis	Serotonin agonists (?)
Phencyclidine receptor action (high affinity)	Stereotyped, drunken, excited behavior; PCP discrimination	Phencyclidine-induced psychosis, anesthesia, analgesia	No specific antagonist
Sigma receptor action (low affinity)	Backwards walking, sideways jumping	Unknown	Haloperidol, rimcazole
NMDA noncompetitive inhibition	Inhibition of NMDA, CNS stimulation, anesthesia; brain protection	Sensory isolation; psychosis; brain protection	
Ionic channels, potassium blockade			Calcium-channel blockers, verapamil

Note. NMDA = *N*-methyl-D-aspartate. CNS = central nervous system.

experimental compound, +SKF-10,047, shows a high affinity for the sigma receptor site and a low affinity for the PCP receptor site. The pharmacologic effects of sigma site agonists are not well known; PCP receptor agonists have phencyclidine-like activity (see Domino 1991).

PHARMACOKINETICS

Domino et al. (1982) compared a two- and three-compartment model of phencyclidine pharmacokinetics in humans based on the data of Wall et al. (1981), who gave 100 μg of ^{3}H-phencyclidine to three human volunteers and followed its plasma disappearance for over 72 hours. Phencyclidine revealed complex kinetics involving an initial pi half-life of 5.5 minutes, an alpha half-life of 4.6 hours, and a beta half-life of 22 hours. The volume of distribution of phencyclidine was large, varying from 2.2 to 2.4 liter/kg for each compartment. This suggests significant tissue binding. The data are summarized in Table 8-4.

The practical importance of this information is that phencyclidine is present in different body tissues for varying periods of time, with a prolonged terminal half-life of about 1 day. Some reports in the literature suggest that phencyclidine may remain in some human fluid samples for as long as 2 weeks. There are considerable individual human differences in phencyclidine biotransformation (Pohorecki et al. 1989). Environmental and possibly genetic factors seem to be involved. The biotransformation of phencyclidine is extremely complex (Gole et al. 1988), involving an overwhelming number of metabolites, most of which are less active than phencyclidine. However, there is good evidence that phencyclidine is biotransformed to a highly reactive iminium ion (Hoag et al. 1984; Law and Farquharson 1980), which leads to inactivation of specific liver microsomal P-450 cytochromes (Osawa and Coon 1988). There are obvious serious clinical implications of irreversible tissue binding of an iminium phencyclidine metabolite.

CHRONIC USE AND ABSTINENCE SYNDROME

Phencyclidine and its derivatives have been ingested chronically (i.e., for months and years) by humans. However, the best information regarding an abstinence syndrome is based on animal data. The fact that very large amounts of phencyclidine (100–1,000 mg/day) have been consumed by some human users without coma and death argues for marked tolerance development to phencyclidine, at least in humans. Balster and Chait (1978), Balster and Wessinger (1983), Balster and Woolverton (1979, 1980a, 1980b), and Flint and Ho (1980) summarized the conflicting data and their own research in animals

Table 8-4. Pharmacokinetic parameters of ^{3}H-phencyclidine given 1.3 μg/kg iv in normal volunteers: comparison of two- and three-compartment models

			Two-compartment model	Three-compartment model
1	P_{bol} pg/ml		—	260
	π hour^{-1}		—	7.5
	π t ½ hour		—	.092
2	A_{bol} pg/ml		190	160
	α hour^{-1}		3.0	.15
	α t ½ hour		.23	4.6
3	B_{bol} pg/ml		240	120
	β hour^{-1}		.056	.032
	β t ½ hour		12	22
First-order rate parameters	k_{12} hour^{-1}		1.2	3.5
	k_{21} hour^{-1}		1.7	3.9
	k_{13} hour^{-1}		—	.078
	k_{31} hour^{-1}		—	.084
	k_e hour^{-1}		.097	.11
Distribution parameters	V_{d1}	liter/kg	3.0	2.4
	V_{d2}	liter/kg	2.2	2.2
	V_{d3}	liter/kg	—	2.2
	V_{dss}	liter/kg	5.2	6.8
	V_d area	liter/kg	5.3	8.3
	Cl_{plasma}	liter/kg/hour	.29	.27

Note. Standard pharmacokinetic abbreviations are used.

for tolerance and dependence. Balster and Wessinger reported that in the rhesus monkey daily injections of phencyclidine given once a day for 7 days over a 4-month period caused a shift in the dose-effect curve for suppression of food-reinforced operant behavior. This shift was as great as fourfold in some, but not all, monkeys. In the squirrel monkey, they reported a twofold shift in the dose-effect curve of phencyclidine given once (0.2 mg/kg) to four times (2.4 mg/kg) per day over an 82–126-day period. No good evidence of a withdrawal syndrome was obtained, but more vigorous dosage schedules were not studied. It is unknown whether this two- to fourfold shift in the dose-effect curve is due to drug metabolism, tissue adaptation, or behavioral changes. That the monkey is a suitable model of phencyclidine dependence was reported by Balster and Woolverton (1979, 1980a, 1980b). They found that continuous access to phencyclidine via self-administration by rhesus monkeys led to tolerance and a mild physical dependence syndrome. Some very interesting cross-tolerance between phencyclidine derivatives and muscarinic cholinergic antagonists like atropine have been reported (Pinchasi et al. 1978a, 1978b), which may help delineate the pharmacologic details of phencyclidine tolerance and cross-tolerance.

PROTOCOLS FOR DETOXIFICATION AND TREATMENT ISSUES

Detoxification of patients taking phencyclidine should be considered in two separate categories. The first is detoxification and treatment of the acute overdose of phencyclidine. The second is detoxification and treatment of the chronic phencyclidine abuser.

The therapy of a patient with an acute overdose of phencyclidine is largely symptomatic in that classic general principles of care of a psychiatric or comatose patient apply. Severe intoxication from phencyclidine and its congeners induces coma and respiratory, cardiovascular, and renal complications (Domino 1978a). The latter are secondary to rhabdomyolysis (Cogen et al. 1978), resulting from an interaction of phencyclidine skeletal muscle exertion and limb restraints (which should be used with great caution). Centrally and peripherally acting anticholinesterase agents have been used but are of little value. In dogs severely poisoned with phencyclidine, I have been unable to show any global improvement using tetrahydroaminoacridine or another cholinesterase inhibitor, physostigmine (Domino

1978b). Patients who have recently ingested large amounts of phencyclidine should have a stomach tube passed and the gastric contents removed (lavage). The oral administration of adsorbents such as charcoal may be helpful (Picchioni and Consroe 1979).

Patients who are comatose usually require tracheal intubation, a stomach tube in place for continuous drainage of its contents, and intravenous fluids (to ensure adequate urine flow). An indwelling urinary catheter should also be inserted to maintain continuous flow. Vital signs should be monitored throughout the period of danger.

At the present time, urine acidification by any convenient means (see below) appears useful to facilitate phencyclidine excretion. The pKa of phencyclidine has been estimated by various techniques to be between 8.5 and 9.5. Hence, at a pH of about 3 units lower (5.5–6.5), most of the phencyclidine is ionized. This physical-chemical fact means that acidic fluids like the contents of the stomach and urine will contain mostly ionized phencyclidine. The charged ionic form of phencyclidine does not readily pass lipophilic tissue membranes. Hence, charged phencyclidine molecules will accumulate in the acid secretion of the stomach and in an acid urine.

Initial experience with the effects of urine acidification on plasma and urine phencyclidine levels in human overdosage have been encouraging (Domino 1978a; Domino and Wilson 1977). Very rapid urine acidification can be achieved in comatose patients with an intravenous infusion of highly diluted 0.1 normal hydrogen chloride. About 10 ml of the acid solution is diluted 1:10 (to 100 ml) with 0.9% sodium chloride and infused slowly. This technique should be used only by skilled persons in patients who are in dire need of rapid treatment. Careful monitoring of the status of the patient and blood and urinary pH is essential. Aronow and colleagues (Aronow and Done 1978; Aronow et al. 1978; Done et al. 1978) have reported extensively on the pharmacokinetics of phencyclidine overdosage and treatment using acidification to form ionized phencyclidine. Hence, the term *ion-trapping*.

A variety of methods of urine acidification have been used, including ascorbic acid, large volumes of cranberry juice, and ammonium chloride. Ascorbic acid, 500–2,000 mg, added to the intravenous fluids every 6 hours and ammonium chloride orally (75–125 mg/kg via stomach tube) or intravenously (1–2% in 0.9% sodium chloride in a dose of 2.76 mEq/kg) have been used. When the urine pH is very acid (around pH 5), a diuretic-like furosemide (0.5–1.0

mg/kg) should be given to facilitate urinary excretion. Adequate hydration and electrolyte balance must be maintained to ensure a urine flow of 1–2 ml/kg/hour. The fact that the acidic fluid of the stomach will also concentrate ionized phencyclidine means that gastric secretions should be removed by continuous drainage via a stomach tube. The use of oral charcoal as a means of absorbing phencyclidine has been recommended (Picchioni and Consroe 1979). Generally, USP activated charcoal is given in doses of 5–20 times that which it is expected to absorb. A 15–30 g slurry of charcoal in water can be prepared and passed down the stomach tube, and continuous drainage shut off for a variable period of time.

During phencyclidine coma, the patient may convulse periodically. It is not known what anticonvulsant, if any, is best to use. Additional central nervous system depression may occur from administering anticonvulsants. Hence, a conservative approach is recommended unless continued seizures indicate that a drug like diazepam should be given temporarily. Intravenous diazepam (10–15 mg) followed by phenytoin has also been used.

As described above, phencyclidine blocks the uptake of catecholamines into adrenergic nerve terminals and also releases catecholamines. As a result, in some patients, there can be a severe phencyclidine-induced hypertensive crisis. Diazoxide, phentolamine, and hydralazine have been used to lower blood pressure. Generally, severe hypertension is not a problem, and good clinical judgment should prevail as to whether any antihypertensive therapy is indicated. Antipsychotic (neuroleptic) agents like the phenothiazines do little to antagonize the phencyclidine confusional state and may prolong it. In addition, wide-spectrum neuroleptics such as chlorpromazine may induce severe hypotension. Thus these agents do not seem to be helpful. A quiet, supportive environment is best. Sometimes diazepam is indicated to sedate hyperactive patients who cannot be controlled in a supportive environment, but no specific antagonism occurs.

The "bottom line" is that phencyclidine intoxication is a difficult management problem in which classic symptomatic therapeutic measures and urine acidification help. Further experimental and clinical research is needed to develop more specific therapies. After the patient recovers from acute phencyclidine intoxication, it is extremely important that follow-up psychiatric, social, and educational therapies be undertaken to prevent recurrence.

The treatment of a chronic phencyclidine abuser is very difficult.

Appropriate psychiatric care and pharmacotherapy should be used as indicated. Tennant et al. (1981) described a very interesting case of chronic phencyclidine dependence in a man treated with desipramine. A working hypothesis is that phencyclidine causes the release and blockage of catecholamine reuptake, particularly norepinephrine, and that the effect can be mimicked by desipramine. Additional studies need to be done systematically to evaluate this approach.

Finally, the reader is referred to an excellent review of phencyclidine by Aniline and Pitts (1981), who provide a great deal of information to both complement and supplement the material presented herein.

REFERENCES

Aniline O, Pitts FN Jr: Phencyclidine (PCP): a review and perspectives. Critical Reviews in Toxicology 10:145–177, 1981

Aronow R, Done AK: Phencyclidine overdose: an emerging concept of management. Journal of American College of Emergency Physicians 7:56–59, 1978

Aronow R, Miceli JN, Done AK: Clinical observations during phencyclidine intoxication and treatment based on ion trapping. Natl Inst Drug Abuse Res Monogr Ser 21:218–228, 1978

Balster RL, Chait LD: The behavioral effects of phencyclidine in animals. Natl Inst Drug Abuse Res Monogr Ser 21:53–65, 1978

Balster RL, Wessinger WD: Central nervous system depressant effects of phencyclidine, in Phencyclidine and Related Arylcyclohexylamines: Present and Future Applications. Edited by Kamenka J-M, Domino EF, Geneste P. Ann Arbor, MI, NPP Books, 1983, pp 291–309

Balster RL, Woolverton WL: Intravenous phencyclidine self-administration by rhesus monkeys leading to physical dependence. Natl Inst Drug Abuse Res Monogr Ser 27:205–211, 1979

Balster RL, Woolverton WL: Continuous-access phencyclidine self-administration by rhesus monkeys leading to physical dependence. Psychopharmacology (Berlin) 70:5–10, 1980a

Balster RL, Woolverton WL: Tolerance and dependence to phencyclidine. Psychopharmacol Bull 16:76–77, 1980b

Burns RS, Lerner SE: The effects of phencyclidine in man: a review, in PCP (Phencyclidine): Historical and Current Perspectives. Edited by Domino EF. Ann Arbor, MI, NPP Books, 1981, pp 449–469

Castellani S, Bupp SJ: Molecular mechanisms in phencyclidine-induced psychosis and its treatment, in *Sigma* and Phencyclidine-like Compounds as Molecular Probes in Biology. Edited by Domino EF, Kamenka J-M. Ann Arbor, MI, NPP Books, 1988, pp 521–539

Chen G: The neuropharmacology of phencyclidine, in PCP (Phencyclidine):

Historical and Current Perspectives. Edited by Domino EF. Ann Arbor, MI, NPP Books, 1981, pp 9–16

Cogen FC, Rigg G, Simmons JL, et al: Phencyclidine-associated acute rhabdomyolysis. Ann Intern Med 88:210–212, 1978

Di Maggio DA, Contreras PC, O'Donohue TL: Biological and chemical characterization of the endopsychosins: distinct ligands for PCP and *sigma* sites, in *Sigma* and Phencyclidine-like Compounds as Molecular Probes in Biology. Edited by Domino EF, Kamenka J-M. Ann Arbor, MI, NPP Books, 1988, pp 157–171

Domino EF: Neurobiology of phencyclidine: an update. Natl Inst Drug Abuse Res Monogr Ser 21:18–43, 1978a

Domino EF: Some aspects of the pharmacology of phencyclidine, in The Psychopharmacology of Hallucinogens. Edited by Stillman RC, Willette RE. New York, Pergamon, 1978b, pp 105–117

Domino EF (ed): PCP (Phencyclidine): Historical and Current Perspectives. Ann Arbor, MI, NPP Books, 1981

Domino EF (ed): Status of Ketamine in Anesthesiology. Ann Arbor, MI, NPP Books, 1990

Domino EF: Summary and Future Directions: *Sigma* and PCP Receptor Systems (Technical Review Meeting Publication). Rockville, MD, National Institute on Drug Abuse, 1991

Domino EF, Kamenka J-M: *Sigma* and Phencyclidine-like Compounds as Molecular Probes in Biology. Ann Arbor, MI, NPP Books, 1988

Domino EF, Wilson AE: Effects of urine acidification on plasma and urine phencyclidine levels in overdosage. Clin Pharmacol Ther 22:421–424, 1977

Domino SE, Domino LE, Domino EF: Comparison of two- and three-compartment models of phencyclidine in man. Substance and Alcohol Actions/Misuse 2:205–211, 1982

Done AK, Aronow R, Miceli JN: Pharmacokinetics of phencyclidine (PCP) in overdosage and its treatment. Natl Inst Drug Abuse Res Monogr Ser 21:210–217, 1978

Flint BA, Ho IK: Tolerance development to phencyclidine by chronic administration. Progress in Neuro-psychopharmacology 4:233–239, 1980

Gole DJ, Pirat J-L, Domino EF: New aspects of phencyclidine (PCP) metabolism, in *Sigma* and Phencyclidine-like Compounds as Molecular Probes in Biology. Edited by Domino EF, Kamenka J-M. Ann Arbor, MI, NPP Books, 1988, pp 625–641

Hoag MKP, Trevor AJ, Asscher Y, et al: Metabolism-dependent inactivation of liver microsomal enzymes by phencyclidine. Drug Metab Dispos 12:371–375, 1984

Law FCP, Farquharson TE: Metabolism and irreversible binding of phencyclidine by rabbit lung and liver microsomes, in Microsomes, Drug Oxidations, and Chemical Carcinogenesis. Edited by Coon MJ, Conney AH, Estabrook RW, et al. New York, Academic, 1980

Lindgren JE, Holmstedt B: Guide to the analysis of phencyclidine and its metabolites in biological material. Arch Toxicol (suppl) 6:61–73, 1983

Luby ED: Phencyclidine revisited, in PCP (Phencyclidine): Historical and

Current Perspectives. Edited by Domino EF. Ann Arbor, MI, NPP Books, 1981, pp 25–30

Maddox VH: The historical development of phencyclidine, in PCP (Phencyclidine): Historical and Current Perspectives. Edited by Domino EF. Ann Arbor, MI, NPP Books, 1981, pp 1–8

McCarthy DA: History of the development of cataleptoid anesthetics of the phencyclidine type, in PCP (Phencyclidine): Historical and Current Perspectives. Edited by Domino EF. Ann Arbor, MI, NPP Books, 1981, pp 7–23

Osawa Y, Coon MJ: Metabolism of phencyclidine and its oxidation product, the iminium compound, leads to destruction of specific rabbit liver microsomal P-450 cytochromes, in *Sigma* and Phencyclidine-like Compounds as Molecular Probes in Biology. Edited by Domino EF, Kamenka J-M. Ann Arbor, MI, NPP Books, 1988, pp 619–624

Picchioni AL, Consroe PF: Activated charcoal: a phencyclidine antidote, or hog in dogs. N Engl J Med 300:202, 1979

Pinchasi I, Maayani S, Sokolovsky M: On the interaction of drugs with the cholinergic nervous system, I: tolerance to phencyclidine derivatives in mice: pharmacological characterization. Psychopharmacology (Berlin) 56:27–36, 1978a

Pinchasi I, Maayani S, Sokolovsky M: On the interaction of drugs with the cholinergic nervous system, II: cross-tolerance between phencyclidine derivatives. Psychopharmacology (Berlin) 56:37–40, 1978b

Pohorecki R, Rayburn W, Coon WW, et al: Some factors affecting phencyclidine biotransformation by human liver and placenta. Drug Metab Dispos 17:271–274, 1989

Quirion R, Chicheportiche R, Contreras PC, et al: Classification of nomenclature of phencyclidine and *sigma* receptor sites, in *Sigma* and Phencyclidine-like Compounds as Molecular Probes in Biology. Edited by Domino EF, Kamenka J-M. Ann Arbor, MI, NPP Books, 1988, pp 601–606

Tennant FS Jr, Rawson RA, McCann M: Withdrawal from chronic phencyclidine (PCP) dependence with desipramine. Am J Psychiatry 138: 845–847, 1981

Wall ME, Brine DR, Jeffcoat AR, et al: Phencyclidine metabolism and disposition in man following a 100 μg intravenous dose. Research Communications on Substance Abuse 2:161–172, 1981

Zukin RS, Zukin SR: Phencyclidine, *sigma* and NMDA receptors: emerging concepts, in *Sigma* and Phencyclidine-like Compounds as Molecular Probes in Biology. Edited by Domino EF, Kamenka J-M. Ann Arbor, MI, NPP Books, 1988, pp 407–424

Chapter 9

Inhalants

Charles W. Sharp, Ph.D.
Luis Fornazzari, M.D.

The abuse of solvents subsumes a broad area of toxicology because of the diversity of substances inhaled. In this chapter, we will consider those substances most commonly known to be abused. It is very important to keep in mind that there are many different solvents that have different physiologic effects as well as different chemical properties. Also, most commercial products contain several distinctly different solvents with distinct toxicologic end points. In addition, most "inhalant abusers" have inhaled a variety of products to excess before they appear in a treatment facility. One exceptional case would be a novice experiencing an overdose, usually resulting in anoxia and possibly death.

Thus it is important to determine as precisely as possible not only the solvent(s) but all the contributing factors (including other drugs, such as alcohol, cigarettes, or marijuana; malnutrition; and respiratory irritants, such as fumes or viruses) before beginning the treatment of primary inhalant abusers. These interrelating factors are often more important for some groups of inhalant abusers in that they use more drugs, are less well nourished, and live in more "polluted" areas than other types of drug abusers. There are also other inhalant abusers who come from more affluent surroundings. Some of those who use the organic nitrites (poppers) or nitrous oxide (laughing gas) would often fit into the latter group. Some of the most affluent include the dentists, anesthesiologists, and other health professionals who inhale anesthetics such as halothane and nitrous oxide and those who use organic nitrites.

NATURE OF THE PROBLEM

The extent of this drug problem is greater than most realize. It is a worldwide problem. Although most countries do not systematically evaluate the abuse of solvents, many reports and meetings on the problem have identified inhalant (solvent) abuse as a problem of serious proportion (Cohen 1977; Crider and Rouse 1988; National Institute on Drug Abuse 1985; 1990). This is a problem not only of developed countries but also of underdeveloped countries. The pattern of inhalant abuse is exemplified by two national studies in the United States: the National Institute on Drug Abuse (1990) national household survey and the annual "High School Students and Young Adults" survey (Crider and Rouse 1988). The household survey reported that the category of 12–17-year-old whites (as compared to blacks or Hispanics) showed the highest use "ever," "in past year," and "in past month" of 9.9, 5.8, and 4.0%, respectively. The pattern of reported use for Hispanics and blacks was much lower, especially in the used "in past month" category, which was about 1%. By region, the South and West (as compared to Northeast and Northcentral) reported the highest patterns of use.

According to the high school survey of senior students in the United States, 1 in 5 have tried inhalants, 3% have used in the past month, and 0.4% use daily. Regional studies (e.g., New York State or the province of Ontario) show similar patterns of use (see Crider and Rouse 1988). As with any drug use, there are regions of higher density. National surveys have not clearly delineated all those regions where high-use inhalant populations may occur, such as in some inner cities that include impoverished or ethnic minorities or other isolated communities, especially those of Native Americans. The extent of the use in these groups is difficult to determine as many of the individuals abusing inhalants are not accessed by survey systems. However, Beauvais and Oetting (1988) have comprehensively studied many Native American groups (Oetting et al. 1988).

For further reading on the nature of the problem, especially the sociocultural conditions, we refer the reader to several reviews of this area (Beauvais and Oetting 1987; Cohen 1977; Crider and Rouse 1988; Ramsey et al. 1989; Sharp and Korman 1981).

GENERAL CONSIDERATIONS

Although treatments are usually not specific or designed for different solvents, it is important to identify the major contributing factors in understanding the prognosis and recovery of the individual and in the design of treatment. This is not easy as it is difficult to identify the causative agents even if one obtains the container or product most often used. Labels are often insufficient to identify even the major element, let alone any minor elements, that could be contributory to the disease state. It is also common for the labels to identify toluene and some other solvents yet ignore other substances. For example, one of the more toxic agents affecting the peripheral nervous system, hexane, has been identified in products that did not list this on the product's label. Only through an analysis of the products used (e.g., by quantitative gas-liquid chromatography) will it be possible to determine most of the volatile solvents.

In anticipation that the physician, forensic toxicologist, or others will be able to identify the major substances contributing to the disease state, we will attempt herein to delineate the symptoms most often encountered in inhalant abusers and hopefully on a rational basis correlate them where possible with the substances that are most likely to be the cause. We will include where possible any specific treatments that will be of assistance along with providing the usual basic supportive care.

To correlate those specific clinical symptoms that result from exposure to various volatile chemicals is not easy, as suitable animal studies have not corroborated many clinical evaluations. Also months to years of exposure are often necessary for the expression of some disease states. As many of these subjects are not admitted to hospitals or outpatient clinics or placed in any drug treatment program for problems associated with inhalant abuse overdose or dependency, little information has surfaced detailing all of their problems. Therefore, in this review, we will utilize clinical epidemiologic studies of noninhalant abusers as well as retrospective clinical case studies of inhalant abusers and other solvent-related accidents, whether from abuse or occupational exposures, along with the information derived from animal studies, to identify particular hazards that may result from inhalation exposure.

LETHAL EFFECTS

Physicians should be aware of the possible causes of deaths attributed to solvent toxicity (Anderson et al. 1982; Bass 1970, 1978, 1984; DiMaio and Garriott 1978; Garriott and Petty 1980; Kringsholm 1980; Ramsey et al. 1989). This is of particular importance to the community where it has occurred. With the proper attention, measures can be taken to prevent other deaths and potential chronic ailments that result from the abuse of these solvents. As these abusers utilize common household substances, the parent and the physician may need assistance to identify the substances used as indicated by other telltale clues (e.g., odors, stains, empty containers, and unusual paraphernalia). In this way one will be able to identify a serious problem of solvent abuse before it causes death. Unforeseen ventricular fibrillations or induced cardiac arrhythmias following high exposures to identified mixtures of solvents are also serious consequences of this abuse. This aspect of the problem was brought to light by a survey (Bass 1970) showing a high association of these deaths with the abuse of substances containing fluorocarbon propellants and other solvents as well.

Although these types of incidences may have declined in the United States due to the restriction in 1980 of the use of fluorocarbons in aerosols, fluorocarbon-related deaths still appear to be of major concern in England (Anderson et al. 1985; Shepherd 1989), in work-related accidents (Clark et al. 1985), and elsewhere. Although it is not as evident, the results of several cases link fibrillation or other cardiac insufficiencies to the use of other halocarbons (Anderson et al. 1985; Gresham and Treip 1983; Jones and Winter 1983; Kringsholm 1980; McLeod et al. 1987; Nouchi et al. 1984; Spencer et al. 1976; Yamashita et al. 1984). These types of products range from anesthetics (halothane) used by hospital personnel and others to the more common solvents (di-, tri-, and tetrachloroethanes and trichloroethylene) contained in cleaning fluids and typing correction fluid solvent (Troutman 1988). The chlorohydrocarbons derived from correction fluids have been judged the cause of a death (G King et al. 1985). Some cardiac arrhythmias have also been reported following abuse of substances containing toluene as well as a nonfatal respiratory arrest (Cronk et al. 1985). Other anesthetics have also been indicated as the cause of deaths in Denmark (ether) and elsewhere (chloroform parties) (Hutchens and Kung 1985).

Respiratory complications are not often encountered but have been noted in inhalant abusers who died (Lecomte et al. 1983; Mee and Wright 1980). Respiratory ailments in some cases are likely exacerbated or caused by smoking and other factors; pulmonary complications related to inhalant abuse have not been supported by animal studies. Despite the identification of the direct or indirect cardiotoxic effects noted above, most deaths are likely the result of asphyxia directly (such as a bag over the head) or indirectly by solvent displacement or by aspiration of stomach contents (Anderson et al. 1985; Ramsey et al. 1989). In a limited number of cases, liver toxicities occur following the repeated inhalation of halogenated hydrocarbons and may lead to death (Garriott and Petty 1980). A final but not unimportant cause of death can be fatal accidents that are directly related to or the result of a sniffing episode.

The use of rags soaked in solvent and applied to oral cavities (a practice common in the United States) rather than through inhalation from bags and the setting of outdoor areas, as contrasted with closets or closed spaces, may lead to a lower number of deaths; yet it is still difficult to determine just how many deaths result from solvent inhalation. Recent information derived from reported deaths (Litovitz et al. 1990) indicates that deaths still occur from the use of fluorocarbons in the United States. The source of the fluorocarbon is primarily car refrigerant replenisher. Other new substances being used are butane derived from cigarette lighters and propane from canisters; these practices also can result in death (Krause and McCarthy 1989; Mathew et al. 1989). Thus it will benefit the medical community if medical examiners more rigorously pursue the cause of death—for example, include measures of solvents or metabolites in the body where possible; check for telltale signs of solvent abuse; examine the vicinity for labeled containers or residual solvents for clues of inhalant use; and question acquaintances to substantiate the nature of any substances likely to be responsible for the death.

NEPHROTOXICITY

Condition

Of greatest concern are the debilitating disease states that arise from inhalant abuse. Some of the currently most widely abused substances, at least in the United States, are the spray paints. The abuse of these substances occurs not only within polydrug users but by painters as well. The exposure to these and similar substances has resulted in the hospitalization of inhalant abusers (Baerg and Kimberg 1970; Bennett and Forman 1980; Marjot and McLeod 1989; Patel and Benjamin 1986; Ravnskov 1978; Sarmiento-Martinez et al. 1989; Streicher et al. 1981; Will and McLaren 1981). A 32-year-old woman has been identified to have renal disease after sniffing spray paint (Patel and Benjamin 1986). One of the primary conditions leading to hospitalization has been severe muscle cramps to the point that some subjects are nearly paralyzed. These subjects often have associated gastrointestinal involvement, including nausea, vomiting, and severe abdominal cramps.

Streicher et al. (1981) identified the occurrence of distal renal acidosis in groups of paint and/or glue sniffers from the Southwest and Hawaii. Although these were not the first reports of renal dysfunction associated with solvent abuse, it was endemic to these groups, and the disease state reoccurred in many individuals who returned to their habit. Their symptoms include hyperchloremic metabolic acidosis, hypokalemia, hypocalcemia, and other electrolyte imbalances. Solvents usually cause a unique distal-type tubular acidosis, but proximal tubules are also affected. Although the distal one is responsible for the known electrolyte and metabolic imbalances, the proximal type is responsible for the loss of amino acids and other proteins. Despite this tubular damage being reversible, other organs, particularly brain, are the target of repetitive acidosis, plus a depletion of important amino acids. A significant increase in glutamine and other amino acids has been found in the cerebrospinal fluid in a group of chronic inhalant abusers (Fornazzari et al., unpublished data, 1988). Glomerulonephritis has also been identified in workers using solvents (Harrison et al. 1986), especially in painters (Ravnskov 1978).

Several kinds of solvent mixtures are correlated with symptoms of either glomerulonephritis or distal renal tubular acidosis, although these somewhat different diseases do not usually occur in the same individuals. Although metallic spray paints are frequently used by these subjects, they also use paint thinners and glues. With this diverse arsenal of inhalants being used, there has been no good clue as to which of the chemicals in these products is responsible for these kidney diseases. Attempts to reproduce these symptoms in animals following exposure to toluene (one of the more common chemicals found in these products) have not been successful. It is very possible that these symptoms are due to a combination of toxicants, possibly including the metals contained in the spray paint, such as cadmium and lead, which are nephrotoxic (Wedeen 1984), or concurrent alcohol use (Jone and Wu 1988; Sarmiento-Martinez et al. 1989) and/or infections (see Farrell et al. 1985; Ravnskov 1978; Yamaguchi et al. 1985). Thus it is important that individuals exposed to high doses of solvents be checked for renal changes and metabolic imbalance.

Treatment

For most of these subjects, electrolyte repletion usually restores the kidney function and eliminates the muscle spasms, even in the more severely affected patients, in a few days. Correction of salts and electrolytes, including potassium, calcium, magnesium, and chloride, should be considered in the treatment of solvent abusers for muscle fatigue, even in the absence of more severe kidney disorders. Although some have employed neuroleptics in acute situations, such as delirium, hallucinations, and outbursts of rage, we do not think psychotropics have a role in the management of inhalant abuse. In most cases, a short (30–60 minute) rest period in a quiet room and reassurance are enough to control the most agitated cases. One should avoid disturbing and threatening situations.

Although most subjects with electrolyte imbalance have responded to treatment (Marjot and McLeod 1989), there was one report of a subject who died despite a reasonable period of electrolyte replenishment (Kirk et al. 1984). Another case report of a "glue sniffer" (Ehyai and Freemon 1983) is of interest in that only minor neurologic and muscular dysfunction was noted on the first examination. However, 2 years later, the same subject showed clinical metabolic acidosis; also, vision and hearing loss were present. It is unfortunate that little is known about the type of solvent and other important environmental factors that may have contributed to the change in conditions from the first visit to the second. In some reports (see Ravnskov 1978; Ravnskov et al. 1983), infections have been observed in subjects exposed to solvents who subsequently exhibit nephrotic changes. Another form of renal toxicity has been reported for the abuse of the anesthetic, methoxyflurane (Brennan et al. 1988; Novak et al. 1988). The former group observed hyperoxaluria as well as retinal crystal deposits in their patient.

CENTRAL NEUROLOGIC DISORDERS

Central neurologic disorders, associated peripheral neuropathies, and neurotoxicities in general are probably the diseases most often identified for inhalant abusers; yet the nature of, or the cause of, these disease states is the least well documented of all the conditions resulting from inhalant abuse. Although in the past, persistent neuropathies have been rarely demonstrated, a few have been more recently described in more detail (Boor and Hurtig 1977; Fornazzari et al. 1983a; Goldbloom and Chouinard 1985; Hormes et al. 1986; King et al. 1981; Lolin 1989; Mikkelsen et al. 1988; Orbaek et al. 1988a, 1988b; Rosenberg et al. 1988a, 1988b; Schikler et al. 1982; Takeuchi et al. 1981). This is partly due to the improved diagnostic and evaluation techniques available in determining the extent of any neurologic deficit (Prockop 1977; Rosen 1984; Wennberg 1984). Even using the best techniques, it is often difficult to associate any specific irreversible neurologic deficit to a specific substance or to inhalant exposure, per se. Recently xylene has been identified as the causative agent in one case (Roberts et al. 1988). It is obvious that during the acute stages of inhalation, central nervous system (CNS) and peripheral nerve conductions are impaired. However, most subjects are greatly improved if not normal a few days after cessation of inhalation of these products. In addition, many other factors—including the environment, genetic variables, dietetic variables, and other drugs—all contribute in distinctly different ways. For example, lead has often been found in inhalant abusers, especially gasoline sniffers. It is not clear whether this form of lead (tetraethyl lead) will cause neuropathies. Therefore, one cannot readily identify specific symptoms as being directly related to a specific solvent, and treatment in those individuals who inhale a variety of solvents should consider other agents and factors. One important variable to consider is the amount of solvent used and the duration of exposure, even though it is difficult to establish this with any degree of reliability. Thus a few days of brief exposure would not be expected to cause serious neurologic impairment, yet months of extensive periods of exposure could cause moderate to severe impairment of different organs, depending on the solvent.

OTOTOXICITY

Inhalants may cause neuropathies of the cranial nerves, peripheral nerves, or both. Cortical and hippocampal dysfunction may be directly related to solvent toxicity. For example, hearing loss was identified in inhalant abusers by Metrick and Brenner (1982) measuring brain-stem auditory responses and by others (Biscaldi et al. 1981; Ehyai and Freemon 1983; Lazar et al. 1983), at nearly the same time as it was observed in rats after toluene exposure (Pryor et al. 1983). There is also a study of painters, printers, and petrol truck drivers that identified audiologic changes derived from chemical exposures in an occupational setting (Bergholtz and Odkvist 1984; Moller et al. 1989). In these cases of a cranial nerve neuropathy, the ototoxicity can be correlated to one specific group of compounds; mono- or dimethylbenzenes. Whether nonmethylated benzene compounds also lead to this toxicity is unknown.

Although some CNS changes were noted for these subjects, no electrolyte imbalances were observed. In one study of subjects with impaired auditory-evoked potential (with learning problems) and other CNS impairments (Lazar et al. 1983), it was indicated that these effects may diminish with time. However, Metrick and Brenner's more detailed studies (1982) as well as the animal studies indicate there is little recovery of the hearing loss over time. Thus this dysfunction does not appear to be reversible if the exposure has reached certain limits.

OTHER CNS EFFECTS

There are some other central effects that may be slowly reversible. In many subjects, enlarged ventricles and cerebral, cerebellar, or brain-stem atrophy—as defined by computed tomography (CT) scans—have been found. Also, electroencephalogram (EEG) abnormalities have been observed. Little is known about the outcome of subjects identified as having cerebral atrophy, with the exception of a follow-up study of housepainters (Bruhn et al. 1981). There was some recovery (as noted by CT scans) observed for some of the painters. Although the exposures to solvent in this group do not usually reach the higher levels experienced by heavy solvent abusers, these painters are exposed for many hours each day and over many years. The older age range of this group may be an indication that an irreversibility of this condition may also be related to the aging process. In a follow-up study of chronic users of cement thinner, a persistent atrophy of cortical and cerebellar structures was observed on CT scan, even after 2 years of abstinence from these inhalants (Fornazzari et al. 1983b). The occurrence of cerebellar and postural tremors may also indicate a more extensive exposure to paint sprays (Hormes et al. 1986; Rosenberg et al. 1988a, 1988b) or the presence of and exposure to other materials; severe symptoms of this type seem to be reported less frequently for "paint spray" inhalant abusers. In milder cases, symptoms may not persist longer than a few weeks in those subjects who no longer inhale and are provided nutritionally balanced diets and maintain good health habits. As stated earlier, the muscle incoordination such as ataxia or tremors may be due to hypokalemia and metabolic acidosis; however, these effects may also result from direct actions of the solvent on the CNS or peripheral nerves. Recently, some direct measures of toluene CNS toxicity have been observed in rats (Pryor et al., in press). Gait and stride width are exacerbated after 2–4 weeks of high-level exposure to toluene.

HALLUCINATIONS OR FEELINGS

Reports of other CNS effects related to glue sniffing include optic neuropathy (Ehyai and Freemon 1983), hallucinations (Chadwick and Anderson 1989; Channer and Stanley 1983; Levy 1986), and aggressive behavior (see Sharp and Korman 1981). Hallucinations are often associated with inhalant abuse. This seldom is seen or identified in studies of groups of inhalant abusers. Thus this may be the expression of susceptible individuals or of a high degree of intoxication. A direct effect of solvents on nerve conduction leading to neurologic discharges that mimic a "crawling insect feeling" (see Goldings and Stewart 1982) may be the basis for the instigation of hallucinations. It is evident that a more comprehensive study of these conditions and individuals is needed. Although aggressive behavior is not usually a problem, there are cases where individuals express strong overt behavior. This has been summarized by Sharp and Korman (1981) from a study of psychiatric emergency room admittants as follows: "Inhalant users differed significantly from matched other drug users in that they displayed significantly more self-directed destructive behavior" (p. 240).

OPTIC EFFECTS

Visual damage is not easy to determine in animals except by visual-evoked responses. However, several studies of human subjects indicate mild to extreme visual (visual-evoked responses verified) anomalies (Berg 1971; Ehyai and Freemon 1983; Keane 1978; Lazar et al. 1983; Malm and Lying-Tunell 1980; Metrick and Brenner 1982). Whether these are related to solvent inhalation or other mitigating factors (e.g., diet, environment, genetic predisposition, other solvents, and other drugs) has yet to be determined. Animal studies have not identified any group of substances that cause these optic neuropathies.

PERIPHERAL NEUROPATHIES

One of the more rigorously studied and now classic examples of solvent toxicity is the neuropathy caused by hexane and its metabolites (see Couri and Milks 1982; Spencer and Schaumburg 1985; Spencer et al. 1980). New individual cases are still being reported (Hall et al. 1986; P King et al. 1985; Tenenbein et al. 1984) as well as those in industrial situations (Passero et al. 1983). This is despite efforts to reduce the hexane and methyl-butyl-ketone contents of many products. Any one brand of substance may change the components of that mixture from time to time. For example, some batches of a certain type (brand) of thinner may contain hexane and related materials, whereas other batches of the same brand may not, as observed by Means et al. (1976). They identified one batch of a thinner that produced a severe peripheral neuropathy in several inhalant abusers. In the final analysis, the symptoms were believed to result from the 15% heptanone and/or 0.5% hexane present in only some of the batches of this thinner. Whether the other chemicals present in the thinner exacerbated the condition or caused other neurologic manifestations is still unknown.

The "hexane" type syndrome has now been well characterized and includes "both sensory and motor neuropathy." "Microscopic examination has revealed axonal swelling, accumulation of neurofilaments in axons, myelin thinning and denudation, and the skeletal muscle changes of neurogenic atrophy" (Prockop 1979, p. 862). When these conditions are apparent, one should be alert for the possibility that the subject may have been exposed to hexane or related ketones (e.g., methyl butyl ketone) even if the original case history does not identify any of these substances. Electromyography and nerve conduction velocities may be utilized in the diagnosis when no overt symptoms are apparent (Arezzo et al. 1985).

In addition to this well-characterized peripheral neuropathy associated with 2-ketones, others have been described. One peripheral neuropathy case was not linked to hexane type compounds, although gasoline (which usually contains a small amount of hexanes) was one of the substances abused (Gallassi et al. 1980). They observed no axonal swelling characteristic of the hexane-type neuropathy. They also found no CNS involvement typical of "leaded" gasoline (with tetraethyl lead) toxicity.

Another solvent, trichloroethane, has been identified as causing a peripheral neuropathy (Liss 1988). This is one of the substituents of correction fluid often inhaled by solvent abusers.

GASOLINE-RELATED TOXICITIES

Another area of solvent abuse, "gasoline sniffing," needs discussion. Although some CNS or peripheral neuropathies may occur due to the solvents in gasoline, other toxicities may result from the tetraethyl lead (or its metabolite triethyl lead) (Coodin et al. 1980; Goldings and Stewart 1982; Hansen and Sharp 1978; Prockop and Karampelas 1981; Remington and Hoffman 1984; Robinson 1978; Valpey et al. 1978). In all cases where high lead levels are observed, hallucinations and disorientation, dysarthria, chorea, and convulsions have been reported. The symptoms also have included moderate to severe ataxia, insomnia, anorexia, slowed peripheral nerve conduction, limb tremors, dysmetria, and sometimes limb paralysis. In most cases, the EEG is normal; in severe states, however, an abnormal to severely depressed cortical EEG is observed. Only in one lethal case was there any kidney damage noted; electrolytes are usually in the normal range. Because many of these symptoms in the early stages of the disease can be reversed by chelation therapy with edetate (EDTA), dimercaprol (BAL), and/or penicillamine, it is important to check the serum lead levels in any chronic inhalant abuser to see if this treatment should be prescribed.

PULMONARY CHANGES

Despite the likelihood that solvents irritate the lungs, there have been few cases noted where the pulmonary system is severely compromised. Solvents have nevertheless been noted to cause pulmonary hypertension, acute respiratory distress, increased residual volume, and restricted ventilation. Increased airway resistance or residual volume may be more clearly noted following an exercise challenge (Reyes de la Rocha et al. 1987). Smoking may have been a contributory factor in one study (Schikler et al. 1984) and was not ruled out in the others. In studies of workers using waterproofing aerosols containing trichloroethane (Woo et al. 1983) or using a paint stripper (Buie et al. 1986), acute respiratory distress has been correlated with the chlorinated hydrocarbon exposure. Although solvents irritate the pulmonary system, it is not at all clear from the limited case studies reported to date how extensive or what types of pulmonary damage occurs that can be primarily due to solvent exposure and not to other inspired substances that are dissolved in the solvents. For example, a report of a homicidal case (a spray paint "sniffer") noted metallic deposition along with hemorrhagic alveolitis (Engstrand et al. 1986).

Any change may be very slow in onset but most likely will be enhanced by the other substances volatilized along with the solvent (e.g., polystyrenes and tars) or utilized by the subject (e.g., tobacco and marijuana). Because of the potential for cause and augmentation by other substances, the amount of smoking should always be considered in any treatment of these individuals.

CARDIOTOXICITY

Most cardiotoxic effects of solvents have been associated with lethality (Mee and Wright 1980). However, several reports have identified ventricular fibrillation and cardiac arrest in hospitalized patients (Boon 1987; Cunningham et al. 1987; McLeod et al. 1987; Ong et al. 1988; Wiseman and Banim 1987; Wodka and Jeong 1989; Wright and Strobl 1984). Some of the subjects had inhaled trichlorethane-containing solvents (McLeod et al. 1987) and were additionally compromised by anesthesia (halothane). Fluorocarbons have been shown to cause arrhythmias in animals (Taylor and Harris 1970). However, the linkage of arrhythmia to glue sniffing is not well supported by animal studies. Glues usually do not contain halocarbons but do contain toluene and other hydrocarbons. However, two reports (Cunningham et al. 1987; Wiseman and Banim 1987) have linked glue sniffing to arrhythmias and dilated cardiomyopathy. The somewhat different cardiotoxicities noted above are not easily explained but congenital or other environmental causes were not ruled out. When observed, antiarrhythmic therapy should be used (McLeod et al. 1987). Exercise exacerbates these cardiotoxicities and should therefore be minimized. Also, anesthesia should not be induced in patients shortly after intoxication, and one should probably avoid the use of halogenated hydrocarbons in other circumstances where heavy solvent exposure is suspected.

HEPATOTOXICITY

Subjects overexposed to chlorohydrocarbons have been known to exhibit hepatorenal toxicities (Baerg and Kimberg 1970; Clearfield 1970; Dossing 1986; Farrell et al. 1985; Hutchens and Kung 1985); this is a well-established phenomenon corroborated by animal studies (see Sharp and Korman 1981). Any individual who is chronically exposed to these compounds would expect to develop hepatorenal toxicities, depending on the dose and time of exposure (Benjamin et al. 1985; Buring et al. 1985). Thus the recent increase in the inhalation of correction fluids that contain trichloroethylene, trichloroethane, and tetrachloroethane increases the likelihood of observing more of these toxicities in inhalant abusers (Greer 1984). This disease state is exemplified in two reports of apparent occupational (poorly ventilated areas) overexposure. Extreme nephronecrosis and associated hepatotoxicity were observed after exposure to mixtures containing methylene chloride and other solvents (Cordes et al. 1988; Miller et al. 1985) and trichloroethane (Hodgson et al. 1989; Keogh et al. 1984). Ketones, including acetone, potentiate haloalkane hepatotoxicity (Plaa 1988). As few cases such as these have been noted for methylene chloride (Cherry et al. 1981; Mizutani et al. 1988), higher concentrations or other factors may have been important in the etiology of the disease condition. So far there have been few inhalant abusers noted to have irreversible liver damage. For example, subjects with altered liver function, as noted by elevated plasma liver enzymes, have recovered in a few weeks (Fornazzari et al., unpublished data, 1988). This low incidence of liver damage so far noted for this group may be due to a less frequent use of chlorinated solvents. The frequent heavy use of alcohol concurrently with inhalants should also be of concern when these subjects are being evaluated. When these patterns of "drug" exposure are known, it would be advisable to conduct liver function tests.

In regard to the combined effects of solvents and alcohol, it is worth noting a problem associated with workers in dry-cleaning establishments. Dry-cleaning operators who intentionally or unintentionally expose themselves to high levels of cleaning fluid (mostly perchlorethylene) are susceptible to a dilation of the superficial skin vessels. The effect has been referred to as "degreasers' flush," especially when alcohol is coadministered (Stewart et al. 1974).

In addition to the aforementioned toxicities, there is increasing evidence that anesthetic chlorinated hydrocarbons (halothane, trichloroethylene, and chloroform) are carcinogenic (Cohen 1979) and have been associated with spontaneous abortions (Buring et al. 1985).

It is premature to state that toluene causes liver damage. However, as it is strongly associated with the onset of renal acidosis and has been identified as the major solvent associated with liver toxicity in the printing industry (Guzelian et al. 1988), it would be prudent to check for liver anomalies in inhalant abusers.

NITROUS OXIDE NEUROPATHIES

Another substance may not be considered when one thinks of inhalants because it is unique both chemically and in its physiologic action, as well as in the primary group using it and also in its marketing. This substance, nitrous oxide, is used as an anesthetic and as a propellant primarily for whipped cream. Laughing gas (N_2O), as it is euphemistically called, was abused soon after it was discovered in the late 19th century. Only in the past decade was it known that central and peripheral nerve damage resulted following high levels of N_2O exposure, even in the presence of adequate oxygen. The symptoms include numbness and weakness in the limbs, loss of dexterity, sensory loss, and loss of balance. The neurologic examination indicates sensorimotor polyneuropathy. There is also a combined degeneration of the posterior and lateral columns of the cord that resembles B_{12} deficiencies (Layzer 1978). Studies focusing on the mechanism of action indicate that cobalamins are inactivated by N_2O; yet vitamin B_{12} does not aid recovery from this disease (Chanarin 1980; Nunn 1987). A review by Brodsky and Cohen (1986) covered many of the medical aspects of the adverse effects of nitrous oxide. Rehabilitation proceeds with abstinence and is relative to the extent of neurologic damage. Despite the widespread distribution of this information to the medical community and the reduced availability of metal cylinders, cases are still being observed (Schwartz and Calihan 1984).

HEMATOLOGIC CHANGES

Microcytic anemia and leukopenia are sometimes found in solvent abusers (Fornazzari et al., unpublished data, 1988). The leukopenia is due to a marked decrease in lymphocytes, leaving the subject immunocompromised and susceptible to infections. This may be related to the recency and extent of exposure and is reversible in most cases.

There are two types of solvent exposure that lead to hemoglobin dyscrasias as the result of the abuse of solvents. Methylene chloride exposure can increase the carboxyhemoglobin levels (Horowitz 1986), a change that also occurs with cigarette smoking. In some instances, high concentrations of methylene chloride exposure can lead to death (Manno et al. 1989). Methylene chloride poisoning and treatment have been reviewed by Rioux and Myers (1988). Recently, these same authors (Rioux and Myers 1989) demonstrated the usefulness of hyperbaric oxygen for the treatment of methylene chloride poisoning. The second group of substances, the organic nitrites, produce methemoglobinemia and hemolytic anemia (Brandes et al. 1989; Wason et al. 1980). This group of substances, the volatile liquid "amyl" (and "butyl" and now isopropyl) nitrites, have also been used in clinical practice as vasodilators to treat angina pectoris, although much less so today. Although they are not usually considered solvents, they are often included in "inhalant abuse." As with nitrous oxide, a different group of individuals inhale isoamyl (amyl) or isobutyl nitrites: in this case, predominately homosexuals. The nitrites are usually not considered toxic during inhalation because of syncope (fainting). However, Guss et al. (1985) noted a dangerously high 37% methemoglobin level in a normal subject who had used isobutyl nitrite (he had also used methaqualone). It has also been reported to produce bradycardia (Rosoff and Cohen 1986), to reduce killer cell activity (Lotzova et al. 1984), and to be potentially carcinogenic (Osterloh and Goldfield 1985). These latter effects are of special concern in the development of acquired immune deficiency syndrome (AIDS) in that there is an association between the development of Kaposi's sarcoma and high amyl-butyl nitrite use (Haverkos et al. 1985; Newell et al. 1984). There is a specific treatment for nitrite overdose. The high and slowly reversible reduction of methemoglobin can be aided by the use of methylene blue (Smith et al. 1980).

The hemotoxicity of benzene has been thoroughly studied and reviewed. This solvent is present in thinners, in varnish removers, and in varying proportions in gasoline. Essentially, benzene has been identified as causing aplastic anemia and leukemia (Austin et al. 1988; Lauwerys et al. 1985).

Also, hematopoietic effects were identified in a subject using glue (trichloroethylene) in his hobby; cessation of the symptoms occurred when he ceased his hobby (Pinkhas et al. 1972). Although this condition may have resulted from different solvents used in his hobby, it also may be a result of the individual's sensitivity.

NEONATAL SYNDROME

There is discussion of a "fetal solvent syndrome." Studies of infants of mothers who chronically abuse solvents have been reported (Hersh 1989; Hersh et al. 1985). This appears similar to other embryopathies (e.g., fetal alcohol syndrome and hydantoin embryopathy). The concomitant influence of undernutrition, other substance abuse, or even genetic predisposition needs to be clarified through further studies.

Goodwin (1988) reported on newborns of five women who showed renal tubular acidosis in their third trimester. On delivery, three of the five newborns showed growth retardation, and two showed renal tubular acidosis.

OTHER INHALANTS

There are two fads that appear to be infrequent, poorly studied, and possibly increasing in many parts of the world. The abuse of ethyl chloride, especially by the homosexual community, has been known about for some time. One report observed dizziness and visual and olfactory disturbances, with succeeding blood pressure fall and grand mal seizure in one case (Nordin et al. 1988). The patient had used ethyl chloride for 30 years. No EEG abnormalities were observed. There was occasional use of benzodiazepines and alcohol.

Another group of substances that have been abused are the various types of cooking gas. Subjects sniff from canisters of propane and cyclopropane or from butane lighters (Hansen and Knudsen 1988). Deaths occur, as reported by Krause and McCarthy (1989) and Siegel and Wason (1990). Another case showed emotional disturbances and hallucinations (Mathew et al. 1989). Neither case provides much insight into whether these substances cause any residual clinical syndromes. However, the clinician should be aware of this form of abuse, because future cases may provide further clarification as to any complications that may result aside from the well-known lethal actions of these gases.

TREATMENT

Some specific treatments have been identified throughout this chapter. However, in general, most subjects will recover from an acute episode or more slowly from a chronic state of intoxication of most volatile substances. That is why most of these solvent abusers are not often seen in emergency rooms. This is aptly summarized by Meredith et al. (1989): "Recovery normally occurs quickly once exposure has ceased but support for respiratory, renal or hepatic failure may be needed as well as treatment for cardiac arrythmias. Therapy with intravenous acetylcysteine should be considered in cases of acute carbon tetrachloride poisoning" (p. 277).

REFERENCES

Anderson HR, Dick B, Mcnair RS, et al: An investigation of 140 deaths associated with volatile substance abuse in the United Kingdom (1971–1981). Hum Toxicol 1:207–221, 1982
Anderson HR, Macnair RS, Ramsey JD: Deaths from abuse of volatile substances: a national epidemiological study. Br Med J 290:304–307, 1985
Arezzo JC, Simson R, Brennan NE: Evoked potentials in the assessment of neurotoxicity in humans. Neurobehavioral Toxicology and Teratology 7:299–304, 1985
Austin H, Delzell E, Cole P: Benzene and leukemia: a review of the literature and a risk assessment. Am J Epidemiol 127:419–439, 1988

Baerg RD, Kimberg DV: Centrilobular hepatic necrosis and acute renal failure in "solvent sniffers." Ann Intern Med 73:713–720, 1970

Bass M: Sudden sniffing death. JAMA 212:2075–2079, 1970

Bass M: Death from sniffing gasoline. N Engl J Med 299:203, 1978

Bass M: Abuse of inhalation anaesthetics. JAMA 251:604, 1984

Beauvais F, Oetting ER: Toward a clear definition of inhalant abuse. Int J Addict 22:779–784, 1987

Beauvais F, Oetting ER: Indian youth and inhalants: an update: inhalant abuse by young children. Natl Inst Drug Abuse Res Monogr Ser 85:30–48, 1988

Benjamin SB, Goodman ZD, Ishak KG, et al: The morphologic spectrum of halothane-induced hepatic injury: analysis of 77 cases. Hepatology 5: 1163–1171, 1985

Bennett RH, Forman HR: Hypokalemic periodic paralysis in chronic toluene exposure. Arch Neurol 37:673, 1980

Berg EF: Retrobulbar neuritis. Ann Ophthalmol 3:1351–1353, 1971

Bergholtz LM, Odkvist LM: Audiological findings in solvent exposed workers. Acta Otolaryngol (suppl) 412:109–110, 1984

Biscaldi GP, Mingardi M, Pollini G, et al: Acute toluene poisoning: electroneurophysiological and vestibular investigations. Toxicological European Research 3:271–273, 1981

Boon NA: Solvent abuse and the heart (editorial). Br Med J 294:722, 1987

Boor JW, Hurtig HI: Persistant cerebellar ataxia after exposure to toluene. Ann Neurol 2:440–442, 1977

Brandes JC, Bufill JA, Pisciotta AV: Amyl nitrite-induced hemolytic anemia. Am J Med 86:252–254, 1989

Brennan RP, Pearlstein AE, Miller SA: Computed tomography of the kidneys in a patient with methoxyflurane abuse. J Comput Assist Tomogr 12:155–156, 1988

Brodsky JB, Cohen EN: Adverse effects of nitrous oxide. Medical Toxicology 1:362–374, 1986

Bruhn P, Arlien-Soborg P, Gyldensted C, et al: Prognosis in chronic toxic encephalopathy: a two-year follow-up study in 26 house painters with occupational encephalopathy. Acta Neurol Scand 64:259–272, 1981

Buie SE, Pratt DS, May JJ: Diffuse pulmonary injury following paint remover exposure. Am J Med 81:702–704, 1986

Buring JE, Hennekens CH, Mayrent SL, et al: Health experiences of operating room personnel. Anesthesiology 62:325–330, 1985

Chadwick OF, Anderson HR: Neuropsychological consequences of volatile substance abuse: a review. Hum Toxicol 8:307–312, 1989

Chanarin I: Nitrous oxide and the cobalamins. Clin Sci 59:151–154, 1980

Channer KS, Stanley S: Persistent visual hallucination secondary to chronic solvent encephalopathy: case report and review of the literature. J Neurol Neurosurg Psychiatry 46:83–86, 1983

Cherry N, Venables H, Waldron HA, et al: Some observations on workers exposed to methylene chloride. Br J Ind Med 38:351–355, 1981

Clark MA, Jones JW, Robinson JJ, et al: Multiple deaths resulting from shipboard exposure to trichlorotrifluoroethane. J Forensic Sci 30: 1256–1259, 1985

Clearfield HR: Hepatorenal toxicity from sniffing spot-remover (trichloroethylene). Dig Dis 15:851–856, 1970

Cohen EN: Inhalation anesthetics may cause genetic defects, abortions and miscarriages in operating room personnel, in Controversy in Anesthesiology. Edited by Eckenhoff JE. Philadelphia, PA, WB Saunders, 1979, pp 47–57

Cohen S: Inhalant abuse: an overview of the problem. Natl Inst Drug Abuse Res Monogr Ser 15:2–11, 1977

Coodin FJ, Dawes C, Dean GW, et al: Riposte to "Environmental lead and young children." Can Med Assoc J 123:469–471, 1980

Cordes DH, Brown WD, Quinn KM: Chemically induced hepatitis after inhaling organic solvents. West J Med 148:458–460, 1988

Couri D, Milks M: Toxicity and metabolism of the neurotoxic hexacarbons n-hexane, 2-hexanone and 2,5-hexanedione. Annu Rev Pharmacol Toxicol 22:145–166, 1982

Crider RA, Rouse BA: Epidemiology of inhalant abuse: an update. Natl Inst Drug Abuse Res Monogr Ser 85:1–203, 1988

Cronk SL, Barkley DE, Farrell MF: Respiratory arrest after solvent abuse. Br Med J 290:897–898, 1985

Cunningham SR, Dalzell GWN, McGirr P, et al: Myocardial infarction and primary ventricular fibrillation after glue sniffing. Br Med J 294: 739–740, 1987

DiMaio VJM, Garriott JC: Four deaths resulting from abuse of nitrous oxide. J Forensic Sci 23:169–172, 1978

Dossing M: Occupational toxic liver damage. J Hepatol 3:131–135, 1986

Engstrand DA, England DM, Huntington RW 3d: Pathology of paint sniffers' lung. Am J Foresic Med Pathol 7:232–236, 1986

Ehyai A, Freemon FR: Progressive optic neuropathy and sensorineural hearing loss due to chronic glue sniffing. J Neurol Neurosurg Psychiatry 46:349–351, 1983

Farrell G, Prendergast D, Murray M: Halothane hepatitis: detection of a constitutional susceptibility factor. N Engl J Med 313:1310–1314, 1985

Fornazzari L, Wilkinson DA, Kapur BM, et al: Cerebellar, cortical and functional impairment in toluene abusers. Acta Neurol Scand 67:319–329, 1983a

Fornazzari L, Wilkinson DA, Carlen PL: Functional but not morphological recovery in chronic solvent abusers. Can J Neurol Sci 10:145, 1983b

Gallassi R, Montagna P, Pazzaglia P, et al: Peripheral neuropathy due to gasoline sniffing: a case report. Eur Neurol 19:419–421, 1980

Garriott J, Petty CS: Death from inhalant abuse: toxicological and pathological evaluation of 34 cases. Clin Toxicol 16:305–315, 1980

Goldbloom D, Chouinard G: Schizophreniform psychosis associated with chronic industrial toluene exposure: case report. J Clin Psychiatry 46: 350–351, 1985

Goldings AS, Stewart RM: Organic lead encephalopathy: behavioral change and movement disorder following gasoline inhalation. J Clin Psychiatry 43:70–72, 1982

Goodwin TM: Toluene abuse and renal tubular acidosis in pregnancy. Obstet Gynecol 71:715–718, 1988

Greer JE: Adolescent abuse of typewriter correction fluid. South Med J 77: 297–298, 1984

Gresham GA, Treip CS: Fatal poisoning by 1,1,1-trichloroethane after prolonged survival. Forensic Sci Int 23:249–253, 1983

Guss DA, Normann SA, Manoguerra AS: Clinically significant methemoglobinemia from inhalation of isobutyl nitrite. Am J Emerg Med 3:46–47, 1985

Guzelian P, Mills S, Fallon HJ: Liver structure and function in print workers exposed to toluene. J Occup Med 30:791–796, 1988

Hall DMB, Ramsey J, Schwartz MS, et al: Neuropathy in a petrol sniffer. Arch Dis Child 61:900–901, 1986

Hansen AC, Knudsen PJ: [Fatal lighter-gas sniffing]. Ugeskr Laeger 150: 867–869, 1988

Hansen KS, Sharp FR: Gasoline sniffing, lead poisoning, and myoclonus. JAMA 240:1375–1376, 1978

Harrison DJ, Thomson D, MacDonald MK: Membranous glomerulonephritis. J Clin Pathol 39:167, 1986

Haverkos HW, Pinsky PF, Drotman DP, et al: Disease manifestation among homosexual men with acquired immunodeficiency syndrome: a possible role of nitrites in Kaposi's sarcoma. Sex Transm Dis 12:203–208, 1985

Hersh JH: Toluene embryopathy: two new cases. J Med Genet 26:333–337, 1989

Hersh JH, Podruch PE, Rogers G, et al: Toluene embryopathy. J Pediatr 106:922–927, 1985

Hodgson MJ, Heyl AE, Van Thiel DH: Liver disease associated with exposure to 1,1,1-trichloroethane. Arch Intern Med 149:1793–1798, 1989

Hormes JT, Filley CM, Rosenberg NL: Neurologic sequelae of chronic solvent vapor abuse. Neurology 36:698–702, 1986

Horowitz BZ: Carboxyhemoglobinemia caused by inhalation of methylene chloride. Am J Emerg Med 4:48–51, 1986

Hutchens KS, Kung M: Experimentation with chloroform. Am J Med 78: 715–718, 1985

Jone CM, Wu AH: An unusual case of toluene-induced metabolic acidosis. Clin Chem 34:2596–2599, 1988

Jones RD, Winter DP: Two case reports of deaths on industrial premises attributed to 1,1,1-trichloroethane. Arch Environ Health 38:59–61, 1983

Keane JR: Toluene optic neuropathy. Ann Neurol 4:390, 1978

Keogh AM, Ibels LS, Allen DH, et al: Exacerbation of Goodpasture's syndrome after inadvertent exposure to hydrocarbon fumes. Br Med J 288:188, 1984

King GS, Smialek JE, Troutman WG: Sudden death in adolescents resulting from the inhalation of typewriter correction fluid. JAMA 253: 1604–1606, 1985

King MD, Day RE, Oliver JS, et al: Solvent encephalopathy. Br Med J 283:663–665, 1981

King PJL, Morris JGL, Pollard JD: Glue sniffing neuropathy. Aust NZ J Med 15:293–299, 1985

Kirk LM, Anderson RJ, Martin K: Sudden death toluene abuse (letter). Ann Emerg Med 13:68–69, 1984

Krause JG, McCarthy WB: Sudden death by inhalation of cyclopropane. J Forensic Sci 34:1011–1012, 1989

Kringsholm B: Sniffing-associated deaths in Denmark. Forensic Sci Int 15: 215–225, 1980

Lauwerys R, Bernard A, Viau C, et al: Kidney disorders and hematotoxicity from organic solvent exposure. Scand J Work Environ Health (suppl) 1:83–90, 1985

Layzer RB: Myeloneuropathy after prolonged exposure to nitrous oxide. Lancet 2:1227–1230, 1978

Lazar RB, Ho SU, Melen O, et al: Multifocal central nervous system damage caused by toluene abuse. Neurology 33:1337–1340, 1983

Lecomte D, Trophilme D, Rudler M, et al: Complications pulmonaires des sniffeurs. Rev Mal Respir 11:713–717, 1983

Levy AB: Delirium induced by inhalation of typewriter correction fluid. Psychosomatics 27:665–666, 1986

Liss GM: Peripheral neuropathy in two workers exposed to 1,1,1-trichloro-ethane (letter). JAMA 260:2217, 1988

Litovitz TL, Schmitz BF, Bailey KM: 1989 annual report of the American Association of Poison Control Centers National Data Collection System. Toxicology 8:394–442, 1990

Lolin Y: Chronic neurological toxicity associated with exposure to volatile substances. Hum Toxicol 8:293–300, 1989

Lotzova E, Savary CA, Hersh EM, et al: Depression of murine natural killer cell cytotoxicity by isobutyl nitrite. Cancer Immunol Immunother 17:130–134, 1984

Malm G, Lying-Tunell U: Cerebellar dysfunction related to toluene sniffing. Acta Neurol Scand 62:188–190, 1980

Manno M, Chirillo R, Daniotti G, et al: Carboxyhaemoglobin and fatal methylene chloride poisoning (letter). Lancet 2:274, 1989

Marjot R, McLeod AA: Chronic non-neurological toxicity from volatile substance abuse. Hum Toxicol 8:301–306, 1989

Mathew B, Kapp E, Jones TR: Commercial butane abuse: a disturbing case. Br J Addict 84:563–564, 1989

McLeod AA, Marjot R, Monaghan MJ, et al: Chronic cardiac toxicity after inhalation of 1,1,1-trichloroethane. Br Med J 294:727–729, 1987

Means ED, Prockop LD, Hooper GS: Pathology of lacquer thinner induced neuropathy. Ann Clin Lab Sci 6:240–250, 1976

Mee AS, Wright PL: Congestive (dilated) cardiomyopathy in association with solvent abuse. J R Soc Med 73:671–672, 1980

Meredith TJ, Ruprah M, Liddle A, et al: Diagnosis and treatment of acute poisoning with volatile substances. Hum Toxicol 8:277–286, 1989

Metrick SA, Brenner RP: Abnormal brainstem auditory evoked potentials in chronic paint sniffers. Ann Neurol 12:553–556, 1982

Mikkelsen S, Jorgensen M, Browne E, et al: Mixed solvent exposure and organic brain damage: a study of painters. Acta Neurol Scand (suppl) 118:1–143, 1988

Miller L, Pateras V, Friederici H, et al: Acute tubular necrosis after inhalation exposure to methylene chloride: report of a case. Arch Intern Med 145:145–146, 1985

Mizutani K, Shinomiya K, Shinomiya T: Hepatotoxicity of trichloromethane. Forensic Sci Int 38:113–128, 1988

Moller C, Odkvist LM, Thell J, et al: Otoneurological findings in psychoorganic syndrome caused by industrial solvent exposure. Acta Otolaryngol (Stockh) 107:5–12, 1989

National Institute on Drug Abuse: National household survey on drug abuse: main findings. Rockville, MD, National Institute on Drug Abuse, 1990

Newell GR, Adams SC, Mansell PWA, et al: Toxicity, immunosuppressive effects and carcinogenic potential of volatile nitrites: possible relationship to Kaposi's sarcoma. Pharmacotherapy 4:284–291, 1984

Nordin C, Rosenqvist M, Hollstedt C: Sniffing of ethyl chloride: an uncommon form of abuse with serious mental and neurological symptoms. Int J Addict 23:623–627, 1988

Nouchi T, Miura H, Kanayama M, et al: Fatal intoxication by 1,2-dichloroethane: a case report. Int Arch Occup Environ Health 54:111–113, 1984

Novak MA, Roth AS, Levine MR: Calcium oxalate retinopathy associated with methoxyflurane abuse. Retina 8:230–236, 1988

Nunn JF: Clinical aspects of the interaction between nitrous oxide and vitamin B12. Br J Anaesth 59:3–13, 1987

Oetting ER, Edwards RW, Beauvais F: Social and psychological factors underlying inhalant abuse. Natl Inst Drug Abuse Res Monogr Ser 85:172–203, 1988

Ong TK, Rustage KJ, Harrison KM, et al: Solvent abuse: an anaesthetic management problem. Br Dent J 164:150–151, 1988

Orbaek P, Rosen I, Svensson K: Electroneurographic findings in patients with solvent induced central nervous system dysfunction. Br J Ind Med 45:409–414, 1988a

Orbaek P, Rosen I, Svensson K: Power spectrum analysis of EEG at diagnosis and follow up of patients with solvent induced chronic toxic encephalopathy. Br J Ind Med 45:476–482, 1988b

Osterloh J, Goldfield D: Uptake of inhaled n-butyl nitrite and in vivo transformation in rats. J Pharm Sci 74:780–782, 1985

Passero S, Battistini N, Cioni R, et al: Toxic polyneuropathy of shoe workers in Italy: a clinical neurophysiological and followup study. Ital J Neurol Sci 4:463–472, 1983

Patel R, Benjamin J Jr: Renal disease associated with toluene inhalation. Clinical Toxicology 24:213–223, 1986

Pinkhas J, Cohen I, Kruglak J, et al: Hobby induced factor VII deficiency. Haemeostasis 1:52–54, 1972

Plaa GL: Experimental evaluation of haloalkanes and liver injury. Fundam Appl Toxicol 10:563–570, 1988

Prockop L: Specific neurological evaluation of inhalant abusers: clinical and laboratory. Natl Inst Drug Abuse Res Monogr Ser 15:81–96, 1977

Prockop L: Neurotoxic volatile substances. Neurology (Minneapolis) 29: 862–865, 1979

Prockop LD, Karampelas D: Encephalopathy secondary to abusive gasoline inhalation. J Fla Med Assoc 68:823–824, 1981

Pryor GT: Toluene-induced motor syndrome in rats resembling that seen in some solvent abusers. Neurotoxicol Teratol (in press)

Pryor GT, Dickinson J, Howd RA, et al: Transient cognitive deficits and high-frequency hearing loss in weanling rats exposed to toluene. Neurobehavioral Toxicology and Teratology 5:53–57, 1983

Ramsey J, Anderson HR, Bloor K, et al: An introduction to the practice, prevalence and chemical toxicology of volatile substance abuse. Hum Toxicol 8:261–269, 1989

Ravnskov U: Exposure to organic solvents: a missing link in post-streptococcal glomerulonephritis? Acta Med Scand 203:351–356, 1978

Ravnskov U, Lundstrom S, Norden A: Hydrocarbon exposure and glomerulonephritis: evidence from patient's occupations. Lancet 2:1214–1216, 1983

Remington G, Hoffman BF: Gas sniffing as a form of substance abuse. Can J Psychiatry 29:31–35, 1984

Reyes de la Rocha S, Brown MA, Fortenberry JD: Pulmonary function abnormalities in intentional spray paint inhalation. Chest 92:100–104, 1987

Rioux JP, Myers RA: Methylene chloride poisoning: a paradigmatic review. J Emerg Med 6:227–238, 1988

Rioux JP, Myers RA: Hyperbaric oxygen for methylene chloride poisoning: report on two cases. Ann Emerg Med 18:691–695, 1989

Roberts FP, Lucas, EG, Mardsen CD, et al: Near-pure xylene causing reversible neuropsychiatric disturbance (letter). Lancet 2:273, 1988

Robinson RO: Tetraethyl lead poisoning from gasoline sniffing. JAMA 240: 1373–1374, 1978

Rosen I: Neurophysiological aspects of organic solvent toxicity. Acta Neurol Scand 70 (suppl 100):101–106, 1984

Rosenberg NL, Spitz MC, Filley CM, et al: Central nervous system effects of chronic toluene abuse: clinical, brainstem evoked response and magnetic resonance imaging studies. Neurotoxicol Teratol 10:489–495, 1988a

Rosenberg NL, Kleinschmidt-DeMasters BK, Davis KA, et al: Toluene abuse causes diffuse central nervous system white matter changes. Ann Neurol 23:611–614, 1988b

Rosoff MH, Cohen MV: Profound bradycardia after amyl nitrite in patients with a tendency to vasovagal episodes. Br Heart J 55:97–100, 1986

Sarmiento-Martinez J, Guardiola Sala JJ, Martinez Vea A, et al: Renal tubular acidosis with an elevated anion gap in a 'glue sniffer' (letter). Hum Toxicol 8:139–140, 1989

Schikler KN, Seitz K, Rice JF, et al: Solvent abuse associated cortical atrophy. J Adolesc Health Care 3:37–39, 1982

Schikler KN, Lane EE, Seitz K, et al: Solvent abuse associated pulmonary abnormalities. Adv Alcohol Subst Abuse 3:75–81, 1984

Schwartz RH, Calihan M: Nitrous oxide: a potentially lethal euphoriant inhalant. American Family Practice 30:171–172, 1984

Sharp CW, Korman M: Volatile substances, in Substance Abuse: Clinical Problems and Perspectives. Edited by Lowinson J, Ruiz P. Baltimore, Williams & Wilkins, 1981, pp 233–255

Shepherd RT: Mechanism of sudden death associated with volatile substance abuse. Hum Toxicol 8:287–291, 1989

Siegel E, Wason S: Sudden death caused by inhalation of butane and propane. N Engl J Med 323:1638, 1990

Smith M, Stair T, Rolnick MA: Butyl nitrite and a suicide attempt. Ann Intern Med 5:719–720, 1980

Spencer D, Raasch FO, Trefny FA: Halothane abuse in hospital personnel. JAMA 235:1034–1035, 1976

Spencer PS, Schaumburg HH: Organic Solvent neurotoxicity: facts and research needs. Scand J Work Environ Health 11 (suppl 1):53–60, 1985

Spencer PS, Schaumburg HH, Sabri MI, et al: The enlarging view of hexacarbon neurotoxicity. CRC Crit Rev Toxicol 3:279–357, 1980

Stewart RD, Hake CL, Peterson JE: "Degreasers' flush," dermal response to trichloroethylene and ethanol. Arch Environ Health 29:1–5, 1974

Streicher HZ, Gabow PA, Moss AH, et al: Syndromes of toluene sniffing in adults. Ann Intern Med 94:758–762, 1981

Takeuchi Y, Hisanaga N, Ono Y, et al: Cerebellar dysfunction caused by sniffing of toluene-containing thinner. Ind Health 19:163–169, 1981

Taylor GJ, Harris WS: Cardiac toxicity of aerosol propellants. JAMA 214: 81–85, 1970

Tenebein M, deGroot W, Rajani KR: Peripheral neuropathy following intentional inhalation of naphtha fumes. Can Med Assoc J 131:1077–1079, 1984

Troutman WG: Additional deaths associated with the intentional inhalation of typewriter correction fluid. Vet Hum Toxicol 30:130–132, 1988

Valpey R, Sumi SM, Copass MK, et al: Acute and chronic progressive encephalopathy due to gasoline sniffing. Neurology 28:507–510, 1978

Wason S, Detsky AS, Platt OS, et al: Isobutyl nitrite toxicity by ingestion. Ann Intern Med 92:637–638, 1980

Wedeen RP: Occupational renal disease. Am J Kidney Dis 111:241–257, 1984

Wennberg A: A neuropathy index based on motor-sensory electroneurography (ENeG). Acta Neurol Scand 70 (suppl 100): 107–111, 1984

Will AM, McLaren EH: Reversible renal damage due to glue sniffing. Br Med J 283:525–526, 1981

Wiseman MN, Banim S: Glue sniffer's heart? Br Med J 294:739, 1987

Wodka RM, Jeong EW: Cardiac effects of inhaled typewriter correction fluid (letter). Ann Intern Med 110:91–92, 1989

Woo OF, Healey KM, Sheppard D, et al: Chest pain and hypoxemia from

    inhalation of a trichloroethane aerosol product. J Toxicol Clin Toxicol
    20:333–341, 1983

Wright MF, Strobl DJ: 1,1,1-Trichloroethane cardiac toxicity: report of a
    case. J Am Osteopath Assoc 84:285–288, 1984

Yamaguchi K, Shirai T, Shimakura K, et al: Pneumatosis cystoides intesti-
    nalis and trichloroethylene exposure. Am J Gastroenterol 80:753–757,
    1985

Yamashita M, Matsuki A, Oyama T: Illicit use of modern volatile anesthet-
    ics. Canadian Anaesthetists Society Journal 31:76–79, 1984

Chapter 10

Tobacco

Reese T. Jones, M.D.

Health-related problems from tobacco dependence surpass those posed by the other drugs in this volume with the possible exception of alcohol. In the mid-1980s, America's 55 million tobacco addicts purchased 623 billion cigarettes. Since each puff is one dose, that is about 6.2 trillion doses of nicotine. Compulsive use of nicotine consumed in the form of tobacco occurs in almost every culture where tobacco is available. In much of the Western world, most smokers would like to quit but find they cannot stop smoking. Tobacco smokers behave in every way as if they are addicted.

It has taken a surprisingly long time for compulsive tobacco use to be generally accepted as drug dependence to nicotine even though well-known investigators came to the conclusion in the early part of this century (Lewin 1931). Relatively small numbers of earlier researchers studying tobacco dependence who concluded "cigarette smoking is probably the most addictive and dependence-producing form of object specific, self-administered gratification known to man" (Russell 1976, p. 1) finally have been joined by the Surgeon General of the U.S. Public Health Service, whose 20th report was entitled "The Health Consequences of Smoking: Nicotine Addiction" (U.S. Department of Health and Human Services 1987). The specific exclusion of tobacco use as a disorder not worthy of diagnosis in DSM-II (American Psychiatric Association 1968) has evolved to the well-characterized diagnostic category of nicotine dependence in DSM-III-R (American Psychiatric Association 1987).

Why term compulsive tobacco use an addiction rather than "a matter of personal choice" (to use the words of tobacco industry spokespersons) or merely a habit like jogging or nail biting? A majority, 50–97%, of people who smoke cigarettes would like to quit smoking if they could (Orleans 1985). More than 90% of all people and 60–80% of all tobacco smokers believe tobacco use to be harmful to health (Fielding 1985; Orleans 1985). More than 60% of regular smokers have on one occasion attempted to stop smoking before returning to tobacco use (Garvey et al. 1989; Russell 1976). True, even long-standing tobacco addicts do stop smoking on their own, and a relatively small group of chronic tobacco users smoke only occasionally and not compulsively (Shiffman 1989). However, spontaneous self-motivated quitting and long-standing but only occasional use occur with other addicting drugs as well.

All the elements of a drug addiction exist in tobacco use. The behavior of a tobacco smoker is controlled by seeking and taking the psychoactive drug nicotine. A two-pack-a-day cigarette smoker throughout the waking day must on average locate and light a cigarette every 26 minutes and then spend approximately 10 minutes in repetitive dosing (called puffs). The frequent dosing is to avoid the intense withdrawal syndrome that appears 1–2 hours after the last dose. Tolerance to many nicotine effects is marked and rapid. Tobacco that does not contain nicotine is not reinforcing and is not accepted by smokers. The package insert for prescribed nicotine properly warns about nicotine dependence.

DIAGNOSIS AND PREVALENCE

Unlike illicit drug use, diagnosis of tobacco dependence is relatively easy since most tobacco addicts openly describe their behavior. One can imagine situations in the future when increasing social stigma associated with tobacco smoking might lead patients not to admit to it unless questioned. Smokers who quit then relapse, particularly those helped by therapeutic programs, may minimize or deny return to tobacco use. In such instances, saliva, urine, or plasma assay of cotinine, the major metabolite of nicotine, is useful as a marker of nicotine intake (Jarvis et al. 1987a).

During the 25 years since the first Surgeon General's report on smoking and health, prevalence of cigarette smoking by adults has decreased each year. Per capita cigarette sales have decreased each year. Total cigarette sales have decreased about 2% yearly during the past 6 years despite increased population. Increasingly, smoking is no longer socially acceptable and is prohibited in public places.

Who Are Tobacco Users?

In 1985, an estimated 33% of men and 28% of women smoked cigarettes regularly. Overall prevalence of smoking in the United States decreased from 37% in 1976 to 30% in 1985 (Marcus et al. 1989; U.S. Department of Health and Human Services 1987). This consequence of a considerable public health effort should give hope when dealing with problems of illicit drug use since the addiction liability of nicotine is judged as great, if not greater, than any other psychoactive drug, and progress is being made without markedly altering supply or punishing users.

Despite the overall decline in numbers of tobacco smokers, rates differ depending on socioeconomic and educational status, gender, and race. Smoking is more common in lower socioeconomic, unemployed, less educated, and lower income groups. For example, the 1985 smoking prevalence for people without a high school diploma was 35% compared with 17% for people with postgraduate college education (Pierce et al. 1989). Young men have been quitting more rapidly than young women, but relatively more young women have initiated smoking, leading to a converging rate of smoking prevalence among men and women (Fiore et al. 1989). However, education has replaced gender as the main sociodemographic predictor of smoking status, and the gap is widening. Regardless of gender, a person who has not attended college is more than twice as likely to be a smoker. Blacks in the United States have consistently smoked at higher rates than whites, although the decline in smoking prevalence has been similar. Predicted prevalence rates for the year 2000 are 34% for blacks and 29% for whites (Fiore et al. 1989; Novotny et al. 1988). The disparity between smoking prevalence among blacks and whites may grow, particularly in view of aggressive cigarette advertising and marketing campaigns targeting minorities.

Psychiatric patients are more likely to be smokers. In a group of 227 outpatients, 52% were smokers, with 88% of the patients diagnosed as having schizophrenia and 70% of patients diagnosed as manic (Hughes 1986a).

Approximately 22 million people in the United States have used smokeless tobacco (Cullen et al. 1986). Current prevalence in adults is 2.2% for men and 0.5% for women. Estimates of 3–26% of adolescent males and less than 3% of adolescent females use smokeless tobacco. However, certain groups (e.g., American Indians) have prevalence of regular smokeless tobacco use ranging from 24% to 64% in some areas (Schinke et al. 1989).

Who Are the New Smokers?

Children dependent on tobacco are a problem (Greydanus 1989). Of the 23 million people in the United States aged 12–17 years, 3.5 million use tobacco products. Tobacco is the gateway psychoactive drug used daily by more young people than any other drug. Nearly 3 million adolescents smoke marijuana. One million use various stimulants, and 6 million drink alcohol. Among adolescents, 16% of boys and 20% of girls smoke cigarettes daily; 12% smoke more than 10 cigarettes per day.

About 50% of high school seniors who report daily smoking began before the age of 14 years (Johnston et al. 1987). More than half of high school seniors who smoke 10 cigarettes or more per day made at least one serious but unsuccessful attempt to stop smoking. Forty-seven percent say they would like to stop, but 75% of daily smokers in high school still smoke 7–9 years later even though while in high school only 5% of them thought they would be daily smokers 5 years later.

New Populations of Potential Addicts

Although tobacco markets are shrinking in Western industrialized countries, tobacco consumption in developing countries is increasing 2% per year, more than outstripping population growth (Mackay 1989). Conservative estimates are that sales in Asia will increase by 18% by the year 2000. China is the largest producer and consumer of cigarettes in the world. A 1984 survey reported that 61% of men and 7% of women smoke in China. Throughout Asia, the Middle East, and in Eastern Europe as trade channels open, multinational tobacco companies are expanding markets by setting up joint ventures and mounting aggressive advertising campaigns with little competition from health education and treatment organizations.

ETIOLOGIC THEORIES

How Does Tobacco Dependence Begin?

Why do people start smoking? Important factors are peer pressure to smoke and psychological influences such as tobacco company advertising glamorizing smoking in young adults. The pharmacology of nicotine or tobacco does not explain why someone first begins to smoke, even though it accounts for continuation of smoking. A person must learn to smoke. In the United States, beginning smokers are typically in their early teens. More than 90% of tobacco smokers begin to smoke as teenagers (McGinnis et al. 1987; Shopland and Brown 1987). Tobacco effects are initially aversive. The lack of tolerance and inability to control dose cause the first cigarette smoked commonly to produce dizziness, nausea, vomiting, and other effects to which the smoker rapidly becomes tolerant (Benowitz 1988).

In recent years, the number of children and adolescents who try cigarettes and then go on to become regular cigarette smokers has declined. However, since still as many as 90% of high school students try at least one cigarette, prevalence of tobacco use still remains high. Prevention programs specifically addressing social influences that initiate smoking onset decrease tobacco experimentation during preadolescent years (Glynn 1989; Hansen et al. 1988; Silvis and Perry 1987).

After learning to manipulate dose and establishing a regular smoking pattern, pharmacologic considerations become primary in maintaining nicotine dependence (McNeill et al. 1986). The transition from experimentation and intermittent smoking to regular, intensive, compulsive tobacco use and nicotine dependence takes less than 2–3 years and by some estimates only a few months or weeks (U.S. Department of Health and Human Services 1987). Gradually, a host of associated elements, or conditioned factors (e.g., social, psychological, tobacco flavor, and aroma) become part of the smoking behavior. Even a one-pack-a-day smoker spends approximately 3 hours of the waking day seeking, lighting up, puffing, and disposing of the drug.

Thus a structured ritual associated with drug-taking behavior occupies as much or more time as almost any other waking behavior.

Tobacco Industry Smoker Education and Economics

Important in the etiology of tobacco dependence are advertising and promotion by the tobacco producers amounting to almost 3 billion dollars per year (Fielding 1985). What might be viewed by a cynic as an educational program for smokers and would-be smokers is specifically designed to enhance secondary associations so that psychological and social aspects of tobacco-using behavior are linked to physiologic and pharmacologic considerations. The secondary associations and the ancillary stimuli probably are what make nicotine the powerful reinforcer that it is for humans (Goldberg and Henningfield 1988; Henningfield and Goldberg 1983), even though nicotine only seems to be a relatively weak primary reinforcer for animals.

　　Important when considering etiology are the economics of tobacco dependence. With the possible exception of cocaine dependence, tobacco use and its consequences have economic impact exceeding any other psychoactive drug. Producing, marketing, and advertising tobacco ranks that industry in the top five of all United States industries (Fielding 1985). Tobacco users spent approximately 25 billion dollars on tobacco products in 1982. Tobacco use contributes about 60 billion dollars to the national economy or 2.5% of the gross national product. The cigarette industry remains one of the most profitable and powerful businesses in America.

PHARMACOLOGY AND PHARMACOKINETICS

Brain Sites of Action

Nicotine is an alkaloid like opium and cocaine. Since nicotine is a weak base at physiologic pH, about 31% is nonionized and thus easily crosses cell membranes. Nicotine readily enters the brain and is rapidly distributed throughout the brain (Hansson and Schmiterlow 1962). Binding to brain tissue is greatest in hypothalamus, hippocampus, thalamus, midbrain, and brain stem and in cerebral cortex as well (London et al. 1985, 1986). Nicotine is bound to dopaminergic neurons, particularly in nigrostriatal and mesolimbic systems. Nicotine effects may be so diffuse because stimulation of nicotinic receptors on presynaptic sites can result in activation of multiple central nervous system pathways with release of acetylcholine, norepinephrine, dopamine, serotonin, vasopressin, growth hormone, adrenocorticotropic hormone, and a variety of central nervous system active peptides (Balfour 1982; Chesselet 1984).

Pharmacokinetics

Nicotine's pharmacokinetics make it an ideal psychoactive drug for self-administration (Benowitz 1988; Busto et al. 1989). Nicotine is carried from burning tobacco as a fine aerosol (0.1–1.0 μ droplets), inhaled, and deposited in distal airways and alveoli. Cigarette smoke from flue-cured tobaccos is acidic (pH 5.5), thus the nicotine is primarily ionized with little buccal absorption. In contrast, nicotine from alkaline (pH 8.5) smoke from air-cured pipe, cigar, and some European cigarettes is readily absorbed from buccal membranes with no need for inhalation. When tobacco smoke reaches the 70 m^2 membrane of lung alveoli and small airways, 80–90% of the nicotine is rapidly absorbed regardless of smoke pH (Armitage et al. 1975).

What Is Special About Smoking a Psychoactive Drug?

Only carotid artery or direct intracerebral injections offer more efficient ways of delivering a drug to the brain than does smoking (Benowitz 1988). Nicotine reaches the brain within 7 seconds after inhalation. Brain levels of nicotine rise rapidly and decline as rapidly because of distribution to skeletal muscle and other tissues. Although the elimination half-life of nicotine is approximately 2 hours and variable (range, 1–4 hours), the time course of central nervous system effects during smoking is more determined by the distribution half-life of 8 minutes.

Metabolism and Excretion

Nicotine is rapidly and extensively metabolized in the liver and to a lesser degree the kidneys and lungs (Benowitz 1988). Renal excretion, dependent on urinary pH, can range from 10% to 35% of a dose. With very acid pH, renal clearance increases enough so that a compensatory increase in nicotine intake occurs during smoking (Benowitz and Jacob 1985). Nicotine's major metabolite, cotinine, is a useful marker of nicotine intake because of its 17-hour half-life and provides an approximate index of daily nicotine consumption (Benowitz and Jacob 1984).

Harmful effects of maternal smoking have been well documented (Mactutus 1989; U.S. Department of Health and Human Services 1987). Nicotine crosses the placenta freely and is in amniotic fluid and umbilical cord blood of neonates (Luck and Nau 1984). Amniotic fluid provides a mechanism for continued exposure of the fetus to nicotine even when maternal levels are relatively low. The sustained exposure of the fetus might contribute to the observed slow growth of the fetus in utero and subsequent lower than average birth weights. Although appearing in breast milk, nicotine concentration is low and unlikely to be physiologically important (Atkinson et al. 1988).

Smokeless Tobacco

Chewing tobacco, snuff, and nicotine gum are buffered to an alkaline pH to maximize absorption from oral mucous membranes. Unlike the almost instantaneous increase in concentration after a puff and inhalation, concentration of plasma nicotine increases more gradually with the use of smokeless tobacco, reaching a plateau in about 30 minutes, with slowly declining levels over 1–2 hours if tobacco remains in contact with the mucous membranes (Benowitz et al. 1988, 1989).

Smoking Behavior

A typical one- to two-pack-a-day smoker takes 200–400 doses of nicotine each 24 hours (Guyatt et al. 1989; Herning et al. 1983; Hughes et al. 1986b; Moody 1984). Each puff is under some degree of control by the smoker, who varies volume, duration, associated inhalation, and exhalation. The ability of the smoker to deliver concentrated doses of nicotine to the brain rapidly by changing puffing and inhalation behavior provides the ideal situation for manipulating mood and arousal.

Considerable variation in plasma nicotine levels occurs during a smoking day in an individual and even greater variability between smokers. For example, smokers living on a research unit averaged 36 cigarettes a day (range, 20–62) and had an average daily intake of 37 mg of nicotine but a range of 10–79 mg (Benowitz and Jacob 1984).

Nicotine intake per cigarette averaged about 1 mg but ranged from 0.37 to 1.56 mg. Thus variability in dosing is a characteristic of nicotine dependence. As might be expected from a drug with a 2-hour half-life, nicotine levels accumulate during the smoking day, decrease overnight, but are still measurable in plasma in the morning (Benowitz et al. 1982). Thus despite intermittent dosing, exposure of the brain to nicotine is 24 hours a day in a smoker. After smoking a single cigarette, peak plasma levels vary from 5 to 30 ng/ml, depending on how the cigarette is smoked. Late afternoon plasma nicotine levels typically range from 5 to 50 ng/ml.

CLINICAL SIGNS AND SYMPTOMS OF INTOXICATION

Dose-dependent Effects

Nicotine in the doses commonly used by tobacco smokers is a versatile and remarkably potent psychoactive drug. Its potency is 5–10 times more than cocaine, in terms of producing discriminable subjective effects. Nicotine intoxication in accidental or suicidal overdose is associated with nausea, vomiting, pallor, weakness, dizziness, lightheadedness, headache, and sweating. Less common are symptoms of abdominal pain, chills, and salivation. At higher doses, seizures, hypotension, and respiratory arrest can develop (Saxena and Scheman 1985).

Dose-response relationships for nicotine are complex. Nicotine at low doses causes ganglionic stimulation and at higher doses ganglionic blockade subsequent to brief stimulation. Thus many dose-response characteristics are biphasic, and the mechanisms are complex. A second pharmacologic factor complicating dose-response relationships is the development of tolerance. Tolerance develops rapidly to nicotine and is lost with equal rapidity (Benowitz et al. 1987b; Porchet et al. 1987, 1988).

Smoking a cigarette activates the sympathetic nervous system (West and Russell 1987), with increased heart rate and blood pressure, cardiac stroke volume and output, and coronary flow. Muscle blood flow increases; peripheral cutaneous vasoconstriction is associated with decreased skin temperature. Norepinephrine and epinephrine levels in plasma increase. Circulating free fatty acids increase (Benowitz 1988).

Desired Effects of Nicotine

For an experienced tobacco smoker, 1 mg of nicotine from a cigarette gives pleasure. It stimulates, relaxes, relieves boredom, and improves cognitive and motor performance (Benowitz 1986, 1988). The first few cigarettes of the day produce arousal and relaxation, most evident in stressful situations. Feelings of enhanced concentration and elevated mood are commonly reported. Particularly evident in abstinent smokers given nicotine under controlled conditions are improved attention, learning, reaction time, and cognition with reduced feelings of anger, tension, depression, and stress (Wesnes and Warburton 1983). Like other cholinergic agonists, nicotine enhances information-processing task performance. Speed and accuracy on visual information-processing tasks are increased. Acquisition and storage of new information is facilitated. Of course, nicotine-induced reversal of performance decrements associated with the abstinence syndrome could account for enhanced performance in dependent smokers given nicotine (Snyder et al. 1989). However, animals and humans not dependent on nicotine show a similar pattern of effect, and thus one must assume that nicotine has such effects independent of reversal of withdrawal abstinence.

The Problem: Abstinence

Within hours when cigarette smoking is stopped or prevented, about 80% of smokers experience a characteristic withdrawal syndrome (Cummings et al. 1985; McNeill et al. 1986; Pickworth et al. 1989; Snyder et al. 1989; West 1984; West et al. 1987, 1989). Irritability, restlessness, impaired concentration, hunger, depression, desire for tobacco, drowsiness, disturbed sleep, impatience, and confusion rapidly appear (Hatsukami et al. 1984; Hughes and Hatsukami 1986). Smokers in withdrawal eat more food and gain weight. Cardiac rate and reaction time are slowed. Most symptoms and signs reach a maximum intensity within 24–48 hours after cessation and gradually decrease over the following 2–3 weeks. However, as with other drugs of dependence, the desire for tobacco, sometimes imprecisely termed *craving*, can recur for years after cessation, particularly in situations where smoking formerly was common.

Similar abstinence symptoms appear after stopping use of smokeless tobacco or nicotine gum and are relieved to some degree by nicotine in any form. Smokers with high nicotine intakes as measured by biochemical indices of drug intake (plasma nicotine, cotinine, or expired breath carbon monoxide levels) experience the most intense withdrawal symptoms (West and Russell 1985). Numbers of cigarettes consumed daily do not predict withdrawal syndrome intensity accurately, reflecting the great variability in inhaled dose, although smokers consuming less than 15 cigarettes a day have less intense withdrawal than those consuming more than 25 cigarettes a day (Killen et al. 1988). Abstinent smokers on average gain 8–10 pounds in body weight a year after smoking (Hall et al. 1989; Perkins et al. 1987).

Nicotine Dependence Compared to Other Drug Dependence

How does the desire for tobacco compare to other dependence-producing drugs? A recent study asked 1,000 outpatients being treated for alcohol and other drug dependence about their tobacco dependence (Kozlowski et al. 1989a). Of these outpatients, 57% said that tobacco would be harder to quit than their other drugs. Alcohol-dependent patients were four times more likely than the drug-dependent patients to say that desire for cigarettes was at least as great as their urge for their "primary" drug. Cigarettes were generally rated as less pleasurable than alcohol or other drugs. Thus a mixed group of drug-dependent individuals judged cigarette dependence as "addictive" but not as pleasurable as other drug use.

MEDICAL AND PSYCHOLOGICAL CONSEQUENCES

The Costs

Tobacco use results in enormous health and economic burdens to individual smokers and to society. Cigarette smoking is the principal cause of preventable morbidity and premature mortality (Fielding 1985; U.S. Department of Health and Human Services 1987). Deaths associated with cigarette dependence exceed 350,000 deaths each year in the United States. Direct health care costs associated with tobacco dependence are approximately 16 billion dollars annually, and indirect costs from lost productivity and wages are an additional 37 billion. Costs from fires and accidents related to tobacco smoking and consequences of passive tobacco smoke inhalation are difficult to assess but are considerable. As smoking becomes less practical in the workplace, it is likely that decreased work output, increased accidents, and, in general, impaired workplace performance will occur in some tobacco-dependent individuals in the early stages of withdrawal in situations where tobacco is not available to them.

Interactions With Other Drugs

Cigarette smoking accelerates the metabolism of other drugs (Benowitz 1988; Busto et al. 1989; Miller 1989), for example, accelerating threefold the metabolism of the active metabolite of diazepam, desmethyldiazepam. Polycyclic hydrocarbons in tobacco smoke stimulate hepatic metabolism and thus should decrease levels of any drugs that share that metabolic path. Imipramine, oxazepam, lorazepam, and caffeine metabolism are accelerated by cigarette smoking. Probably because of pharmacodynamic interactions, cigarette smokers report less sedation than nonsmokers from a number of central nervous system active drugs, including diazepam, chlordiazepoxide, and chlorpromazine (Boston Collaborative Drug Surveillance Program 1974). Tobacco smokers require higher doses of the analgesics pentazocine and propoxyphene for pain relief and consume higher doses of caffeine in coffee (Brown and Benowitz 1989). For reasons unclear, use of amphetamine, heroin, methadone, and alcohol is associated with increased smoking.

TREATMENT CONSIDERATIONS

Most Quit With Little or No Treatment

More than 95% of smokers who quit tobacco smoking do so without any formal treatment (Garvey et al. 1989). As with other drugs of dependence, people who come for treatment when trying to stop are a minority of all users. Unfortunately, even with tobacco dependence, most of the data relevant to treatment and cessation patterns come from the intensive study of the minority of drug users who enter into treatment programs. For tobacco users who stop on their own, it is common for several cycles of quitting then relapse to precede successful smoking cessation (Gunby 1988; Orleans et al. 1989). For medically ill patients, the rate of self-managed quitting is estimated at less than 1% per year, but can be increased severalfold with only minimal intervention from a physician—that is, merely a simple instruction to stop smoking (Cummings et al. 1989b).

Minimal Treatment Intervention

A few minutes of counseling by physicians may be sufficient for many patients to quit smoking (Russell et al. 1987). Although most physicians agree that advising smokers to quit is important (Cummings et al. 1989b), more than half of smokers who had visited a physician during the previous year had not been advised to quit smoking (Anda et al. 1987). Physician counseling about tobacco dependence during routine office visits is as cost-effective as other common medical practices (e.g., monitoring mild hypertension). Between 3% and 10% of smokers are likely to quit as a result of brief advice from a physician or other authority figure. Adequate advice to quit smoking should take less than 4 minutes, and in some studies 1–2 minutes. Cost-effectiveness of counseling alone appears to be similar to that of using nicotine gum and for the patient considerably less expensive. A prescription for nicotine gum may increase cessation rates relative to counseling and advice alone by 1.6% (Cummings et al. 1988). Even if physicians' advice helps only 1% of smokers to quit, it is as cost-effective as many accepted medical practices (Cummings et al. 1989a).

The estimated 2–3% of all smokers who stop smoking each year by their own devices or after participation in organized treatment programs and who remain abstinent are characterized by high levels of motivation, good self-management skills for quitting, and good social supports (Curry et al. 1989; Ershler et al. 1989; Swenson 1989; Tunstall et al. 1985). The more reasons a person has for quitting, the greater the likelihood of success. Lower prequitting nicotine intake and resulting lessened dependence on nicotine may be associated with greater success (Hajek 1989; Killen et al. 1988). Such considerations appear to be general principles as applicable to tobacco dependence as to cocaine and heroin dependence.

Elements Common to All Treatments

Even minimal intervention consisting of physician's advice to stop and no additional treatment results in 10–60% 1-year quit rates among high-risk, medically ill patients. Tobacco-dependence treatment programs typically report 15–25% 1-year quit rates. A few claim 40–50%

success rates (Hall et al. 1985; Orleans 1985). Characteristics of more successful treatments include a combination of behavioral and psychological interventions, often with some variation of so-called aversive rapid smoking exercises. The elements of effective treatment programs, even those placing emphasis on pharmacologic interventions, include skills training, that is, learning how to say no when a cigarette is offered or when the urge to smoke occurs; various levels of group support ranging from spouse to larger groups; and self-reward strategies.

Dealing With the Abstinence Syndrome

Treatment can be more effective by properly managing the abstinence syndrome (Hajek 1989). With lessened physical symptoms of dependence, the withdrawal symptoms might be tolerable enough to require little more than peer support, advice, counseling, and education. Gradual nicotine dose reduction is useful, although not always simple to implement, since careful instructions are required to prevent the inadvertent and unconscious smoking of cigarettes so as to increase or maintain nicotine dose even though numbers of cigarettes per day decrease. For example, in a group of smokers living on a research ward, when the number of cigarettes available was reduced from 39 to 5 per day, the average intake of nicotine per cigarette tripled (Benowitz et al. 1986). Thus if this group had been in treatment and was simply advised to reduce the number of cigarettes smoked by one-half, there would be no effect on nicotine dose. It was not until cigarettes were decreased to 5 per day that the daily nicotine exposure substantially decreased. For similar reasons, switching from what are advertised as high-yield to lower-yield cigarettes will not necessarily decrease nicotine absorbed unless the cigarettes are smoked without resorting to various techniques for artificially increasing the absorbed dose of nicotine (Kozlowski et al. 1989b).

Degree of cigarette dependence can generally be diagnosed with a few simple questions. The most useful information is the number of cigarettes smoked and the time of smoking the first cigarette. Someone who smokes within 30 minutes of awakening has high nicotine dependence. For most people, the within-30-minutes cutoff to define dependent smoking behavior is adequate, but for patients with multiple drug dependencies, even within the 30-minute window faster smokers were more nicotine dependent (Heatherton et al. 1989). Those smokers who smoke the first cigarette of the day within 10 minutes of awakening are more dependent than those who smoke within 11–30 minutes and might benefit from treatment approaches addressing the physical attributes of dependence.

Pharmacologic Treatments

Antagonists or blockade. Pharmacologic therapies include the use of receptor antagonists (mecamylamine) or receptor blockade subsequent to initial sites of action (propranolol or clonidine) (Jarvik and Henningfield 1988). As with antagonist therapy for other drugs of abuse, mecamylamine poses problems in that it reduces the satisfaction and other effects of cigarette smoking to the extent that in short-term trials smoking increases, presumably to overcome the effects of the partial blockade. Other complications of ganglionic blockade (e.g., hypotension, ileus, and urinary retention) also limit its usefulness.

Clonidine in some studies has reduced the intensity of craving for tobacco and diminished tobacco withdrawal symptoms, presumably by actions on alpha$_2$-adrenergic receptors (Glassman et al. 1988), although its effects do not seem robust and vary from study to study. When treating opiate dependence, blockade and behavioral extinction strategies generally have not been satisfactory. For similar reasons, an extinction model of treatment may be less desirable for most tobacco addicts given the multitude of pressures for an ex-smoker to resume. Pharmacologic aversion therapies (e.g., with apomorphine) generally have not been effective.

Nicotine substitution. Nicotine substitution currently is the most useful pharmacologic treatment. In the United States, nicotine gum is the only marketed form of therapeutic nicotine delivery. Alternative approaches under investigation include sustained release transdermal nicotine delivery systems, inhaled nicotine aerosols, nicotine nasal spray, and nicotine-containing tablets or lozenges for sublingual administration. Issues of adequate bioavailability, safety both for the user and for others, and social acceptability vary with route, with all having some limitations. Transdermal delivery produces plasma levels approaching those resulting from nicotine gum, with enough nicotine absorbed to decrease, although not eliminate, the desire to smoke (Abelin et al. 1989). Nicotine aerosols with suitable particle size and consistency should, in principle, produce aveolar absorption similar to the nicotine aerosol produced during smoking (Burch et al. 1989). However, aerosol delivery systems still present dose-regulation problems as well as causing irritation to throat and upper airways after repeated aerosol use. Nasal sprays of nicotine result in plasma nicotine levels similar to those produced by tobacco snuff, but have not been tested extensively under clinical conditions (Jarvis et al. 1987b). The absorption of oral nicotine is slow and erratic, mostly from small bowel, but about 30% of the oral dose reaches systemic circulation (Benowitz 1988).

The best-studied pharmacologic approach for treatment is nicotine-containing chewing gum developed in the early 1970s. Nicotine gum not only provides a controlled, relatively slow delivery of nicotine, but was thought to offer a substitute oral activity believed to be important to some smokers. The latter benefit has not been well substantiated, and, in fact, one of the common complaints of the gum users is that it is difficult and unpleasant to chew. In the United States, the nicotine gum contains 2 mg of nicotine in an ion exchange resin in a gum base. When used regularly and as directed on the package insert, the plasma levels of nicotine average one-third to two-thirds the levels after smoking (Benowitz et al. 1987a; Nemeth et al. 1988). The gum appears to be most effective in people who have stopped smoking. The nicotine withdrawal symptoms are decreased. In continuing tobacco smokers, the gum does not predictably decrease smoking. The gum's utility in situations where tobacco-dependent individuals must remain temporarily abstinent (e.g., at work or on long airplane flights) has not been adequately evaluated.

Nicotine gum is most effective when part of a comprehensive treatment program including behavioral therapy, education, and group support as offered in many smoking cessation clinics. Under those optimal conditions, success rates at 6 months were 27% for those patients receiving the nicotine gum compared to 18% for placebo gum (Lam et al. 1987). The gum is less effective in an office practice setting, with reported 1-year abstinence rates of 9% (Russell et al. 1983). Combined analysis of several trials reported 6-month smoking cessation rates of 11% with the gum compared to 11% after placebo gum, but a slight advantage of 17% cessation with the gum when compared to no gum at all (Lam et al. 1987).

Successful treatment with nicotine gum depends on selecting motivated patients and providing adequate instruction on the gum use. For example, patients must chew intermittently until the characteristic taste or tingling associated with nicotine release appears rather than use continuous chewing, which quickly leads to fatigue of jaw muscles and increased salivation, resulting in swallowing most of the nicotine rather than allowing for buccal absorption. Patients should be warned that the rapid satisfaction obtained from a few puffs on a cigarette just will not happen after chewing the gum and the resulting slower buccal absorption of nicotine. Typically, nicotine gum is prescribed for 3 months, with a gradual tapering of dose to avoid withdrawal symptoms from the nicotine in the gum. Dependence on nicotine gum occurs with reports of 13–38% of treated patients continuing to use the gum for 1 year or more despite firm medical advice to stop (Hughes 1989).

Assessing Treatment Outcome

Treatment program evaluation for other drug dependence might well emulate the outcome criteria and treatment evaluation considerations that now seem to be those minimally acceptable in tobacco-dependence treatment research. Objective biochemical markers of smoking status (breath or blood carbon monoxide levels; blood, saliva, or urinary cotinine; or thiocyanate) provide objective verification of outcome and are expected in any well-controlled treatment research. Reports of 6-month outcome data are properly suspect, and, in general, 1-year outcome results are the expected norm for evaluation of treatments. Much of the current research interest in tobacco-dependence treatment is concerned with reducing the high relapse rates of even the more successful treatments (Stitzer and Gross 1988).

Environments to Treat Tobacco Dependence

Smoke-free medical centers and health care facilities are now broadly supported by patients and staff, and the policy change is relatively easy to implement (Hurt et al. 1989). However, inpatient psychiatric and drug-dependence units often are not included in such a policy. The reasons for this are not always well defended. Pilot programs in a number of adolescent psychiatric units, adolescent drug-dependence units, and adult psychiatric units suggest no unusual problems if proper preparation in planning and implementation takes place (Smith and Grant 1989). Such facilities communicate an unambiguous message to patients and staff concerning health risks of smoking

and are consistent with drug-dependence treatment principles. Tobacco dependence is a treatable disorder and should not be ignored in
psychiatric patients hospitalized for treatment of other psychiatric
disorders. A smoke-free hospital is an important aspect of that treatment.

FINAL THOUGHTS

Lessons may be learned from tobacco dependence that may be useful
in understanding and dealing with other addicting drugs. No one can
say for certain why tobacco use has decreased in the Western countries, especially in the United States. But tremendous gains have been
made during the past 25 years. Probably a combination of public education, special attention to antismoking efforts targeted at young people, increasing price of tobacco products, and a general enhanced
awareness of good health practices by large groups of people are important. However, some populations remain relatively unchanged in
their tobacco use; thus what works for some does not work for all, so
there is much to be learned. The use of nicotine, the most addicting
psychoactive drug (or as addicting as any, if you prefer), can be modified, and nicotine addicts can be treated without draconian policies to
punish the users or the need for Constitution-threatening public policy changes to reduce supply.

REFERENCES

Abelin T, Buehler A, Muller P, et al: Controlled trial of transdermal nico-
    tine patch in tobacco withdrawal. Lancet 1:7–10, 1989
American Psychiatric Association: Diagnostic and Statistical Manual of
    Mental Disorders, 2nd Edition. Washington, DC, American Psychi-
    atric Association, 1968
American Psychiatric Association: Diagnostic and Statistical Manual of
    Mental Disorders, 3rd Edition, Revised. Washington, DC, American
    Psychiatric Association, 1987
Anda RF, Remington PL, Sienko DG, et al. Are physicians advising smok-
    ers to quit? the patient's perspective. JAMA 257:1916–1919, 1987
Armitage AK, Dollery CT, George CF, et al: Absorption and metabolism of
    nicotine from cigarettes. Br Med J 4:313–316, 1975
Atkinson HC, Begg EJ, Darlow BA: Drugs in human milk: clinical phar-
    macokinetic considerations. Clin Pharmacokinet 14:217–240, 1988
Balfour DK: The effects of nicotine on brain neurotransmitter systems.
    Pharmacol Ther 16:269–282, 1982
Benowitz NL: Clinical pharmacology of nicotine. Annu Rev Med 37:21–32,
    1986

Benowitz NL: Drug therapy. Pharmacologic aspects of cigarette smoking and nicotine addiction. N Engl J Med 319:1318–1330, 1988

Benowitz NL, Jacob P III: Daily intake of nicotine during cigarette smoking. Clin Pharmacol Ther 35:499–504, 1984

Benowitz NL, Jacob P III: Nicotine renal excretion rate influences nicotine intake during cigarette smoking. J Pharmacol Exp Ther 234:153–155, 1985

Benowitz NL, Kuyt F, Jacob P III: Circadian blood nicotine concentrations during cigarette smoking. Clin Pharmacol Ther 32:758–764, 1982

Benowitz NL, Jacob P III, Kozlowski LT, et al: Influence of smoking fewer cigarettes on exposure to tar, nicotine, and carbon monoxide. N Engl J Med 315:1310–1313, 1986

Benowitz NL, Jacob P III, Savanapridi C: Determinants of nicotine intake while chewing nicotine polacrilex gum. Clin Pharmacol Ther 41:467–473, 1987a

Benowitz NL, Lake T, Keller KH, et al: Prolonged absorption with development of tolerance to toxic effects after cutaneous exposure to nicotine. Clin Pharmacol Ther 42:119–120, 1987b

Benowitz NL, Porchet H, Sheiner L, et al: Nicotine absorption and cardiovascular effects with smokeless tobacco use: comparison with cigarettes and nicotine gum. Clin Pharmacol Ther 44:23–28, 1988

Benowitz NL, Jacob P III, Yu L: Daily use of smokeless tobacco: systemic effects. Ann Intern Med 111:112–116, 1989

Boston Collaborative Drug Surveillance Program: Drowsiness due to chlorpromazine in relation to cigarette smoking. Arch Gen Psychiatry 31:211–213, 1974

Brown CR, Benowitz NL: Caffeine and cigarette smoking: behavioral, cardiovascular, and metabolic interactions. Pharmacol Biochem Behav 34:565–570, 1989

Burch SG, Erbland ML, Gann LP, et al: Plasma nicotine levels after inhalation of aerosolized nicotine. Am Rev Respir Dis 140:955–957, 1989

Busto U, Bendayan R, Sellers EM: Clinical pharmacokinetics of non-opiate abused drugs. Clin Pharmacokinet 16:1–26, 1989

Chesselet MF: Presynaptic regulation of neurotransmitter release in the brain: facts and hypothesis. Neuroscience 12:347–375, 1984

Cullen JW, Blot W, Henningfield J, et al: Health consequences of using smokeless tobacco: summary of the Advisory Committee's report to the Surgeon General. Public Health Rep 101:355–373, 1986

Cummings KM, Giovino G, Jaen CR, et al: Reports of smoking withdrawal symptoms over a 21 day period of abstinence. Addict Behav 10:373–381, 1985

Cummings SR, Hansen B, Richard RJ, et al: Internists and nicotine gum. JAMA 269:1565–1569, 1988

Cummings SR, Rubin SM, Oster G: The cost-effectiveness of counseling smokers to quit. JAMA 261:75–79, 1989a

Cummings SR, Stein MJ, Hansen B, et al: Smoking counseling and preventive medicine: a survey of internists in private practices and a health maintenance organization. Arch Intern Med 149:345–349, 1989b

Curry S, Thompson B, Sexton M, et al: Psychosocial predictors of outcome in a worksite smoking cessation program. American Journal of Preventive Medicine 5:2–7, 1989

Ershler J, Leventhal H, Fleming R, et al. The quitting experience for smokers in sixth through twelfth grades. Addict Behav 14:365–378, 1989

Fielding JE: Smoking: health effects and control. N Engl J Med 313:491–498, 1985

Fiore MC, Novotny TE, Pierce JP, et al: Trends in cigarette smoking in the United States: the changing influence of gender and race. JAMA 261:49–55, 1989

Garvey AJ, Heinold JW, Rosner B: Self-help approaches to smoking cessation: a report from the normative aging study. Addict Behav 14:23–33, 1989

Glassman AH, Stetner F, Walsh BT, et al: Heavy smokers, smoking cessation, and clonidine. JAMA 259:2863–2866, 1988

Glynn TJ: Essential elements of school-based smoking prevention programs. J Sch Health 59:181–188, 1989

Goldberg SR, Henningfield JE: Reinforcing effects of nicotine in humans and experimental animals responding under intermittent schedules of iv drug injection. Pharmacol Biochem Behav 30:227–234, 1988

Greydanus DE: Routing a modern Pied Piper of Hamelin (editorial). JAMA 261:99–100, 1989

Gunby P: Don't be discouraged if trying to quit tobacco, Surgeon General urges (news). JAMA 260:1511, 1988

Guyatt AR, Kirkham AJ, Baldry AG, et al. How does puffing behavior alter during the smoking of a single cigarette? Pharmacol Biochem Behav 33:189–195, 1989

Hajek P: Withdrawal-oriented therapy for smokers. Br J Addict 84:591–598, 1989

Hall SM, Tunstall C, Rugg D, et al: Nicotine gum and behavioral treatment in smoking cessation. J Consult Clin Psychol 53:256–258, 1985

Hall SM, McGee R, Tunstall C, et al: Changes in food intake and activity after quitting smoking. J Consult Clin Psychol 57:81–86, 1989

Hansen WB, Johnson CA, Flay BR, et al: Affective and social influences approaches to the prevention of multiple substance abuse among seventh grade students: results from project SMART. Prev Med 17:135–154, 1988

Hansson E, Schmiterlow CG: Physiologic disposition and fate of C^{14} labelled nicotine in mice and rats. J Pharmacol Exp Ther 137:91–102, 1962

Hatsukami DK, Hughes JR, Pickens RW, et al: Tobacco withdrawal symptoms: an experimental analysis. Psychopharmacology 84:231–236, 1984

Heatherton TF, Kozlowski LT, Frecker RC, et al: Measuring the heaviness of smoking: using self-reported time to the first cigarette of the day and number of cigarettes smoked per day. Br J Addict 84:791–799, 1989

Henningfield JE, Goldberg SR: Nicotine as a reinforcer in human subjects and laboratory animals. Pharmacol Biochem Behav 19:989–992, 1983

Herning RI, Jones RT, Benowitz NL, et al: How a cigarette is smoked determines blood nicotine levels. Clin Pharmacol Ther 33:84–90, 1983

Hughes JR: Dependence potential and abuse liability of nicotine replacement therapies. Biomed Pharmacother 43:11–17, 1989

Hughes JR, Hatsukami D: Signs and symptoms of tobacco withdrawal. Arch Gen Psychiatry 43:289–294, 1986

Hughes JR, Hatsukami DK, Mitchell JE, et al: Prevalence of smoking among psychiatric outpatients. Am J Psychiatry 143:993–997, 1986a

Hughes JR, Pickens RW, Gust SW, et al: Smoking behavior of type A and type B smokers. Addict Behav 11:115–118, 1986b

Hurt RD, Berge KG, Offord KP, et al: The making of a smoke-free medical center. JAMA 261:95–97, 1989

Jarvik ME, Henningfield JE: Pharmacological treatment of tobacco dependence. Pharmacol Biochem Behav 30:279–294, 1988

Jarvis MJ, Tunstall PH, Feyerabend C, et al: Comparison of tests used to distinguish smokers from nonsmokers. Am J Public Health 77:1435–1438, 1987a

Jarvis MJ, Hajek P, Russell MA, et al: Nasal nicotine solution as an aid to cigarette withdrawal: a pilot clinical trial. Br J Addict 82:983–988, 1987b

Johnston LD, O'Malley PM, Bachman JG: Psychotherapeutic, licit, and illicit use of drugs among adolescents: an epidemiological perspective. J Adolesc Health Care 8:36–51, 1987

Killen JD, Fortmann SP, Telch MJ, et al: Are heavy smokers different from light smokers? a comparison after 48 hours without cigarettes. JAMA 260:1581–1585, 1988

Kozlowski LT, Wilkinson DA, Skinner W, et al: Comparing tobacco cigarette dependence with other drug dependencies: greater or equal 'difficulty quitting' and 'urges to use,' but less 'pleasure' from cigarettes. JAMA 261:898–901, 1989a

Kozlowski LT, Heatherton TF, Frecker RC, et al. Self-selected blocking of vents on low-yield cigarettes. Pharmacol Biochem Behav 33:815–819, 1989b

Lam W, Sze PC, Sacks HS, et al: Meta-analysis of randomised controlled trials of nicotine chewing-gum. Lancet 2:27–30, 1987

Lewin L: Phantastica, Narcotic and Stimulating Drugs: Their Use and Abuse. New York, Dutton, 1931

London ED, Waller SB, Wamsley JK: Autoradiographic localization of [^{3}H]nicotine binding sites in the rat brain. Neurosci Lett 53:179–184, 1985

London ED, Szikszay M, Dam M: Metabolic mapping of the cerebral effects of abused drugs. Natl Inst Drug Abuse Res Monogr Ser 67:26–35, 1986

Luck W, Nau H: Exposure of the fetus, neonate, and nursed infant to nicotine and cotinine from maternal smoking. N Engl J Med 311:672, 1984

Mackay J: Battlefield for the tobacco war. JAMA 261:28–29, 1989

Mactutus CF: Developmental neurotoxicity of nicotine, carbon monoxide, and other tobacco smoke constituents. Ann NY Acad Sci 562:105–122, 1989

Marcus AC, Shopland DR, Crane LA, et al: Prevalence of cigarette smoking in the United States: estimates from the 1985 current population survey. Journal of the National Cancer Institute 81:409–414, 1989

McGinnis JM, Shopland D, Brown C: Tobacco and health: trends in smoking and smokeless tobacco consumption in the United States. Annu Rev Public Health 8:441–467, 1987

McNeill AD, West RJ, Jarvis M, et al: Cigarette withdrawal symptoms in adolescent smokers. Psychopharmacology (Berlin) 90:533–536, 1986

Miller LG: Recent developments in the study of the effects of cigarette smoking on clinical pharmacokinetics and clinical pharmacodynamics. Clin Pharmacokinet 17:90–108, 1989

Moody PM: Human smoking patterns and smoke deliveries. Int J Addict 19:431–439, 1984

Nemeth CR, Benowitz NL, Robinson N, et al: Nicotine gum: chew rate, subjective effects and plasma nicotine. Pharmacol Biochem Behav 29: 747–751, 1988

Novotny TE, Warner KE, Kendrick JS, et al: Smoking by blacks and whites: socioeconomic and demographic differences. Am J Public Health 78:1187–1189, 1988

Orleans CT: Understanding and promoting smoking cessation: overview and guidelines for physician intervention. Annu Rev Med 36:51–61, 1985

Orleans CT, Schoenbach VJ, Salmon MA, et al: A survey of smoking and quitting patterns among black Americans. Am J Public Health 79: 176–181, 1989

Perkins KA, Denier C, Mayer JA, et al: Weight gain associated with decreases in smoking rate and nicotine intake. Int J Addict 22:575–581, 1987

Pickworth WB, Herning RI, Henningfield JE: Spontaneous EEG changes during tobacco abstinence and nicotine substitution in human volunteers. J Pharmacol Exp Ther 251:976–982, 1989

Pierce JP, Fiore MC, Novotny TE, et al: Trends in cigarette smoking in the United States: educational differences are increasing. JAMA 261:56–60, 1989

Porchet HC, Benowitz NL, Sheiner LB, et al: Apparent tolerance to the acute effect of nicotine results in part from distribution kinetics. J Clin Invest 80:1466–1471, 1987

Porchet HC, Benowitz NL, Sheiner LB: Pharmacodynamic model of tolerance: application to nicotine. J Pharmacol Exp Ther 244:231–236, 1988

Russell MA: Tobacco smoking and nicotine dependence, in Research Advances in Alcohol and Drug Problems, Vol 3. Edited by Gibbons RJ, Israel Y, Kalant, et al. New York, John Wiley, 1976, pp 1–48

Russell MA, Merriman R, Stapleton J, et al: Effect of nicotine chewing gum as an adjunct to general practitioner's advice against smoking. Br Med J 287:1782–1785, 1983

Russell MA, Stapleton JA, Jackson PH, et al: District programme to reduce smoking: effect of clinic supported brief intervention by general practitioners. Br Med J 295:1240–1244, 1987

Saxena K, Scheman A: Suicide plan by nicotine poisoning: a review of nicotine toxicity. Vet Hum Toxicol 27:495–497, 1985

Schinke SP, Schilling R II, Gilchrist LD, et al: Native youth and smokeless tobacco: prevalence rates, gender differences, and descriptive characteristics. NCI Monogr 1989:39–42, 1989

Shiffman S: Tobacco "chippers"—individual differences in tobacco dependence. Psychopharmacology (Berlin) 97:539–547, 1989

Shopland DR, Brown C: Toward the 1990 objectives for smoking: measuring the progress with 1985 NHIS data. Public Health Rep 102:68–73, 1987

Silvis GL, Perry CL: Understanding and deterring tobacco use among adolescents. Pediatr Clin North Am 34:363–379, 1987

Smith WR, Grant BL: Effects of a smoking ban on a general hospital psychiatric service. Hosp Community Psychiatry 40:497–501, 1989

Snyder F, Davis FC, Henningfield JE: The tobacco withdrawal syndrome: performance decrements assessed on a computerized test battery. Drug Alcohol Depend 23:259–266, 1989

Stitzer ML, Gross J: Smoking relapse: the role of pharmacological and behavioral factors. Prog Clin Biol Res 261:163–184, 1988

Swenson IE: Smoking habits and smoking cessation among North Carolina nurses. Women Health 15:29–48, 1989

Tunstall CD, Ginsberg D, Hall SM: Quitting smoking. Int J Addict 20: 1089–1112, 1985

U.S. Department of Health and Human Services: The Health Consequences of Smoking: Nicotine Addiction. A Report of the Surgeon General. Rockville, MD, US Department of Health and Human Services, Public Health Service, Centers for Disease Control Office on Smoking and Health, 1987

Wesnes K, Warburton DM: Smoking, nicotine and human performance. Pharmacol Ther 21:189–208, 1983

West RJ: Psychology and pharmacology in cigarette withdrawal. J Psychosom Res 28:379–386, 1984

West RJ, Russell MA: Pre-abstinence smoke intake and smoking motivation as predictors of severity of cigarette withdrawal symptoms. Psychopharmacology (Berlin) 87:334–336, 1985

West RJ, Russell MAH: Cardiovascular and subjective effects of smoking before and after 24 h of abstinence from cigarettes. Psychopharmacology (Berlin) 92:118–121, 1987

West RJ, Hajek P, Belcher M: Time course of cigarette withdrawal symptoms during four weeks of treatment with nicotine chewing gum. Addict Behav 12:199–203, 1987

West R, Hajek P, Belcher M: Time course of cigarette withdrawal symptoms while using nicotine gum. Psychopharmacology (Berlin) 99:143–145, 1989

Chapter 11

Psychotherapy and Chemical Dependence

Lance M. Dodes, M.D.
Edward J. Khantzian, M.D.

PSYCHODYNAMIC FORMULATIONS UNDERLYING
CURRENT PSYCHOTHERAPEUTIC APPROACHES

Recent psychodynamic thinking about substance abuse has focused on its ego psychological basis, specifically in terms of defense function and defense deficit. This thinking has drawn on current understandings of affective dysfunction, object relations, and narcissistic pathology.

Use of substances to manage overwhelming affects has been the most central theme in present understandings of substance abuse. Krystal and Raskin (1970) pointed to a defect in the stimulus barrier, resulting in repeated experiences of traumatization by painful affects that cannot be warded off. A normal developmental process of differentiation, desomatization, and verbalization of affects was described as incomplete in addicts. Substance use could be seen as a prosthetic aid to this defective stimulus barrier. Likewise, Milkman and Frosch (1973), Wurmser (1974), and Khantzian (1978) have pointed to specific affective states of aggression, anxiety, depression, rage, and shame that addicts attempt to control or reverse by use of drugs. Khantzian (1985b) described a self-medication hypothesis for addictive disorders, in which the selection of the particular drug of abuse is based on matching pharmacologic effects with the specific major painful feelings with which the individual abuser suffers.

A second major formulation of substance abuse is that of object substitute. In this view, described by Krystal and Raskin (1970) and referred to by others (Wieder and Kaplan 1969; Wurmser 1974), the drug is treated as a transference object, with ambivalent properties attached to it. Incomplete individuation with yearning for a controllable, available love object is an important basis for this aspect of substance abuse.

Narcissistic issues as an underlying basis for substance abuse represent a third major element in current formulations. Wurmser (1974) described a "narcissistic crisis" leading to drug use. Feelings of rage, shame, and abandonment linked to collapse of a grandiose self or an idealized object provide a basis for drug use as an attempt to ameliorate massive narcissistic frustration.

Another dynamic is a defect in addicts with respect to the bundle of ego functions that have been termed collectively as "self-care" (Khantzian 1978; Khantzian and Mack 1983). This system of functions includes anticipation of dangerous situations and reacting appropriately to protect oneself, as well as caring sufficiently about oneself to do so. As such, "self-care" is related to issues of self-esteem and to the capacity to utilize affects as signals. Substance abusers, who are regularly deficient in taking good care of themselves, seem to be particularly clear examples of this kind of deficit psychopathology.

Related to self-care deficits, as well as to the problem of defensive avoidance of affective flooding, are failures to be aware of affective states in general. This condition, which has been described as "alexithymia" in psychosomatic patients and as "dis-affected" (McDougall 1984), is frequently associated with substance abusers. The origin of this kind of difficulty with experiencing affects has been suggested to be posttraumatic following an adult or childhood catastrophic experience (Krystal 1982) or to be associated with a pervasive early developmental dilemma in which the mother is paradoxically out of touch with the child's feelings yet insists on controlling any expression of them by the child (McDougall 1984).

Another dynamic formulation relevant to substance abusers is that of an unconscious search for mastery over suffering. In this view, the conversion of a passive experience of suffering into an active one is central for many drug abusers. Associated with this is also a conversion of poorly understood, confusing, and undifferentiated feelings, like those in the affectively deficient patients mentioned above, to a drug-induced dysphoria, which is understood.

Finally, Dodes (1990) has recently suggested that a central function of addictive behavior is to manage feelings of helplessness and powerlessness. Use of substances serves, in this view, as an attempt to regain control over one's affective state, thereby reestablishing the ability to control one's own inner experience. This inner control is a central aspect of narcissistic potency. Addicts are described as having a particular narcissistic vulnerability to being traumatized by experiences of helplessness or powerlessness. Their intense drive to remedy, via addictive behavior, the narcissistic blow of this loss of control is described as narcissistic rage. Dodes (1990) said this narcissistic rage gives to addiction some of its principally defining characteristics, namely its insistent, compulsive, unrelenting qualities and its relative unresponsiveness to external factors.

STUDIES ON PSYCHOTHERAPY WITH SUBSTANCE ABUSERS

In their summary of studies of psychotherapy with addicts, Woody et al. (1983) noted that of seven investigations with methadone-treated patients, in which patients were randomly assigned to psychotherapy or another treatment (usually drug counseling), five studies showed better outcome in the psychotherapy group. In their own study, Woody et al. (1983) also found that patients receiving both psychotherapy and drug counseling did better than a drug counseling group alone, in terms of more areas of improvement as well as in less use of illicit opiates and less need (in terms of dosage) for methadone. Brown (1985) also found, studying abstinent alcoholics in Alcoholics Anonymous (AA), that of the 45% of this group who sought psychotherapy, more than 90% found it helpful. Other studies have suggested that there is a high incidence of psychiatric disorders, particularly depression, among addicts (Khantzian and Treece 1985; Rounsaville et al. 1982). Woody et al. (1984) also noted that addicted patients with more severe psychiatric conditions particularly benefited from psychotherapy versus drug counseling alone. This group of investigators also noted that when psychotherapists are integrated in a treatment program, not only does outcome improve, but drug counselors are helped with their more difficult cases, and there is reduced stress on the entire staff via successful management of the most psychiatrically troubled patients (Woody et al. 1986).

When added to paraprofessional drug counseling with drug abusers on an inpatient service, psychotherapy has also been found to improve compliance with treatment measured in terms of discharges against medical advice or disciplinary discharges or unauthorized absences (Rogalski 1984). Rounsaville et al. (1985) also indicated success in a study treating ambulatory cocaine abusers with a modified interpersonal psychotherapy approach in conjunction with medication trials. Finally, a review of 30 studies of group psychotherapy with alcoholics concluded that it was likely a valuable addition to treatment programs (Brandsma and Pattison 1985).

In addition to these quantitative studies, a number of psychodynamic authors have reported on the treatability of substance abusers; these include the writers cited in the preceding section, as well as others (Dodes 1984, 1988; Rosen 1981; Silber 1974).

APPROACHES IN PSYCHOTHERAPY

A few authors have raised concerns about treating substance abusers (alcoholics) with psychotherapy. These concerns have stressed risks to remaining alcohol free if patients are engaged in an exploratory psychotherapy. These concerns have been based on thoughts that the patient is unable to tolerate the strong transference in psychotherapy or will misuse the therapy to increase denial of alcoholism (Vaillant 1981), or the therapist will ignore the life-threatening nature of the substance abuse (Bean-Bayog 1985) or will fail to make the diagnosis (Brown 1985). As suggested above, these concerns are not borne out in an increasing number of studies or in reports by dynamically oriented therapists. (For a discussion of the limitations of certain criticisms of psychotherapy with alcoholic patients see Dodes [in press].) In discussing concerns about therapy with alcoholics, Dodes (1988) suggested a psychodynamic basis for fear of psychotherapy and the fear of loss of sobriety through it. He described an idealizing transference to AA and its "higher power" and transitional object qualities of patients' attachment to both AA and the higher power. In pointing out that examination of these transferences may disrupt the idealization (or the projectively endowed power of the transitional object), he suggested that it is the fear of disruption of these transferences that underlies the fear of psychotherapy among many patients, as well as some treaters. Such a disruption of transferences is in fact a real possibility, bringing with it a potential loss of sobriety, and Dodes urged caution in interpreting the roles and functions of AA in psychotherapy. However, overall, so long as the therapist is attuned to the technical requirements of these patients, psychotherapy is clearly often indicated and appropriate for substance abusers.

In considering psychotherapy with substance abusers, it is clear from recent psychodynamic formulations that it must address a number of critical areas, including affect regulation, self-care, and narcissistic deficits, and the role of substance use in these areas. At the beginning of therapy, however, it is essential to address the emergency condition of the patient's substance abuse. Failure to attend to this has in the past been the source of valid criticism of psychotherapy with addicts, in which a psychotherapy is embarked on without attention to the patient's ongoing substance abuse and consequent destructive course.

It is essential at the start of the treatment, therefore, to deal with the question of abstinence. To do so, it is necessary to clarify the diagnosis with the patient. Although many patients will seek psychotherapy precisely because they are concerned about their drug or alcohol abuse, other patients will come to treatment under pressure (most commonly from work or family) and will not have acknowledged their addiction to themselves. Even those who are genuinely self-referred will often minimize the central aspect of their loss of control of substance use. Patients who have not acknowledged the destructiveness of their substance abuse in their lives, and further have not acknowledged that this abuse has gone beyond their ability to control it, will not have internal reason to abstain.

From a psychodynamic standpoint, in making the diagnosis that the patient is addicted to drugs, or is an alcoholic, one is also confronting the patient with a blow to his or her narcissistic potency. This may itself become in time a route for dynamic investigation of issues of power and control in the patient's psychological life (Dodes 1988, 1990). In addition, as Mack (1981) pointed out, the acknowledgment by the patient of powerlessness over the substance is a first step in the patient's assumption of responsibility. The clarification (or confrontation, if necessary) of the diagnosis, then, provides both the realistic basis for motivation to remain abstinent and a source of important focus for dynamic work around externalization of responsibility and meanings of the loss of control.

Thus far we have been presuming that the patient commences psychotherapy from the point at which he or she seeks treatment. However, as mentioned, a number of authors have taken the position with respect to alcoholics that the treatment should be "staged," with an initial lengthy period of involvement in AA. This phase is intended first to achieve abstinence and develop an identity as an alcoholic before beginning psychotherapy (Bean-Bayog 1985; Brown 1985; Rosen 1981). These concerns about engaging in psychotherapy from the beginning of treatment, as noted above, are based on assumptions of the therapist's failures to address the need for abstinence appropriately, as well as concerns that psychotherapy will shift the patient's focus from the appreciation that he or she is alcoholic. These concerns are readily avoided by appropriate attention to these issues, making postponement of psychotherapy unnecessary (Dodes 1988, in press).

But the issues involved in abstinence in the process of a dynamic psychotherapy may be complex. Writing about alcoholics, Dodes (1984) pointed out that in taking up with the patient his or her hurtfulness to the self through substance abuse, the therapist is simultaneously addressing the internal self-care deficit of the patient and providing an external object. This object may offer a developmentally missing function, in providing appropriate concern for the patient's well-being. The therapist may then be permitted to assume a special position in the patient's intrapsychic life, which has the potential to allow an internalization of self-care. Dodes added, however, that the capacity of the patient to achieve abstinence at the start of a therapy is a complex function, dependent in part on the psychological functions of the substance abuse and in part on the degree of ambivalence around internalizing the therapist's caring concern in the transference. This ambivalence about internalizing an object, he suggested, derives from conflicts and solutions around fear, rage, or mistrust of the early parental figure. Rapid achievement of abstinence may occur via an idealizing or merging transference to the therapist or even via compliant identification with the aggressor, as well as through a positive transference in a true therapeutic alliance. Other patients, however, are not able to abstain because they cannot "view, permit, or create the therapist to be the predominantly good object whose interest and concern can be introjected" (p. 254). Dodes concluded by saying that where abstinence could not be achieved at the start of treatment, psychotherapy could be continued only when the use of alcohol did not create an immediate emergency for the patient and also did not interfere with attending to the process of the therapy. In these cases, therapy could proceed with exploration of the issues of failure to abstain, including the issues in the transference. These issues ultimately involve lifelong problems around certain affective areas (rage, helplessness, fear, and shame) and narcissistic deficits.

It is remarkable that, despite the central importance of these issues for substance abusers, many (perhaps particularly alcoholics) often quickly become abstinent when commencing a psychotherapy (Dodes 1984; Khantzian 1980). Patients may also usefully engage in a variety of therapeutic modalities simultaneously in their attempts to become substance free. When this occurs, it is frequently important for the therapist to serve as a central broker and monitor of all the treatments. Khantzian (1985a) described this role as that of a "primary care therapist." In this role, the therapist first carefully obtains a drug history and empathically explores the drug effects sought and experienced, as well as investigating environmental precipitants, especially in the family. The therapist next takes an active role in decisions about needs for detoxification, confinement, involvement in AA or Narcotics Anonymous (NA), and possible pharmacologic treatment. Likewise, assessment of the possibility of referral for other psychotherapeutic modalities (e.g., group therapy) is a part of the primary care role. Khantzian also pointed out that, with the addict's characteristic difficulties with affect recognition and self-care, the therapist may have to take a considerably more active stance than is usual in traditional psychotherapy. He emphasized that excessive passivity on the part of therapists in the face of the kinds of serious ego deficiencies present in addicts is a technical error, and it is important for the therapist to "appreciate the importance of structure, activity, warmth, flexibility and empathy" (p. 85). This has important advantages as well as a potential problem. As an advantage, Khantzian noted that such an active stance avoids the objection that psychotherapy fosters unworkable transferences and countertransferences. However, he also noted that, having been so active, the therapist may ultimately have to transfer the patient to another therapist; patients may have difficulty permitting their negative feelings toward a therapist who has been so crucial in a reality way in saving their lives.

At this point, we should make note of a controversy in conceptualizing the diagnosis and treatment of substance abuse. This revolves around the "disease" concept. This model has frequently been used as an antidynamic approach, closing off psychodynamic investigation. However, as Dodes (1988) described, it is potentially integrable with a fully psychodynamic psychotherapy. Writing about alcoholics, he described an approach in which the "disease" is defined as an historical and psychological fact rather than an explanation. That is, the "disease" has two elements: a history of alcoholic drinking and a permanent psychological risk of repeating this behavior in the future. Dodes then pointed out that this permanent risk is the same as the regressive potential in any patient in psychotherapy. That is, the potential to resume old pathologic defenses and behaviors is never completely eliminated in any patient in psychotherapy, and this is equally true for addicts. Their permanent risk of renewed abuse can be understood, therefore, without invoking a new or unique theory peculiar to this population. The disease presented and understood in this way does not interfere, and in fact can be integrable, with a fully psychodynamic therapy. (He also noted that this regression model does not apply to the individual with organic brain impairment whose next bout of drinking may have principally to do with chronic physiologic factors.)

Beyond the issues of diagnosis, abstinence, and establishing a treatment plan utilizing appropriate resources, some authors have encouraged a rather directive approach to the psychotherapy of substance abusers. Bean-Bayog (1985) suggested a model for alcoholics in which the first agenda, after drinking is stopped, is a kind of educational process in which patients learn techniques for remaining sober. This is then followed by a grieving process for what has been lost through drinking, as well as for the loss of the alcohol itself. She suggested an actual time period for each stage of this process. This model principally addresses psychopathology that is produced by alcoholism and provides a useful focus on this pathology. However, its directive qualities make it less likely to detect or explore deeper issues that emerge in a more traditional approach, which follows the patient's thoughts.

Other authors have also suggested technical modifications in therapy. In addressing the problems with awareness of affective states commonly found in addicts, Krystal (1982) suggested a number of specific quasi-didactic approaches. These involve explaining to the patient the nature of his or her affect and cognitive problems, helping with practicing affects, taking up inhibition in utilizing affects as signals for self-care, and pointing out impairments in empathy. These modifications are part of a preliminary stage in therapy during which ego functioning and affect tolerance are improved, prior to attempting a more general psychoanalytic psychotherapy. From a somewhat different perspective, McDougall (1984) pointed to the need for an extended holding environment for such patients, possibly for a number of years, before they will have the capacity to permit themselves to see and know their own emotional lives. Rather than suggest specific modifications of technique, McDougall suggested awareness of the characteristic countertransference produced by such patients, namely boredom, disinvestment, and hopelessness. These reactions may be understood as a primitive communication of the experience of the patient as an infant, projected into the analyst.

In a related manner to Krystal's (1982) approach with alexithymics, Khantzian (1986) addressed the problems in treating self-care deficits in addicts. He emphasized the importance of "empathically identifying self-defeating and self-destructive consequences of their self-care deficits, and how this vulnerability has left them susceptible to addictive involvement" (p. 217). He linked their failures in self-protection to historical roots, as well as examining in detail current life situations to help patients learn to identify their feelings and use them as signals, rather than triggers of impulsive action.

Finally, it follows from an understanding of the psychodynamic factors cited earlier that attention will need to be paid to whatever meanings and roles of the addictive behavior apply in a given case. These may involve, for instance, the response to certain affective states (Khantzian 1985b), narcissistic vulnerabilities such as Wurmser (1974) described, the object role of drugs (Krystal and Raskin 1970), or the active nature of addictive behavior in correcting a sense of helplessness (Dodes 1990).

Once the substance-abusing patient has clearly acknowledged the diagnosis, has embarked on abstinence, and, where necessary, has begun to learn to identify and verbalize his or her affects and use them as signals, it becomes appropriate to expand the therapy to all areas of the patient's feelings and conflicts. The therapy becomes essentially the same as that with nonaddicts, although the therapist must always remain alert to the possibility of resumed substance abuse. For instance, dreams about previously abused substances in an abstinent patient in psychotherapy should be explored in the usual manner, investigated as possible sources of further understanding of the patient's use of substances, and also serve as a signal to patient and therapist to be mindful of a possible increased risk of resumed abuse. In addition, the therapy should address, as the issues arise, various meanings of the substance abuse as outlined previously. Ultimately, the place of the substance abuse in the patient's total psychological functioning should become more clear.

PSYCHOTHERAPY AND AA

Combination of individual psychotherapy and AA is very common in treatment of alcoholics (or combination with NA for other addicts). As noted above, a number of authors have suggested a primary role for AA, with psychotherapy serving as a supportive adjunct, and they have generally suggested beginning the therapy only after a lengthy initial period of time in AA (Bean-Bayog 1985; Brown 1985). This model also assigns to AA the tasks of dealing with the patient's alcoholism and abstinence, while assigning other personality factors to the psychotherapy. Rosen's (1981) view, while also assuming this "staging" model, takes a different position about the role of psychotherapy. He viewed patients' attachment to AA as "symbiotic" and sees psychotherapy as an opportunity to help patients separate from AA via a new attachment to the therapist. In the psychotherapy, a termination process can occur (unlike with AA, which does not provide any mechanism for termination). Patients thereby have the opportunity to work through unresolved issues of separation-individuation, which according to Rosen is particularly important for alcoholic patients.

Dodes (1988) examined the psychology of combined treatment of psychoanalytically oriented psychotherapy with AA. He described a phenomenon of splitting off of elements of the narcissistic transference in this combined approach. In this split, some aspects of the idealizing and mirroring transference are assigned by the patient to AA, and its "higher power." Other aspects of the patient's transference, which may also include some elements of the idealizing transference, are assigned to the therapist. While this split produces a technical modification of the treatment, Dodes noted that it "is no different from the practice of psychotherapy with many patients who present with a mix of narcissistic deficit and structural conflict" (p. 287). That is, as in such treatments in general, interpretive work proceeds simultaneously with positive attachments, which supply needed valuing or affirmation; in the combined therapy, these multiple levels of engagement occur, but with some narcissistic aspects of the transference created outside of the individual therapy. Dodes suggested that this combination is quite workable, although caution must be exercised by the therapist to be aware of the idealizing and transitional object nature of these transferences to AA and the higher power and to be careful not to examine them in the therapy prematurely. This would endanger the patient's sobriety that, he suggested, has been achieved through "willing surrender of the option to drink in exchange for the nurturance and protection of an idealized object" (p. 289).

GROUP THERAPY AND OTHER MODALITIES

Among the psychotherapeutic modalities employed with substance abusers, group approaches are by far the most common. They are a mainstay of inpatient treatments and the backbone of most outpatient clinics for substance abusers. However, as Khantzian (1980) noted, group psychotherapy is not a panacea, and there is "no evidence to substantiate the widely held belief that group therapy in and of itself is the treatment of choice" (p. 8). However, as Khantzian (1985a, 1986) also noted, groups do provide particular advantages. Patients may be helped by other group members to appreciate their failures in being adequately cautious, or adequately anxious about dangerous situations, especially those situations associated with drug use. Groups with a task orientation or behavioral-cognitive techniques may be particularly helpful with these self-care and self-regulating deficits (Khantzian 1985a). In addition, professionally led groups have, as do AA and NA, the benefit of a common history among the members. The commonality of shared experience with a sense of being understood facilitates a safe holding environment. In turn, this provides a base for tolerable confrontation.

Brown (1985) emphasized difficulties in attempting to treat patients who are still abusing (drinking) in the same group with abstainers. She expressed concern that the drinkers monopolize the group process, and that abstinent members assume responsibility for them and will avoid issues that they think are likely to increase anxiety, and hence increase the risk of drinking, of other members.

In addressing the problem of drinking among group members,

some clinicians temporarily exclude patients from the group, with a "reapplication" process. Many clinics design groups according to whether they are for "early sobriety" patients or for more firmly established abstinent patients. In general, as a parallel with individual work, groups for firmly established abstinent patients may expand their focus to address psychodynamic issues without restriction.

Most substance abuse inpatient programs, and many outpatient clinics, also utilize couples and family therapy. These modalities readily allow for addressing the interpersonal current meanings of substance abuse (e.g., its role in patterns of interpersonal struggling), as well as permitting investigation of ways that family members may unwittingly contribute to the patient's abuse. The latter characteristically involve protecting the patient from the consequences of the substance abuse (e.g., calling in to work to say the patient is sick when the patient is actually drugged or withdrawing). Such protection interferes with the patient's perception of the diagnosis and the reality costs to him or her of the substance abuse, and thereby postpones confrontation with the narcissistic blow of his or her loss of control, and ultimately postpones needed treatment. Finally, in family and couples work, in addition to recognizing interpersonal aspects of the substance abuse and the family pathology that may contribute to it, there may be an important educational component to the work, informing family members about substances, the risks of relapses, and the need to support other ongoing treatment.

SUMMARY AND CONCLUSIONS

In this chapter, we have attempted to identify from a contemporary psychodynamic perspective vulnerabilities in psychological structure and object relationships that predispose individuals to depend on substances of abuse. Substance abusers suffer with problems in recognizing and tolerating painful affects, disturbances in narcissistic areas and object relations, and deficits in self-care.

We have reviewed evidence that supports the utility and efficacy of psychotherapy with substance abusers. Our review suggests that substance abusers' vulnerabilities can be effectively targeted and treated through a combination of active and traditional approaches that allow for an unfolding of the patient's vulnerabilities and conflicts in an individual treatment relationship. Technical considerations are reviewed for addressing, early in treatment, the importance of abstinence as a condition for psychotherapy, as well as therapeutic modifications necessary to help patients with disturbances in affect recognition/tolerance and self-care, which may interfere with the work of psychotherapy.

Finally, we have tried to consider how individual psychotherapy may work in complementary ways with AA and NA, group psychotherapy, and other treatment modalities.

REFERENCES

Bean-Bayog M: Alcoholism treatment as an alternative to psychiatric hospitalization. Psychiatr Clin North Am 8:501–512, 1985

Brandsma JM, Pattison EM: The outcome of group psychotherapy with alcoholics: an empirical review. Am J Drug Alcohol Abuse 11:151–162, 1985

Brown S: Treating the Alcoholic: A Developmental Model of Recovery. New York, John Wiley, 1985

Dodes LM: Abstinence from alcohol in long-term individual psychotherapy with alcoholics. Am J Psychother 38:248–256, 1984

Dodes LM: The psychology of combining dynamic psychotherapy and Alcoholics Anonymous. Bull Menninger Clin 52:283–293, 1988

Dodes LM: Addiction, helplessness, and narcissistic rage. Psychoanal Q 59: 398–419, 1990

Dodes LM: Psychotherapy is useful, often essential, for alcoholics. Psycho

Khantzian EJ: The ego, the self and opiate addiction: theoretical and treatment considerations. International Review of Psychoanalysis 5:189–198, 1978

Khantzian EJ: The alcoholic patient: an overview and perspective. Am J Psychother 34:4–19, 1980

Khantzian EJ: Psychotherapeutic interventions with substance abusers: the clinical context. J Subst Abuse Treat 2:83–88, 1985a

Khantzian EJ: The self-medication hypothesis of addictive disorders: focus on heroin and cocaine dependence. Am J Psychiatry 142:1259–1264, 1985b

Khantzian EJ: A contemporary psychodynamic approach to drug abuse treatment. Am J Drug Alcohol Abuse 12:213–222, 1986

Khantzian EJ, Mack J: Self-preservation and the care of the self. Psychoanal Study Child 38:209–232, 1983

Khantzian EJ, Treece C: DSM-III psychiatric diagnosis of narcotic addicts. Arch Gen Psychiatry 42:1067–1071, 1985

Krystal H: Alexithymia and the effectiveness of psychoanalytic treatment. International Journal of Psychoanalytic Psychotherapy 9:353–378, 1982

Krystal H, Raskin H: Drug Dependence: Aspects of Ego Function. Detroit, MI, Wayne State University Press, 1970

Mack J: Alcoholism, AA, and the governance of the self, in Dynamic Approaches to the Understanding and Treatment of Alcoholism. Edited by Bean MH, Zinberg NE. New York, Free Press, 1981, pp 128–162

McDougall J: The "dis-affected" patient: reflections on affect pathology. Psychoanal Q 53:386–409, 1984

Milkman H, Frosch WA: On the preferential abuse of heroin and amphetamines. J Nerv Ment Dis 156:242–248, 1973

Rogalski CJ: Professional psychotherapy and its relationship to compliance in treatment. Int J Addict 19:521–539, 1984

Rosen A: Psychotherapy and Alcoholics Anonymous: can they be coordinated? Bull Menninger Clin 45:229–246, 1981

Rounsaville BJ, Weissman M, Kleber H, et al: Heterogeneity of psychiatric diagnosis in treated opiate addicts. Arch Gen Psychiatry 39:161–166, 1982

Rounsaville BJ, Gawin F, Kleber H: Interpersonal psychotherapy adapted for ambulatory cocaine abusers. Am J Drug Alcohol Abuse 11:171–191, 1985

Silber A: Rationale for the technique of psychotherapy with alcoholics. International Journal of Psychoanalytic Psychotherapy 3:28–47, 1974

Vaillant GE: Dangers of psychotherapy in the treatment of alcoholism, in Dynamic Approaches to the Understanding and Treatment of Alcoholism. Edited by Bean MH, Zinberg NE. New York, Free Press, 1981, pp 36–54

Weider H, Kaplan E: Drug use in adolescents. Psychoanal Study Child 24: 399–431, 1969

Woody GE, Luborsky L, McLellan T, et al. Psychotherapy for Opiate Addicts. Arch Gen Psychiatry 40:639–645, 1983

Woody GE, McLellan T, Luborski L, et al: Severity of psychiatric symptoms as a predictor of benefits from psychotherapy: The Veterans Administration–Penn study. Am J Psychiatry 141:1172–1177, 1984

Woody GE, McLellan AT, Luborsky L, et al: Psychotherapy for substance abuse. Psychiatr Clin North Am 9:547–562, 1986

Wurmser L: Psychoanalytic considerations of the etiology of compulsive drug use. J Am Psychoanal Assoc 22:820–843, 1974

Chapter 12

Alcoholics Anonymous

Margaret Bean-Bayog, M.D.

Although most psychiatrists endorse the idea of self-help groups like Alcoholics Anonymous (AA), they are often distrustful of the language, style, and assumptions of such groups. Their own training and thinking proceeds from a different frame of reference. They often do not understand the process of recovery from addiction, how these groups and their Twelve-Step system work to facilitate recovery, and how their own skills complement these processes.

This chapter is intended as a brief guide to AA as a resource in the treatment of alcoholic people. What is it? What does it do? How does it work? How can we use it? When and how do psychotherapy and AA complement and strengthen one another, and when do they conflict? What can we do to protect the patient when this happens?

WHAT IS AA?

AA is the single most often recommended "treatment" for alcoholism. It is a lay self-help fellowship. AA does not conceive of itself as a "treatment" of alcoholism at all, but it has been credited with the recovery of many alcoholics. Developed and run by alcoholics for alcoholics, it has solved a number of dilemmas that continue to make problems for other methods of treatment. AA has developed a program of recovery from alcoholism emphasizing the disease concept of alcoholism and the necessity for abstinence for recovery. In the "Preamble" read at the beginning of most meetings, AA (AA World Services 1952a) describes itself as

> A fellowship of men and women who share their experience, strength, and hope with each other that they may solve their common problems and help others to recover from their alcoholism. The only requirement for membership is a desire to stop drinking.
>
> There are no dues or fees for A.A. membership; we are self-supporting through our own contributions. A.A. is not allied with any sect, denomination, politics, organization, or institution; does not wish to engage in any controversy, neither endorses or opposes any causes. Our primary purpose is to stay sober and help other alcoholics to achieve sobriety.

Different observers see different things in AA. Sociologists see it as a means of reeducation or relabeling, anthropologists as a subculture, religious professionals as a means of spiritual conversion and change, psychiatrists as psychotherapy, and physicians as a treatment for alcoholism. The variety of descriptions attests to the richness and diversity of this organization that facilitates a process of personal change (Bean 1975a, 1975b). It has become a model for many subsequent self-help groups, such as Overeaters, Gamblers, and Parents Anonymous (Norris 1976).

Membership estimates are uncertain, since there are no rosters of members or attendance taking, and membership is anonymous, voluntary, and subjectively and personally defined, the only requirement being a desire to stop drinking. In 1972, AA estimated its membership at 250,000 (AA World Services 1972). It has grown steadily (Norris 1978), especially among women and those under age 30. In 1989, estimated membership had risen to over 1,600,000 (AA World Services 1989). Increasingly, members come referred by a professional person. Although it includes diverse ages, religions, ethnic and social groups, occupations, and social classes, AA members are probably not a random sample of alcoholics. Only a small fraction of alcoholics are in AA or other treatments. Baekeland and Lundwall (1977) estimated that "taken together, AA and medical and psychiatric treatment sources thus reach about 6.7% of the alcoholic population, for the most part briefly" (p. 162). A major obstacle to recovery is getting the alcoholic diagnosed early and engaged in any kind of treatment.

DEVELOPMENT

Except for expensive inpatient sanitariums, mental hospitals, and religion, AA was one of the earliest efforts to help people with alcoholism. It was begun in 1935. Before AA's development, alcoholism was not accepted as a disease, and the medical profession did not have a clear and widely accepting understanding and treatment for it. Alcoholics were often considered hopeless and were thought to have a moral rather than a medical problem (Kurtz 1979). Serious professional efforts to treat alcoholism, such as the Yale Plan Clinics, behavioral treatment, group and family therapy, and disulfiram, appeared some years after, probably as a result of AA's early work with alcoholics.

AA was founded by two active alcoholics. One, Bill Wilson, was an investment broker who had been influenced by the Oxford Movement, a nondenominational program of spiritual self-improvement. The other was an Akron, Ohio, surgeon. They used parts of the Oxford Group program—started by Frank Buchman, a Philadelphian, in the 1920s—to form an effective metaphor for recovery from alcoholism (Kurtz 1979).

The two newly sober alcoholics found others, and the tiny group struggling to help each other stay sober slowly grew. They had no idea whether what they were trying to do could be done. Professionals, families, and employers had given up on them. Gradually, they empirically developed a battery of ideas and techniques that could be used to grapple with most of the dangers of a return to drinking. AA's most basic assumptions and principles emerged: recovery could be assured only if the sober alcoholic did not take the first drink. This was best accomplished "one day at a time." They also found that they were better able to stay sober if they helped other active alcoholics. Helping others get sober is called Twelfth-Step work. Recovery from alcoholism is enormously difficult, but AA members were learning to do it and to transmit the methods they developed to new members.

Early newspaper accounts of the discovery of a program of recovery from alcoholism increased interest, and participation in meetings grew. In 1939, a group of sober AA members wrote descriptions of their experiences under the title "Alcoholics Anonymous." The group also caught the imagination of a writer for the *Saturday Evening Post*; after his article appeared in 1941, the spread of groups accelerated (Alexander 1941). Now there are AA groups all over the world. Today urban areas in most countries are likely to have AA meetings available.

ADMINISTRATIVE PHILOSOPHY

AA has been determined not to run aground on extraneous issues, as an earlier alcoholism self-help group, the Washington Society, had done over the question of abolition. So the members run it themselves, not taking stands on political issues or accepting contributions from any member in excess of $2,000 per year. AA's sole focus is on the members' drinking problem. Policies to preserve the organization are enshrined in the Twelve Traditions, which include such ideas as that leaders serve but do not govern, rules for anonymity (no one is to identify him- or herself as an AA member in the media), and other administrative guidelines to protect the function of this informal and decentralized organization (AA World Services 1952b).

AA MEETINGS

AA has a loosely organized system of group meetings of many kinds and an even more informal network of relationships with different meanings and functions: rescue work, outreach, support, shared spiritual growth, education, friendship, and fun. Groups in different areas elect members to represent them at policy-making sessions, including a yearly national meeting. Local AA groups retain a great deal of autonomy to make decisions and structure their meetings. Active alcoholics get most of their help within local groups. Each member may individually interpret AA's philosophy or ignore it altogether.

There are several types of meetings. At speaker meetings, a few members describe their drinking, their suffering, how they used AA, and their lives now without alcohol. These meetings are usually "open," which means that nonalcoholics can attend. Small group discussions are places where people ask questions and talk about their alcohol problems and their lives. Step meetings are organized to break down the process of recovery into small units, based on the

Table 12-1. The Twelve Steps of Alcoholics Anonymous

1. We admitted that we were powerless over alcohol . . . that our lives had become unmanageable.
2. Came to believe that a Power greater than ourselves could restore us to sanity.
3. Made a decision to turn our will and our lives over to the care of God *as we understood Him.*
4. Made a searching and fearless moral inventory of ourselves.
5. Admitted to God, to ourselves and to another human being the exact nature of our wrongs.
6. Were entirely ready to have God remove all these defects of character.
7. Humbly asked Him to remove our shortcomings.
8. Made a list of all persons we had harmed, and became willing to make amends to them all.
9. Made direct amends to such people wherever possible, except when to do so would injure them or others.
10. Continued to take personal inventory, and when we were wrong promptly admitted it.
11. Sought through prayer and meditation to improve our conscious contact with God, *as we understood Him*, praying only for knowledge of His will for us and the power to carry that out.
12. Having had a spiritual awakening as the result of these steps, we tried to carry this message to alcoholics, and to practice these principles in all our affairs.

Source. Alcoholics Anonymous (1952b).

Twelve Suggested Steps (see Table 12-1), which are worked and reworked by each person in his or her own way. Discussion and step meetings are often "closed," for alcoholics only, as protection from shame and stigma. There are also orientation meetings for beginners (usually people less than 2 years sober).

AA meetings are enormously diverse. They may have from as few as two to as many as several thousand members. They may last from 30 minutes to several hours. While technically any meeting is open to any alcoholic, there are groups for physicians, homosexuals, women, youth, and so on. Meetings may be held in churches, hospitals, prisons, members' homes, at sea, or almost anywhere. They may be highly structured and ritualized or unstructured and flexible. In addition to meetings, AA members may participate in conferences, conventions, retreats, and social functions.

FELLOWSHIP

The informal networks include small clusters of people who socialize after or outside of meeting and sponsorship. This extensive caring web of sober people performs a crucial protective function and builds hope of recovery in the new member by example and identification.

SPONSORSHIP

Sponsorship is usually an informal one-on-one partnership in which a person who has been sober a long time is asked by a new member for personal help in getting and staying sober. The sponsor keeps in close touch with the new member, teaching protection from acting on craving to drink, sharing experience, giving advice, encouraging good self-care, supporting, clarifying and arguing about the things the person needs to do to stay sober, interpreting and explaining what has happened to the new member, and being accessible. Each sponsor works in his or her own way. Techniques are empirically developed out of each sponsor's own experience of recovery.

For the sponsor, sponsorship provides a model of memory of the suffering of active drinking and early stages of getting sober and deeply important affirmation of the power of the process, the fact of hope, which ensures the sponsor's own continuing sobriety. When a new member stays sober, there is joy for the rest of the group. Each person's recovery is a symbol of the capacity to use help to master, transcend, and integrate the suffering, fear, self-hatred, loss, and destruction of love that result from alcoholism. One alcoholic caring for another in the program is considered a healing agent.

THE TWELVE STEPS

Another major tool in the recovery program is the suggested Twelve Steps for recovery from alcoholism (Table 12-1). They are a distillation of a large number of processes and include many mechanisms for maturation. The original religious wording has been softened by the use of the steps as "suggestions" only and the idea of God *"as we understand Him,"* which can mean whatever the new member chooses. For example, some agnostics will define the collective strength of their AA group as their "Power greater than ourselves." Boiled down, these steps include: 1) an admission of alcoholism (i.e.,

inability to control the drinking, which implies the need for abstinence); 2) change of the personal context from isolation to social, personal, and spiritual relationships, with dependence on some resource
other than the self, transforming narcissism, grandiosity, and omnipotence (Galanter 1979; Tiebout 1949, 1954); 3) self-examination, ca-
tharsis, and personal change; 4) improvement of self-esteem and reso-
lution of guilt; and 5) work with other alcoholics. The Twelve Steps
not only help the person achieve sobriety, but also facilitate psychological maturation.

MORE TOOLS AND TECHNIQUES

AA views alcoholism as damaging the sufferer in three areas of life:
physical, mental, and spiritual. During recovery, improvement usually
occurs in that order.

Physically, there may be acute and longer-term withdrawal. Disturbances of sleep and dreaming (Williams and Rundell 1981), perceptual abnormalities (Porjesz and Begleiter 1981), and cognitive impairment (Parsons and Leber 1981) may last for several months to
years after the last drink. Clinically, the mood swings and anxiety of
early abstinence commonly improve over time. AA handles symptoms
of protracted subclinical withdrawal by controls, supports, reassurance, understanding, tolerance, and caretaking relationships. In AA,
the power of the craving to drink is respected. It is called a compul-
sion. The new member is given short, simple instructions: "Don't
drink." "Go to meetings." "Join a group." "Get a sponsor." "Ask for
help." The person's experience is usually chaotic and painful. The
new member may have substantial neurologic impairment. The person is preoccupied with inner feelings. It is hard to get and keep the
new member's attention. Short, simple, repeated suggestions are
adapted to his or her level of function.

New members are advised not to attempt to revise their whole
life too quickly, not to stop smoking, change jobs, or make other major changes. They are instructed to take good care of themselves.
Alcoholics do not do so from disorganization and feeling they deserve
punishment. They need to be told to get enough food, sleep, and care.
"H.A.L.T.—Don't get hungry, angry, lonely, tired." Feelings of physical fatigue, hunger, thirst, and emotional upset all mimic withdrawal,

a state the alcoholic knows will be alleviated by a drink, so they are risky for the new sober alcoholic. (This is one reason psychotherapy, with its increased anxiety, is not recommended in early sobriety.)

Later, when the new member is better, more complex ideas will be conveyed. One study of sponsorship found that sponsors intuitively and systematically worked differently with newcomers who were less than 2 months sober (Alibrandi 1978). New members were given specific prescriptions for sobriety, supportive contacts with AA members, and help accepting their alcoholism. With increasing length of sobriety, the focus of the work shifted to changing oneself.

Most members do not begin to work through the Twelve Steps in detail until some safety and structure have been restored to their lives. This takes varying periods of time. After the person has passed through the early phase of tenuous control with surging moods and physical symptoms, AA provides a framework for maturation through primitive to more advanced levels of psychological functioning. Several of the Twelve Steps provide specific and systematic methods to facilitate the construction of mature psychological coping mechanisms and to abandon, refine, or add to more primitive ones.

Denial gradually begins to be given up, starting with the First Step, as more of reality can be tolerated by the new member. Magical thinking, wishing, avoidance, blaming others, intellectualization, and rationalization all characterize active drinking, and all are modified by participation in AA, especially by working the middle steps. They are replaced first by repression, reaction formation (love of sobriety, and not drinking), and undoing (e.g., helping other alcoholics stay sober to undo one's past drinking). Later, with further development, they may be replaced by anticipation, humor, altruism, and sublimation.

PSYCHOTHERAPY AND AA

Despite all these familiar processes, many psychiatrists reading the Twelve Steps will balk at them. They may react to the explicit religious aspect or they may run aground on a fundamental difference in the assumptions underlying recovery from alcoholism in AA and psychological growth in psychotherapy: the issue of loss of control. Most psychotherapists see patients as able to learn to control behavior. AA insists that alcoholics cannot control their drinking, but must relinquish the struggle for control and stop drinking altogether. This is the root of the abstinence controversy (Brown 1985). Sophisticated writers have shown how the metaphors of powerlessness and dependence in AA paradoxically help patients resolve narcissism, grandiosity, and omnipotence (Mack 1981), but if the psychotherapist does not understand how recovery works in AA, there will be a conflict between the two value systems, resulting in a split with the patient caught in the middle.

Patients, often psychiatrically mismanaged before recovery, do not trust the therapist to understand and protect the abstinence. Therapists may devalue the focus on alcohol if they interpret continued dependence on AA as a sacrifice of independence (Brown 1985; Gerard et al. 1962).

Therapists who are untrained to handle alcoholism issues may listen in perplexity to alcoholism workers' insistence that psychiatrists cannot treat alcoholism or that therapists must be alcoholic to treat alcoholics. Demoralized, they may agree that their skills do not pertain. I see this as a loss. What is needed, it seems to me, is translation or consultation to surmount this language barrier. Recovering alcoholics often wish for psychotherapy but distrust it as dangerous to their recovery from alcoholism. Therapists can learn what occurs in recovery from alcoholism so that they can modify their approach to complement rather than undercut the recovery process.

For instance, only 16% of alcoholics who had psychotherapy *before* they established abstinence found it to be of help, whereas 64% of those in psychotherapy *after* abstinence found it helpful (Brown 1985).

Recovery from alcoholism in AA involves a series of complex cognitive and behavioral processes in which the person: 1) identifies the alcohol as a problem; 2) establishes a focus on the drinking; 3) grasps the concept of loss of control, leading to abstinence; 4) learns the tools and techniques to maintain abstinence; 5) labels himself or herself as alcoholic; 6) heals from the psychological damage of active alcoholism; and 7) then is in a position to pursue further mastery integration and psychological growth (Bean-Bayog 1985; Brown 1985).

At certain points in this process, attempted psychotherapy will sabotage the alcoholism treatment and vice versa. In other circumstances, however, psychotherapeutic skills may be crucial.

For instance, in the undiagnosed alcoholic, psychiatric exploration of the drinking, the refusal to label the alcohol as a problem, and the resistance to entry into alcoholism treatment may all facilitate establishment of a safe sobriety from which framework the patient can later pursue an exploratory psychotherapy. Psychotherapy would be contraindicated, at this time, if the therapist believes the patient can learn to control the drinking, because the patient will not be kept safe.

The psychotherapist unused to collaborating with AA may react to the patient's dependence on a sponsor as a transference split and try to wean the patient away. The psychotherapist knowledgeable about alcoholism will usually not compete, but may use the patient's experience of the sponsor as a transference displacement, which can be supportively explored. The roles are different. Most psychotherapists do not want to take over the educative, nurturing, and emergency functions of the sponsor (e.g., 3 A.M. phone calls) and may delegate with relief, understanding that the intense dependence on the sponsor in early recovery is a means to an end and attenuates as learning consolidates and recovery proceeds. Patients are usually intensely relieved to be given permission, or better yet support, for AA participation and use of a sponsor.

PROBLEMS WITH AA

Psychiatrists are sometimes distressed about other aspects of AA, pointing out that it can be uneven, sometimes archaic, rigid, or doctrinaire. There is no quality control. It is important to remember that AA consists of people, some still sick from alcoholism and variable in their ability to help others, usually with no formal training, and with different amounts of personal kindness, skill, and altruistic commitment.

Some AA members may transmit the idea to a newcomer that AA is the only thing that works, undermining the use of other resources, such as a physician, psychotropic drugs or disulfiram (Antabuse), and group or family therapy. Most AA members do not take this position. The new member who encounters this usually responds to professional reassurance and clarification.

Referral to AA may be difficult. This results from resistance to accepting the diagnosis and treatment of alcoholism, which is very painful. Patients may interpret the recommendation that they go to AA as a rejection by their psychiatrists. But they are also likely to refuse to go because they cannot bear to think of themselves as alcoholic and feel humiliated that the psychiatrist does.

It is important to note that self-labeling as an alcoholic is *not* necessary for membership in AA. The patient can be encouraged to have a look, see for himself, get some alcohol education, and not to decide whether he is alcoholic immediately. Avoiding the requirement of labeling is an excellent short-term solution to the problem of stigma, shame, and denial.

Although AA can be flexible and varied, it is sometimes global, applying one formula to all incoming alcoholics, which may be a serious problem for patients with more than one illness, such as major affective disorder and alcoholism.

Some members do not differentiate between classes of drugs. Since such drugs as minor tranquilizers and other sedatives interfere with recovery of alcoholics and may cause relapse, AA members may tell people to stop *all* drugs as crutches, including lithium, major tranquilizers, disulfiram, and antidepressants, with all drugs considered alike. Patients who run into this difficulty will need clarification and support.

Some consider AA to produce and maintain dependence, since members never "graduate" and are expected to participate indefinitely. This does not necessarily imply a limited view of the alcoholic's capacity for growth. AA provides an antidote to the prevailing cultural insistence that it is good to drink. It reminds alcoholics that drinking *for them* is not only not good, but not safe. This repetitive reiteration may be helpful in the face of repetitive cultural and media urging of alcohol use (Mack 1981; Zinberg 1981). Continuing participation in a treatment or recovery program is important for the recovery of many alcoholics. A "slip," or return to drinking, by an abstinent AA member often follows cessation of attendance at AA meetings.

Some people have trouble attaching themselves to AA. Women, blacks, gay people, young people, polydrug users, and ex-offenders may feel a double stigma. But such members can form AA groups of their own, since it takes only two members to start a new group. The difficulty these people have in joining AA may be simply a variant on the rationalization used by nearly all members at the beginning: to avoid acknowledgment of membership, because of the pain of accepting the diagnosis of alcoholism and treatment of it.

ADVANTAGES OF AA

Many alcoholics use AA to recover from an entrenched disorder that has resisted many efforts at treatment. By looking at AA, it is possible to see the working of an effective treatment for alcoholism. Zinberg (1977) wrote

> A.A. tenets are very successful. They attack the individual's denial of alcoholism without insisting upon an extensive rearrangement of other elements in the personality structure. They help alleviate the loneliness and depression of the alcoholic without gratifying him unbearably, and they refuse to abandon or judge him. A.A. tenets help to keep him in a subtle balance between the twin fears of sobriety and drunkenness, and provide a dynamic balance for a wide range of personality conflicts. Finally, and perhaps most important, the alcoholic's feeling of guilt about drinking is rendered less devastating by the disease concept. (p. 93)

AA is free. There are no dues or fees, although people may make small donations at meetings.

Meetings are available daily in all major metropolitan areas of the United States. Most medium-sized communities have at least weekly meetings. The greater Boston area has more than 400 meetings a week. Meetings are also available in foreign countries in larger cities.

The AA literature is a resource. As of this writing, 3 million copies of the "Big Book" or "Alcoholics Anonymous" have been sold (AA World Services 1989). Newcomers are advised to read the stories of recovery in it. Information about AA and pamphlets are available from the General Service Office of Alcoholics Anonymous, Box 459, Grand Central Station, New York, New York 10163.

AA offers patients a nondrinking peer group in an otherwise drinking society, friendship and support, problem-solving techniques, a kind of group therapy and resocialization, education, and examples of the possibility of recovery.

HOW TO REFER TO AA

Since the Twelfth Step specifies helping alcoholics as a central function of AA, most professionals attempting to work with alcoholics will find willing allies in AA members (Curle 1974). The psychiatrist can decidedly increase the chance that a patient will be able to join and remain in AA. To get an alcoholic to go to an AA meeting, it is helpful to call an AA member who will arrange to go with the patient. *Most people*, both professional and potential members, *have great*

difficulty going to their first meeting, and it is important to understand their resistances.

The referral should be made thoughtfully and seriously. It is important for the therapist to speak positively and respectfully about
AA. First discuss AA in a general way, exploring the patient's knowledge and reactions to it. This often faces the patient with humiliating
or frightening feelings. Do not be discouraged by a negative response.
Persist in encouraging the patient to start to find out about AA. Most
alcoholics have heard about AA and may think they know all about
it, even though they have never been to a meeting, or to only a few.
Often they present reasons why they could not possibly go and why it
will not help. If the professional knows how and why AA is useful, the
referral will be easier. Use reasonable powers of persuasion and make
it as easy as possible for the patient to go to that first meeting. I may
explore the resistance by suggesting that a patient "shop" or preview
a half dozen meetings and then come tell me what he or she disliked
the most.

It may help to arrange for telephone or personal contact with an
individual AA member. The psychiatrist can suggest that an AA
member will phone and arrange this. Recovering alcoholic physicians
in the area are often very helpful in facilitating such contacts. They
can encourage the patient to phone AA, or, better, call the AA number, introduce themselves, and then hand the patient the telephone. A
number for AA is listed in almost every city telephone directory.
Many cities have a 24-hour answering service and can provide an experienced and knowledgeable member to speak to a newcomer on
short notice.

Suggest that the newly identified alcoholic go to a local AA
meeting. Since this involves personal exposure, it is usually more difficult than to go to a far away meeting. AA groups vary considerably
in class and subculture, so it is helpful if the psychiatrist can direct
the patient to a particular group matched for education and social
class. Some physicians offer to take a patient themselves. Although
patients surprisingly rarely take the doctor up on this, the offer diminishes resistance to the idea of going.

Provide the patient with a directory of local meetings. Telephone
your local AA answering service to obtain these.

Suggest attendance at another AA meeting, even for patients
who say they have tried AA before. There is a tendency for drinking
alcoholics to feel hopeless about every treatment they have previously

tried, since they have not yet been helped. It is also useful to ask about this despair.

After the patient has attended the first meeting, he or she can be encouraged to participate. There is a saying that "AA does not work as a spectator sport." It is useful for the members to become involved in it, especially in the first few months, when the hazard of relapse is high. Some recommend "90 meetings in 90 days" as protective. The new member should be encouraged to join a group, get a sponsor, and go to discussion and step meetings.

ATTENDANCE BY THE PSYCHIATRIST

The psychiatrist can go to an open AA meeting. Most groups are delighted to have such visitors. Anyone can call the AA number in the telephone book and ask how to go to a meeting. If one has been to one or more AA meetings and can speak knowledgeably about groups in the area, the chances of successfully completing the referral are improved. Unless someone has actually seen a meeting, it is difficult to grasp what the process is about, and what your patient may be experiencing or reacting to. It is easier to refer a patient when one knows something about what to expect.

Visiting AA meetings can help us compensate for the fact that almost none of us received supervised clinical work with alcoholic people in our training. Alcoholics in AA meetings are often amazingly candid about their experience, and watching how AA members respond to them, support, educate, and intervene can be a bit like watching a seasoned therapist see a patient through a one-way mirror. I suggest to medical students going to an AA meeting that they compare how their house officers in the emergency room react to alcoholics ("Oh no, not a drunk") with the reaction in AA ("Boy, do you look sick. Well, we know what will help. If you want what we've got, come along with us.") Think about which helper feels better about *themselves* and why. There is no reason not to identify with and imitate clinical competence, confidence, and compassion, even if it is going on in an unfamiliar language and without the benefit of credentials.

Seeing sober, formerly drinking alcoholics enjoying life without alcohol reminds us of the hope of recovery. Most people identify only actively drinking alcoholics as alcoholics, and since most recovering alcoholics are hidden because of stigma, a psychiatrist may not realize it when the patient in his or her office is a sober alcoholic. Clinicians working with active alcoholics will have a skewed sample of those who have not responded to AA or other treatments. This perpetuates the stereotype of the alcoholic as hopeless. Physicians may treat medical complications in hundreds of alcoholics, yet not see a single recovered alcoholic until they visit their first AA meeting.

A visit to a large middle-class AA meeting is also good for eroding class stereotypes. Most trainees and professionals are careful to avoid stereotyping patients, but after a visit to such an AA meeting, such comments as "so many of them are kids," or "so many women," or "I thought they'd all be depressed, middle-aged men" are common. It is easier to suspect the possibility of alcoholism in, for example, a 20-year-old college girl after one has seen some young, middle-class women in AA.

The speakers at AA meetings are generally interesting and may be profoundly moving. The friendliness, optimism, and kindness is infectious, best felt to be appreciated. It is also useful to see alcoholics treated with consideration, understanding, and respect. Some AA members intuitively recognize alcoholism, even at early stages. They pick up subtle distortions of thinking that distinguish an alcoholic fighting to look and act like a normal, healthy drinker from a truly normal, healthy drinker. They recognize that alcoholic because they, in order to become sober, have been forced to identify and eradicate in themselves exactly those subtle distortions. They are like astute clinical observers who have a sixth sense of the dynamics of the phenomenon.

They also know, by experience, how painful it is for an alcoholic to have the protective cover removed, to be stripped of defenses, and faced with this disorder. But even more, by experience of suffering, they intuitively and empathically know what the price will be if the alcoholic cannot be helped to face the pain of diagnosis and recovery. Unless the alcoholic can be brought to acknowledge the problem, he or she will be left to the catastrophe of continuing or worsening alcoholism; therefore, in AA, they confront, empathize, and offer hope and help.

AA members also differ from professionals in that they have a different perspective, which rises out of different experience. Every person in AA has the experience that alcoholism is a treatable disease, since they have gotten sober themselves. They know how to oppose the hopelessness of the drinking alcoholic. They have collectively hammered out a set of techniques for establishing and maintaining freedom from alcoholic drinking that are helpful and effective in a wide variety of people with a range of alcohol problems. They have taken what ought to be, but often are not, professional attitudes: that people with alcoholism are human, suffering, and can be helped. They have developed a set of concepts that allows difficult work to be sustained over a long time. The rest of us can work with them and learn from them.

REFERENCES

AA World Services: AA Preamble. New York, AA World Services, 1952a

AA World Services: Twelve Steps and Twelve Traditions. New York, AA World Services, 1952b

AA World Services: Alcoholics Anonymous, the Fellowship of Alcoholics. New York, AA World Services, 1972

AA World Services: Alcoholics Anonymous. New York, AA World Services, 1989

Alexander J: Alcoholics Anonymous. Saturday Evening Post, March 1, 1941

Alibrandi LA: The folk psychotherapy of Alcoholics Anonymous, in Practical Approaches to Alcoholism Psychotherapy. Edited by Zimberg S, Wallace J, Blume SD. New York, Plenum, 1978, pp 239–256

Baekeland F, Lundwall LK: Engaging the alcoholic in treatment and keeping him there, in The Biology of Alcoholism, Vol 5: Treatment and Rehabilitation of the Chronic Alcoholic. Edited by Kissin B, Begleiter H. New York, Plenum, 1977, pp 161–195

Bean M: Alcoholics Anonymous, part I. Psychiatric Annals 5(2):7–61, 1975a

Bean M: Alcoholics Anonymous, part II. Psychiatric Annals 5(3):7–57, 1975b

Bean-Bayog M: Alcoholism treatment as an alternative to psychiatric hospitalization. Psychiatr Clin North Am 8:501–512, 1985

Brown S: Treating the Alcoholic: A Developmental Model of Recovery. New York, John Wiley, 1985

Curlee J: How a therapist can use Alcoholics Anonymous. Ann NY Acad Sci 233:133–143, 1974

Galanter M: Religious conversion: an experimental model for affecting alcoholic denial, in Currents in Alcoholism. Edited by Galanter M. New York, Grune & Stratton, 1979, pp 69–78

Gerhard DH, Saenger G, Wile R: The abstinent alcoholic. Arch Gen Psychiatry 6:83–95, 1962

Kurtz E: Not God: A History of Alcoholics Anonymous. Center City, MN, Hazelden Educational Services, 1979

Mack J: Alcoholism, AA, and the governance of the self, in Dynamic Approaches to the Understanding and Treatment of Alcoholism. Edited by Bean M, Zimberg N. New York, Free Press, 1981, pp 128–162

Norris JL: Alcoholics Anonymous and other self-help groups, in Alcoholism: Interdisciplinary Approaches to an Enduring Problem. Edited by Tarter RE, Sugarman AA. Reading, PA, Addison-Wesley, 1976, pp 131–150

Norris JL: Analysis of the 1977 survey of the membership of AA. Paper presented at the 32nd International Congress on Alcohol and Drug Dependence, Warsaw, Poland, September 3, 1978 (Available from AA World Services)

Parsons OA, Leber WR: The relationship between cognitive dysfunction and brain damage in alcoholics: causal, interactive or epiphenomenal? Alcoholism: Clinical and Experimental Research 5:326–343, 1981

Porjesz B, Begleiter H: Human evoked brain potentials and alcohol. Alcoholism: Clinical and Experimental Research 5:304–317, 1981

Tiebout HM: The act of surrender in the therapeutic process. Quarterly Journal of Studies on Alcohol 10:48–58, 1949

Tiebout, HM: The ego factors in surrender in alcoholism. Quarterly Journal of Studies on Alcohol 15:610–621, 1954

Williams HL, Rundell OH: Altered sleep physiology in chronic alcoholics: reversal with abstinence. Alcoholism: Clinical and Experimental Research 5:318–325, 1981

Zinberg N: Alcoholics Anonymous and the treatment and prevention of alcoholism. Alcoholism: Clinical and Experimental Research 1:91–102, 1977

Zinberg N: Alcohol addiction: toward a more comprehensive definition, in Dynamic Approaches to the Understanding and Treatment of Alcoholism. Edited by Bean M, Zinberg Z. New York, Free Press, 1981, pp 97–127

Chapter 13

Relapse Prevention

Genell G. Sandberg, Ph.D.
G. Alan Marlatt, Ph.D.

In this chapter, we present an overview of the relapse prevention model of treatment for substance use disorders, emphasizing practical applications of the assessment and treatment techniques presented. Background research and theory leading to the development of this model can be found in earlier publications on the relapse prevention approach (Marlatt 1979, 1982; Marlatt and George 1984; Marlatt and Gordon 1985; Marlatt and Parks 1982). Much of the material presented in this chapter is drawn from those sources.

WHAT IS RELAPSE PREVENTION?

Relapse prevention is a self-control program that combines behavioral skill-training procedures with cognitive intervention techniques to assist individuals in initiating and maintaining desired behavioral changes. Based on the principles of social learning theory (Bandura 1977), relapse prevention uses a psychoeducational approach that combines both behavioral and cognitive components that aid clients to learn new coping responses (alternatives to addictive behavior), to modify maladaptive beliefs and expectancies concerning substance use, and to change personal life-styles. This focus on both cognitions and behavior is similar to that of other cognitive-behavioral approaches developed recently as an outgrowth of more traditional behavioral therapy programs. Cognitive-behavioral treatment approaches to a variety of clinical problems have been described elsewhere (Beck et al. 1979; Kendall and Hollon 1979; Mahoney 1974; Meichenbaum 1977).

Initially, the relapse prevention model was developed as a behavioral maintenance program for use in the treatment of addictive behaviors (Marlatt and Gordon 1980). In the addictions, the typical treatment goals are either to refrain totally from performing a target behavior (e.g., to abstain from drug use) or to impose regulatory limits or controls over the occurrence of a behavior (e.g., to control food intake by dieting). Although the material presented in this chapter is directed toward substance use disorders, the relapse prevention model may have applications that extend beyond traditional substance abuse problems. Problems such as excessive drinking, smoking, overeating, or substance abuse may be considered collectively as a subclass of a larger set of what we refer to as addictive behaviors. These behaviors include those acts leading to a state of immediate gratification. With many addictive behaviors (especially substance abuse), the experience of immediate gratification (the pleasure, "high," tension-reduction, or release of energy associated with the act itself) is followed by delayed negative consequences, such as physical discomfort or disease, social disapproval, financial loss, and decreased self-esteem. Other examples of addictive behaviors may include such "impulse-control" problems as compulsive gambling, certain sexual disorders (e.g., exhibitionism, pedophilia, and fetishisms), and impulsive aggressive acts (e.g., child abuse and rape). Because many treatment programs for these kinds of problems require clients to abstain totally from engaging in the target behavior, the relapse prevention model has been applied to an increasingly broader range of addictive behaviors.

TREATMENT GOALS AND PHILOSOPHY

Relapse prevention procedures can be applied as a specific maintenance strategy to prevent relapse or as a more general program of lifestyle change. The aim of a specific maintenance strategy is to anticipate and prevent the occurrence of a full-blown relapse following treatment or a period of improvement (e.g., to prevent a recent drug abuser from returning to habitual drug use). These procedures are designed to enhance the maintenance of behavior change and may be applied regardless of the theoretical orientation or intervention methods used during the initial treatment phase. One important difference between initial treatment procedures and those designed to enhance maintenance effects over time is that the former techniques are usually administered to the client by a therapist, whereas maintenance procedures are often self-administered by the client. The goal of teaching the client self-administered maintenance techniques is to train the client to become his or her own therapist and thus carry on the thrust of the intervention program after the termination of the formal therapeutic relationship. This self-control orientation is characteristic of the relapse prevention approach to maintenance. The relapse prevention model is fundamentally a self-control program in which clients are taught how to anticipate and cope effectively with problems as they arise during the posttreatment or follow-up period. Because self-control procedures employed during the maintenance phase may be relatively independent in their effects from the externally administered techniques in the initial treatment phase, the relapse prevention approach may be applied regardless of the approach used during treatment. Once an alcoholic has stopped drinking, for example, relapse prevention methods can be applied toward the effective maintenance of abstinence, regardless of the methods used to initiate abstinence (e.g., Alcoholics Anonymous [AA] meetings, disulfiram [Antabuse], group therapy, aversion therapy, or voluntary cessation).

As a more general program of life-style change, the relapse prevention model is used to facilitate changes in personal habits and lifestyle to reduce the risk of physical disease or psychological stress. Here the aim of the relapse prevention program is much broader in scope: to teach the individual how to achieve a balanced life-style and to prevent the formation of unhealthy habit patterns. A balanced lifestyle is characterized by a harmonious balance between work and play activities and the development of "positive addictions" (Glasser 1976), such as physical exercise and meditation. Thus the central motif of this approach is one of moderation, a balanced life-style being centered between the opposing extremes of behavioral excess and restraint. Viewed from this more global perspective, relapse prevention can be considered as a component of the developing movement in "health psychology" or holistic medicine (Pelletier 1979; Stone et al. 1979).

In the following sections, we will present an overview of the relapse prevention model for both the specific and global applications described above. We begin with a general discussion of the relapse process and the theoretical model as it applies specifically to the treatment of substance abuse. First, we outline the immediate precipitating events that precede a relapse and the cognitive and affective reactions associated with its occurrence. Second, we describe predispositional factors or covert antecedents that may set the stage for relapse or increase the probability that a relapse will occur. In the final sections, we discuss assessment and intervention strategies derived from the relapse prevention model that can be used either to prevent the occurrence of relapse or to cope with the aftermath of a relapse should one occur.

DEFINITION OF RELAPSE

In the self-control model of relapse prevention, relapse is defined as any discrete violation of a self-imposed rule or set of rules governing the rate or pattern of a selected target behavior. Total abstinence, the most stringent rule one can adopt, is violated by a single occurrence of a target behavior. Viewed from this absolute perspective, a single slip may be equated with a total relapse. Although violation of the abstinence rule is the primary form of relapse we have studied in our research, other forms of relapse would also be included within the above definition. Violation of rules governing caloric intake imposed by a diet would also constitute a relapse, as would exceeding alcohol-consumption limits imposed in a controlled-drinking program. Within this general definition of relapse, we are distinguishing between the first violation of the rules (the initial lapse) and the subsequent secondary effects in which the behavior may increase in the direction of the original pretreatment baseline level (a full-blown relapse—e.g., when the first drink or first use of a particular drug is followed by a binge or uncontrolled usage).

In the relapse prevention approach, relapse is viewed as a transitional process, a series of events that may or may not be followed by a return to pretreatment baseline levels of the target behavior. It is possible to view the alcoholic who takes a single drink after a period of abstinence as someone who has made a slight excursion over the border between abstinence and relapse. Whether this first excursion is followed by a return to abstinence depends considerably on the personal expectations and attributes of the person involved. One of the goals of relapse prevention is to provide an individual with the necessary skills and cognitive strategies to prevent the single occurrence of a lapse from escalating into a total relapse. Rather than looking pessimistically on a lapse as a dead-end failure, the relapse prevention approach views each lapse as a fork in the road, one path returning to the former problem behavior (relapse) and the other continuing in the direction of positive change. Instead of being viewed as an indication of failure, a lapse can be viewed more optimistically as a challenge, an opportunity for new learning to occur.

OVERVIEW OF DETERMINANTS OF THE RELAPSE

In the following overview of determinants of relapse, only the highlights of the model are presented. Further details on background research and theory leading to the development of this model can be found elsewhere (Cummings et al. 1980; Marlatt 1978, 1979; Marlatt and Gordon 1980, 1985). A schematic representation of the relapse model is presented in Figure 13-1.

To begin, we are assuming that the individual experiences a sense of perceived control while maintaining abstinence (or complying with other rules governing the target behavior). The target behav-

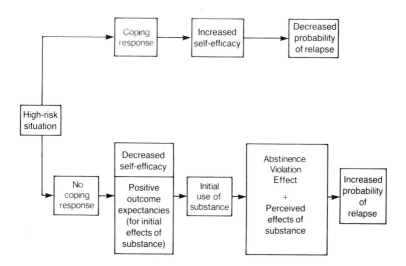

Figure 13-1. Cognitive-behavioral model of the relapse process.

ior is "under control" so long as it does not occur. For example, the longer the period of successful abstinence, the greater the individual's perception of self-control. This perceived control will continue until the person encounters a high-risk situation. A high-risk situation is defined broadly as any situation that poses a threat to the individual's sense of control and increases the risk of potential relapse. In an analysis of 311 initial relapse episodes obtained from clients with a variety of problem behaviors (problem drinking, smoking, heroin addiction, compulsive gambling, and overeating), we identified three primary high-risk situations that were associated with almost three-quarters of all the relapses reported (Cummings et al. 1980). A brief description of the three categories associated with the highest relapse rates follows.

Negative Emotional States

Negative emotional states (35% of all relapses in the sample) are situations in which the individual is experiencing a negative (or unpleasant) emotional state, mood, or feeling (e.g., frustration, anger, anxiety, depression, and boredom) prior to or simultaneously with the first lapse. For example, a smoker in the sample gave the following description of a relapse episode:

> It had been raining continually all week. Saturday I walked down to the basement to do laundry and I found the basement filled with a good three inches of water. To make things worse, as I went to turn on the light to see the extent of the damage, I got shocked from the light switch. Later that same day I was feeling real low and knew I had to have a cigarette after my neighbor, who is a contractor, assessed the damage at over $4,000. I went to the store and bought a pack.

Interpersonal Conflict

Interpersonal conflict (16% of the relapses) situations involve an ongoing or relatively recent conflict associated with any interpersonal relationship (e.g., marriage, friendship, family members, and employer-employee relations). Arguments and interpersonal confrontations occur frequently in this category. A gambler who had been abstaining from betting on the horses described his relapse in the following terms:

> I came home late from a horrible day on the road, and I hadn't stepped in the house five minutes before my wife started accusing me of gambling on the horses. Racetrack, hell! I told her if she didn't believe me I'd give her a real reason to file for divorce. That night I spent $450 at the Longacres Track.

Social Pressure

Social pressure (20% of the sample) situations are those in which the individual is responding to the influence of another person or group of people who exert pressure on the individual to engage in the taboo behavior. Social pressure may be either direct (direct interpersonal contact with verbal persuasion) or indirect (being in the presence of others who are engaging in the same target behavior, even though no direct pressure is involved). Here is an example of direct social pressure given by a formerly abstinent problem drinker in our sample:

> I went to my boss's house for a surprise birthday dinner for him. I got there late and as I came into the living room everyone had a drink in hand. I froze when my boss's wife asked me what I was drinking. Without thinking, I said "J&B on the rocks."

Discussion of the Three Categories

In our analyses of relapse episodes (Cummings et al. 1980; Marlatt and Gordon 1980), we have found that there are more similarities than differences in relapse categories across the various addictive behaviors we studied. These same three high-risk situations are frequently found to be associated with relapse, regardless of the particular problem involved (problem drinking, smoking, gambling, heroin use, or overeating). This pattern of findings lends support to our hypothesis that there are common triggers that frequently initiate the relapse process for a variety of different addictive behaviors.

If a person is able to execute an effective coping response in a high-risk situation (e.g., is assertive in counteracting social pressures), the probability of relapse decreases significantly. A person who copes successfully with a high-risk situation is likely to experience a sense of mastery or perception of control. Successful mastery of one problematic situation is often associated with an expectation of being able to cope successfully with the next challenging event. The expectancy of being able to cope with successive high-risk situations as they develop is closely associated with Bandura's (1977) notion of self-efficacy, defined as the individual's expectation concerning the capacity to cope with an impending situation or task. A feeling of confidence in one's abilities to cope effectively with a high-risk situation is associated with an increased perception of self-efficacy, a kind of "I know I can handle it" feeling. As the duration of the abstinence (or period of controlled use) increases, and a person is able to cope effectively with more and more high-risk situations, perception of control increases in a cumulative fashion; the probability of relapse decreases accordingly.

What happens if a person is unable or unwilling to cope successfully with a high-risk situation? Perhaps the person has never acquired the coping skills involved, or perhaps the appropriate response has been inhibited by fear or anxiety. Perhaps the individual fails to recognize and respond to the risk involved before it is too late. Whatever the reason, if a coping response is not performed, the person is likely to experience a decrease in self-efficacy, frequently coupled with a sense of helplessness and a tendency to give in passively to the situation. "It's no use, I can't handle this" is a common reaction. As self-efficacy decreases in the precipitating high-risk situation, one's expectations for coping successfully with subsequent problem situations also suffer. If the situation also involves the temptation to engage in the prohibited behavior (substance abuse) as a means of attempting to cope with the stress involved, the stage is set for a probable relapse. The probability of relapse is enhanced if the individual holds positive expectancies about the effects of the substance involved. Often the person will anticipate the immediate positive effects of the substance, effects based on past experience, while simultaneously ignoring or not attending to the delayed negative consequences involved. The lure of immediate gratification looms dominantly as the reality of the full consequences of the act recedes. For many persons, smoking a marijuana cigarette or taking a drink has long been associated with coping with stress. "A drink would sure help me get through this," or, "If only I could have a joint, I would feel more relaxed" are commonly held beliefs. Positive outcome expectancies are a primary determinant of alcohol and drug abuse (Marlatt and Rohsenow 1980). Expectancies figure prominently as determinants of relapse in our model.

The combination of being unable to cope effectively in a high-risk situation coupled with positive outcome expectancies for the effects of the habitual coping behavior (drug or alcohol abuse) greatly increases the probability that an initial lapse will occur. On the one hand, the individual is faced with a high-risk situation with no coping response available; self-efficacy decreases as the person feels less able to exert control. On the other hand, there is the lure of the old coping response: the drink or the drug. At this point, unless a last-minute coping response or a sudden change of circumstances occurs, the individual may cross over the border from abstinence (or controlled use) to relapse. Whether the first lapse is followed by a total relapse to a large extent depends on the individual's attributions as to the "cause" of the lapse and the reactions associated with its occurrence.

The requirement of abstinence is an absolute dictum. Once someone has crossed over the line, there is no going back. From this all-or-none perspective, a single drink or use of a drug is sufficient to violate the rule of abstinence: once committed, the deed cannot be undone. Unfortunately, most people who attempt to stop a habit, such as using drugs or drinking, perceive quitting in this "once and for all" manner. To account for the reaction to the transgression of an absolute rule, we have postulated a mechanism called the abstinence violation effect (AVE) (Curry et al. 1987; Marlatt and Gordon 1980). The AVE is postulated to occur under the following conditions. Prior to the first lapse, the individual is personally committed to an extended or indefinite period of abstinence. The intensity of the AVE will vary as a function of several factors, including the degree or prior commitment or effort expended to maintain abstinence, the duration of the abstinence period (the longer the period, the greater the effect), and the subjective value or importance of the prohibited behavior to the individual. We hypothesize that the AVE is characterized by two key cognitive-affective elements: cognitive dissonance (conflict and guilt) and a personal attribution effect (blaming the self as the cause of the relapse).

COVERT ANTECEDENTS OF RELAPSE

In the foregoing discussion of the immediate determinants and reactions to relapse, the high-risk situation is viewed as the precipitating or triggering situation associated with the initial lapse or first "slip" following a period of abstinence or controlled use. In many of the relapse episodes we have studied, the first lapse is precipitated in a high-risk situation that the individual unexpectedly encounters. In most of these instances, the person is not expecting the high-risk situation to occur and/or is generally ill-prepared to cope effectively with the circumstances as they arise. Quite often, the person will suddenly find himself or herself in a rapidly escalating situation that cannot be dealt with effectively. For example, one of our clients who had a serious drinking problem experienced her first lapse after several weeks · of abstinence when she treated a new friend to lunch. A last-minute change of plans led them to eat at a restaurant that served alcoholic beverages. Just moments after their arrival, a cocktail waitress approached their table and asked for drink orders. Our client's friend ordered a cocktail first, and then the waitress turned to the client saying, "And you?" She too ordered a drink, the first of a series of events that culminated in a full-blown relapse. As the client said later, "I didn't plan it and I wasn't prepared for it." Suddenly confronted with a high-risk situation (a social pressure situation, in which the client was influenced both by her friend's ordering a drink and by the waitress' asking her for an order), she was unable to cope effectively.

In other relapse episodes, however, the high-risk situation appears to be the last link in a chain of events preceding the first lapse. For example, another client was a compulsive gambler who came to us for help in controlling his habit, a habit that had caused him numerous marital and financial problems. Before coming to us, he had managed to abstain from all gambling for about 6 months, followed by a relapse and an inability to regain abstinence. We asked the client, a resident of Seattle, Washington, to describe this last relapse episode. "There's nothing much to talk about," he began. "I was in Reno and I started gambling again." Obviously, Reno, Nevada, is a high-risk city for any gambler trying to maintain abstinence. We then asked him to describe the events preceding his arrival in Reno. A close analysis of this chain of events led us to conclude that this client had covertly set up or "planned" his relapse. Although he strongly denied his responsibility in this covert planning process, there were clearly a number of choice-points (forks in the road) preceding the relapse where the client "chose" an alternative that led him closer to the brink of relapse. He finally ended up in downtown Reno shaking hands with a one-armed bandit, an event that triggered a weekend-long binge of costly gambling. It was as if he had placed himself in a situation so risky that it would take a "moral Superman" to resist the temptation to resume gambling.

Why do some clients appear to "set up" their own relapse? From a cost-benefit perspective, a relapse can be seen as a rational choice for many individuals. The benefit is swift in coming: a payoff of immediate gratification. For many, the reward of instant gratification far outweighs the cost of potential negative effects that may or may not occur sometime in the distant future. Why not take the chance when this time it might be different, and perhaps it could be done with impunity? Cognitive distortions such as denial and rationalization make it much easier to set up one's own relapse episode; one may deny both the intent to relapse and the importance of long-range negative consequences. There are also a number of excuses one can use to rationalize the act of indulgence.

One of the most tempting rationalizations is that the desire to indulge is justified. Our research findings and clinical experience in working with a variety of addictive behavior problems suggest that the degree of balance in a person's daily life-style has a significant impact on the desire for indulgence or immediate gratification. Here, we are defining balance as the degree of equilibrium that exists in one's daily life between those activities perceived as external demands (or "shoulds") and those perceived as activities engaged in for pleasure or self-fulfillment (the "wants"). Paying bills or performing routine chores or menial tasks at work would count highly as shoulds for many individuals. At the other end of the scale are the wants, the activities the person likes to perform and from which he or she gains gratification (e.g., going fishing, taking time off for lunch with a friend, or engaging in a creative work task). Other activities represent a mixture of wants and shoulds. We find that a life-style encumbered with a preponderance of perceived shoulds is often associated with an increased perception of self-deprivation and a corresponding desire for indulgence and gratification. It is as if the person who spends his or her entire day engaged in activities high in external demand (often perceived as "hassling" events) attempts to balance this disequilibrium by engaging in an excessive wants or self-indulgence at the end of the day (e.g., drinking to excess in the evening). To justify the indulgence, the client may rationalize it by saying, "I owe myself a drink or two—I deserve a break today!"

The desire for indulgence as an attempt to restore balance or equilibrium is often mediated by both affective and cognitive processes. On the affective side, the desire for indulgence may be experienced on a somatic level as an urge or craving for the prohibited substance. Both urges and cravings manifest themselves primarily as nonverbal impulses or emotional-affective states. We are defining an urge as a relatively sudden impulse to engage in an act (e.g., an impulse to smoke a cigarette) and craving as the subjective desire to experience the effects or consequences of a given act. Craving for alcohol, for example, is defined as a desire for the rewarding or satisfying effects of drinking, rather than for the alcohol itself (Marlatt 1978). Both urges and craving experiences are assumed to be mediated by the anticipated gratification (immediate pleasure or enjoyment) associated with the indulgent act and its affective consequences.

To comprehend the cognitive antecedents of a relapse episode, three constructs are of central importance: rationalization, denial, and decisions or choices associated with the chain of events preceding the first lapse. A rationalization is a cognitive rationale or an ostensibly legitimate excuse to engage in a particular behavior. This conceptualization is similar to traditional psychodynamic theory. According to this position, rationalization is defined as a defense mechanism in which the individual attributes rational or credible motives for a proposed act without a full analysis of the "true" or underlying reasons for this behavior. Denial is a similar mechanism: the individual denies or refuses to recognize selected aspects of the situation or set of events. The person may deny the existence of any motive to engage in a relapse, for example, or may deny awareness of the delayed negative consequences of such behavior. Denial and rationalization are cognitive distortion mechanisms that often go hand in hand in the covert planning of a relapse episode. These two cognitive distortion mechanisms may combine to influence the individual to make certain choices or decisions as part of a chain of events leading ultimately to a relapse. We currently hypothesize that a person headed for a relapse makes a number of mini-decisions over time, each of which brings the individual closer to the brink of succumbing to or creating a high-risk situation. An example is that of the abstinent drinker who buys a bottle of sherry to take home, "just in case guests drop by." In our gambler case study, a decision was made to expand a driving trip to California to include a visit to the blue waters of Lake Tahoe, just a few miles down the road from Reno, Nevada. The term *apparently irrelevant decisions* is used to describe these choices. It is as though the person begins slowly to set the stage for a possible relapse by making a series of apparently irrelevant decisions, each moving a person one step closer to relapse. A final advantage in setting up a relapse in this manner is that the individual may be able to avoid assuming personal responsibility for the relapse episode itself. By putting oneself in an impossibly tempting high-risk situation, one can claim being "overwhelmed" by external circumstances that make it "impossible" to resist a relapse. We call this informally the "downtown Reno effect." There is almost nothing a gambler can do to resist the temptation of a downtown Reno high-risk situation, but he or she can accept responsibility for the chain of events that led him or her there in the first place. One of the primary goals of the relapse prevention program to be presented in the following sections is to train a person to recognize the early warning signals that may precede a relapse and to plan and execute a series of intervention strategies before it is "too late" to do anything and the person ends up in a downtown Reno situation.

ASSESSMENT AND SPECIFIC INTERVENTION STRATEGIES

In this section, we present highlights of the relapse prevention assessment and intervention strategies. We first discuss strategies designed to teach the client how to anticipate and cope with the possibility of relapse: to recognize and cope with high-risk situations that may precipitate a lapse and to modify cognitions and other reactions to prevent a single lapse from developing into a full-blown relapse. Explicitly focused on the immediate precipitants of the relapse process, these procedures are referred to collectively as specific intervention strategies. Second, we go beyond the micro-analysis of the initial lapse and present strategies designed to modify the client's life-style and to identify and cope with covert determinants of relapse. We refer to these procedures as global relapse prevention self-control strategies. In selecting techniques from the material to be presented in the remaining sections, it should be kept in mind that the relapse prevention model can be applied either as an "add-on" program, in which techniques are introduced as an addition to an already existing substance abuse treatment program, or as a general self-control approach designed to develop and maintain a balanced life-style. A complete application of the relapse prevention model would include both global (life-style) and specific intervention techniques.

Both specific and global relapse prevention strategies can be grouped in three main categories: skill training, cognitive reframing, and life-style intervention. Skill-training strategies include both behavioral and cognitive responses to cope with high-risk situations. Cognitive reframing procedures are designed to provide the client with alternative cognitions concerning the nature of the habit-change process (i.e., to view it as a learning process), to introduce coping imagery to deal with urges and early warning signals, and to reframe reactions to the initial lapse (restructuring of the AVE). Finally, life-style intervention strategies (e.g., relaxation and exercise) are designed to strengthen the client's global coping capacity and to reduce the frequency and intensity of urges and craving that are often the product of an unbalanced life-style.

Which of the various intervention techniques should be applied with a particular client? It is possible to combine techniques into a standardized "package," with each subject receiving identical components, if the purpose is to evaluate the effectiveness of a package relapse prevention program. Most readers, however, will be applying the relapse prevention model with clients in an applied clinical setting. In contrast with those who deal with the demands of treatment outcome research, those working in the clinical area typically prefer to develop a tailor-made program of techniques for each client. The individualized approach is the one we recommend for implementation of relapse prevention with most client problems. Particular techniques should be selected, based on a carefully conducted assessment program (Donovan and Marlatt 1987). Therapists are encouraged to select intervention procedures based on their initial evaluation and their assessment of the client's substance abuse problem and general lifestyle pattern.

The relapse prevention model can be applied in the treatment of clients who abuse any substance for which total abstinence is the goal of treatment. It should be noted, however, that when the model is applied to certain other problem behaviors, such as the eating disorders, the goal of treatment becomes moderation ("controlled") intake of food, not abstinence. The possibility of controlled drinking as an alternative to abstinence is the single-most controversial issue associated with treatment planning. Because this is a complex and difficult issue, a complete discussion of the controversy is beyond the scope of this chapter, and the reader is referred elsewhere (Heather and Robertson 1987; Marlatt 1983; Marlatt and Nathan 1978; Miller 1976; Miller and Caddy 1977; Pattison et al. 1977; Sobell and Sobell 1978). As a general rule of thumb, selection of controlled drinking as a treatment goal is not recommended for treatment with individuals who have a long-standing physical dependence on alcohol and who have developed serious life problems associated with their drinking. As a form of secondary prevention, controlled drinking may work best for those who are beginning to develop problems with their drinking, rather than as a remedial treatment program for individuals who have developed a long-term dependence on alcohol. Marlatt (1979) provided a detailed discussion of assessment and treatment techniques with the relapse prevention approach and controlled drinking.

When abstinence has been identified as the goal of treatment, the overall aim of the specific intervention procedures is to teach the client to anticipate and cope with the possibility of relapse: to recognize and cope with high-risk situations that may precipitate a slip, and to modify cognitions and other reactions to prevent a single lapse from developing into a full-blown relapse. Figure 13-2 provides a schematic overview of the specific intervention techniques described. The first step in the prevention of relapse is to teach the client to recognize the high-risk situations that may precipitate or trigger a relapse. Here, the earlier one becomes aware of being involved in a chain of events that increases the probability of a slip or lapse, the

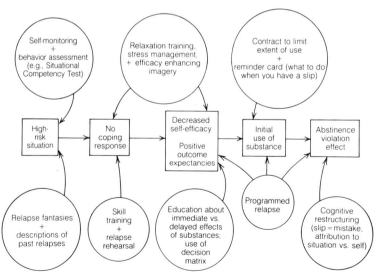

Figure 13-2. Relapse prevention: specific intervention strategies.

sooner one can intervene by performing an appropriate coping skill
and/or recognizing and responding to the discriminative stimuli associated with "entering" a high-risk situation and using cues both as
warning signals and as reminders to engage in alternative or remedial
action.

An essential aspect of teaching clients to handle high-risk situations is to help them identify and anticipate these situations. Earlier
we discussed prototypic kinds of high-risk situations. However, ultimately the identification of high-risk situations is an individualized
question requiring idiographic assessment procedures. Self-monitoring procedures offer an effective method for assessing high-risk situations whenever it is possible to have clients keep a record of their
addictive behavior for a baseline period prior to treatment. As little as
2 weeks of self-monitoring data can often highlight the situational influences and skill deficits that underlie an addictive behavior pattern.

Determining the adequacy of preexisting coping abilities is a
critical assessment target. In a treatment outcome investigation
aimed at teaching alcoholics to handle situational temptations,
Chaney et al. (1978) devised the Situational Competency Test to
measure coping ability. In this technique, the client is presented with
a series of written or audiotaped descriptions of potential relapse situations. Each description ends with a prompt for the client to respond.
Later, the client's responses to the scenes can be scored on a number
of dimensions, including response duration and latency, degree of
compliance, and specification of alternative behaviors. A similar technique involves the use of self-efficacy ratings, in which the client is
presented with a list of potential relapse situations (Annis and Davis
1987). For each situation, the client uses a rating scale to estimate his
or her subjective expectation of successful coping. Ratings across a
wide range of situations enable the individual to identify both problematic situations and skill deficits in need of remedial training. Results from these types of assessment tools can later dictate the focus
of skill-training procedures.

Carefully executed assessment procedures will enable the individual to identify many high-risk situations. The client must then
learn an alternative approach for responding to these situations. A
first step in this new approach is to recognize that high-risk situations
are best perceived as discriminative stimuli signaling the need for behavior change in the same way that road signs signal the need for
alternative action. When viewed in this way, these situations can be

seen as junctures where choices are made rather than as inevitable and uncontrollable challenges that must be endured. In this light, the choice simply to avoid or take a detour around risky situations becomes more available to the individual. However, routine avoidance of particular high-risk situations is unrealistic. Therefore, clients must acquire skills that enable them to cope with these situations as they arise. The specific coping skills to be taught will depend on whether the existing deficiencies are due to actual skill deficits or to response inhibition. A person who has never learned or mastered the skills required to cope with the high-risk situation needs remedial skill training. In response inhibition, a person has already acquired the skills needed to cope with the situation, but is unable to execute them because of inhibiting anxiety or conflicted motivation. In this instance, skill training focuses on interventions designed to disinhibit the appropriate behavior, either by reducing anxiety (e.g., systematic desensitization) or by working on motivational resistance to active coping.

Remedial skill training necessitated by identification of coping skill deficits is the cornerstone of the relapse prevention treatment program. When the individual lacks coping skills, a variety of remedial skills can be taught. The content of the skill-training program is variable and will depend on the needs of the individual. Possible content areas include assertiveness, stress management, relaxation training, anger management, communication skills, and general social or dating skills. In addition to these specific content areas, the relapse prevention approach routinely includes training in additional general problem-solving skills (Goldfried and Davison 1976). Along with education about the long-range negative effects of excessive substance use on physical health and social well-being, a decision matrix, by which clients examine both the immediate and delayed effects of substance use, may help counter the tendency of clients to think only of the initial pleasant short-term effect, which we label the problem of immediate gratification (or the PIG phenomenon). In skill training, the actual teaching procedures are based on the work of McFall (1976) and other investigators. The range of methods includes behavior rehearsal, instruction, coaching, evaluative feedback, modeling, and role playing. In addition, methods introduced by Meichenbaum (1977) on cognitive self-instruction have proven especially valuable for teaching clients constructive self-statements. For troubleshooting and consolidating the newly acquired skills, regular homework assignments are an essential ingredient in skill training.

To reiterate, implementation of a specific skill-training program
will be dictated by the client's unique profile of high-risk situations. If
the individual typically drinks or overdrinks after arguments with a
spouse or significant other, communication or anger management
skills are indicated. If risky encounters revolve around contact with
the opposite sex, dating and social skills may be recommended. In
some instances, it will be impractical to rehearse the new coping skills
in real-life situations. This problem can be surmounted through relapse rehearsal methods. In this procedure, the client is instructed to
imagine being in actual high-risk situations and performing more
adaptive behaviors and thinking more adaptive thoughts. The emphasis here is on coping rather than mastery imagery. That is, the client
is encouraged to visualize that he or she is successfully handling the
difficult situation through effective coping instead of exercising will-
power. To emphasize self-efficacy enhancement, the client can be instructed to imagine the rehearsed experience is accompanied by
mounting feelings of competence and confidence. As a consequence,
the person experiences heightened expectations of successful coping
in future real-life situations, and thereby reduces the probability of
relapse. The relapse rehearsal procedure can be easily carried out as
an intersession homework assignment.

That the client may fail to employ these coping strategies effectively and experience a slip must be anticipated. The client's postslip
reaction is a pivotal intervention point in the relapse prevention model
because it determines the degree of escalation from a single, isolated
slip to a full-blown relapse. The first step in anticipating and dealing
with this reaction is to devise an explicit therapeutic contract to limit
the extent of use if a slip occurs. The actual specifications of the contract should be worked out individually with the client. However, the
fundamental method of intervention after a slip is the use of cognitive
restructuring to counteract the cognitive and affective components of
the AVE. It may be helpful in this regard to have the client carry a
wallet-sized reminder card with instructions to read and follow in the
event of a slip. The text of this card should include the name and
phone number of a therapist or treatment center to be called, as well
as the cognitive reframing antidote to the AVE.

GLOBAL SELF-CONTROL STRATEGIES

The final thrust in the relapse prevention self-management program is
the development of global intervention procedures for life-style

change. It is insufficient to teach clients mechanistic skills for handling high-risk situations and regulating consumption. A comprehensive self-management program must also improve the client's overall life-style to increase the capacity to cope with more pervasive stress factors serving as antecedents to the occurrence of high-risk situations. To accomplish this training, a number of treatment strategies have been devised to short-circuit the covert antecedents to relapse and promote mental and physical wellness. A schematic representation of the global self-control strategies employed in the relapse prevention approach is indicated in Figure 13-3.

As we discussed previously, a persistent and continuing disequilibrium between shoulds and wants can pave the way for relapse by producing a chronic sense of deprivation. As these feelings mount, the individual will experience a growing desire to treat himself or herself to an immediately gratifying indulgence. For most clients, substance use has come to be viewed as a source of immediate gratification and as a method for restoring balance to an "unfairly" lopsided equation. This desire for indulgence translates into urges, cravings, and distortions that permit one "unintentionally" to meander closer to the brink of relapse.

An effective way to induce clients to view the disequilibrium of wants and shoulds as a precursor of relapse is by having them self-monitor the wants and shoulds that prevail in their lives. By keeping a daily record of duties and obligations on one hand and indulgences on

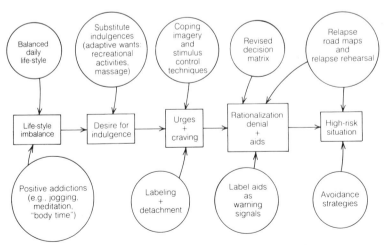

Figure 13-3. Relapse prevention: global self-control strategies.

the other, the client can soon become aware of any imbalance between his or her shoulds and wants. Next, the client should be encouraged to seek a restoration of balance by engaging daily in healthy lifestyle habits or "positive addictions." The advantage of this shift from negative (substance abuse) to positive addiction lies in the latter's capacity to contribute toward the person's long-term health and wellbeing while also providing an adaptive coping response for life stressors and relapse situations. As long-range health benefits accrue, the person begins to develop more self-confidence and self-efficacy.

Despite the efficacy of these techniques for counteracting feelings of deprivation that would otherwise predispose the individual toward relapse, occasional urges and cravings may still surface from time to time. As indicated in Figure 13-3, various urge control procedures are recommended. Sometimes urges and cravings are directly triggered by external cues (e.g., the sight of one's favorite beer mug in the kitchen cabinet). The frequency of these externally triggered urges can be substantially reduced by employing simple stimulus control techniques aimed at minimizing exposure to these cues. In some instances, avoidance strategies offer the most effective way of reducing the frequency of externally triggered urges. The client may need temporarily to avoid certain events or situations, such as the wine section of the local grocery store, until he or she develops more coping skills. Generally, avoidance strategies can often come in handy for dealing with unexpected high-risk situations that emerge. A selection of viable avoidance strategies can enhance the individual's sense of choice when confronted with dangerous situations. The relapse road map is an imagery technique that enables the client both to predict the occurrence of potential high-risk situations well in advance of their actual occurrence and to plan alternative "routes" or strategies to cope with these exigencies.

In teaching clients to cope with urge and craving experiences, it is important to emphasize that the discomfort associated with these internal events is natural. Often, people undergoing cravings have a tendency to feel as though the discomfort will continue to mount precipitously until their resistance collapses under the overwhelming weight of a ballooning urge. In working with this concern, we stress that urges and cravings are triggered by environmental or endogenous cues, and they rise in intensity, reach a peak, and then subside. Indeed, urges can be likened to waves in the sea: they rise, crest, and fall. Using this metaphor, we encourage the client to wait out the urge, to look forward to the downside, and to keep his or her balance when the urge wave is peaking. Extending this metaphor, we refer to this strategy as urge surfing. The client presumably learns to ride out urges just as the surfer learns to maintain balance without wiping out as the wave swells and crests.

Recall that urges and cravings may not always operate at a conscious level, but may become masked by cognitive distortions and defense mechanisms. As such they still exert a potent influence by allowing for apparently irrelevant decisions that inch the person closer to relapse. To counter this, we train the client to see through these self-deceptions by recognizing their true meanings. Explicit self-talk can help in making apparently irrelevant decisions seem more relevant. By acknowledging to oneself that certain mini-decisions (e.g., keeping a bottle of wine at home for friends dropping over) actually increase the risk of relapse, one becomes able to use these experiences as early warning signals. An important objective in these urge control techniques is to enable the individual to externalize urges and cravings and to view them with objective detachment. Another way to achieve this detachment is to encourage the client to label the urge deliberately as soon as it registers into consciousness. Urges should be viewed as natural occurrences in response to environmental and lifestyle forces rather than as signs of treatment failure and indicators of future relapse.

CONCLUSIONS

The empirical underpinnings of the relapse prevention model outlined in this chapter have been reviewed elsewhere (Marlatt and Gordon 1985). However, only a few outcome studies have appeared in the literature to date that have compared the relapse prevention model with other approaches to the treatment of addiction or the prevention of relapse (Brownell et al. 1986). Even so, research is currently underway on the treatment efficacy of relapse prevention. The few outcome studies that have appeared, along with research on the role of expectancies (self-efficacy and outcome expectancies) and coping skills in the habit-change process, have provided general support for the relapse prevention model. We refer other clinicians and researchers who wish more detailed information on research support and clinical application of the relapse prevention model to the Marlatt and Gordon (1985) text.

REFERENCES

Annis HM, Davis CS: Assessment of expectancies in alcohol dependent clients, in Assessment of Addictive Behaviors: Behavioral, Cognitive, and Physiological Procedures. Edited by Donovan DM, Marlatt GA. New York, Guilford, 1987

Bandura A: Self-efficacy: toward a unifying theory of behavioral change. Psychol Rev 84:191–215, 1977

Beck AT, Rush AJ, Shaw BF, et al: Cognitive Therapy of Depression. New York, Guilford, 1979

Brownell KD, Marlatt GA, Lichtenstein E, et al: Understanding and preventing relapse. Am Psychol 41:765–782, 1986

Chaney EF, O'Leary MR, Marlatt GA: Skill training with alcoholics. J Consult Clin Psychol 46:1092–1104, 1978

Cummings C, Gordon JR, Marlatt GA: Relapse: strategies of prevention and prediction, in The Addictive Behaviors. Edited by Miller WR. Oxford, England, Pergamon, 1980

Curry SJ, Marlatt GA, Gordon JR: Abstinence violation effect: validation of an attributional construct with smoking cessation. J Consult Clin Psychol 55:145–149, 1987

Donovan DM, Marlatt GA (eds): Assessment of Addictive Behaviors. New York, Guilford, 1988

Glasser W: Positive Addiction. New York, Harper & Row, 1976

Goldfried MR, Davison GC: Clinical Behavior Therapy. New York, Holt, Rinehart & Winston, 1976

Heather N, Robertson I (eds): Controlled Drinking, 2nd Edition. London, Methuen, 1987

Kendall PC, Hollon SD (eds): Cognitive-Behavioral Interventions: Theory, Research and Procedures. New York, Academic, 1979

Mahoney MJ: Cognition and Behavior Modification. Cambridge, MA, Ballinger, 1974

Marlatt GA: Craving for alcohol, loss of control and relapse: cognitive-behavioral analysis, in Alcoholism: New Directions in Behavioral Research and Treatment. Edited by Nathan PE, Marlatt GA, Loberg T. New York, Plenum, 1978

Marlatt GA: Alcohol use and problem drinking: a cognitive-behavioral analysis, in Cognitive-Behavioral Interventions: Theory, Research and Procedures. Edited by Kendall PC, Hollon SD. New York, Academic, 1979

Marlatt GA: Relapse prevention: a self-control program for the treatment of addictive behaviors, in Adherence, Compliance and Generalization in Behavioral Medicine. Edited by Stuart RB. New York, Brunner/Mazel, 1982

Marlatt GA: The controlled drinking controversy: a commentary. Am Psychol 38:1097–1110, 1983

Marlatt GA, George WH: Relapse prevention: introduction and overview of the model. Br J Addict 79:261–273, 1984

Marlatt GA, Gordon JR: Determinants of relapse: implications for the maintenance of behavior change, in Behavioral Medicine: Changing Health Lifestyles. Edited by Davidson PO, Davidson SM. New York, Brunner/Mazel, 1980

Marlatt GA, Gordon JR (eds): Relapse Prevention: Maintenance Strategies in the Treatment of Addictive Behaviors. New York, Guilford, 1985

Marlatt GA, Nathan PE: Behavioral Approaches to Alcoholism. New Brunswick, NJ, Rutgers Center of Alcohol Studies, 1978

Marlatt GA, Parks GA: Self-management of addictive disorders, in Self-Management and Behavior Change. Edited by Karoly P, Kanfer FH. Elmsford, NY, Pergamon, 1982

Marlatt GA, Rohsenow DR: Cognitive processes in alcohol use: expectancy and the balanced placebo design, in Advances in Substance Abuse, Vol 1. Edited by Mello NK. Greenwich, CT, JAI Press, 1980

McFall RM: Behavioral Training: A Skill-Acquisition Approach to Clinical Problems. Morristown, NJ, General Learning Press, 1976

Meichenbaum D: Cognitive-Behavior Modification. New York, Plenum, 1977

Miller PM: Behavioral Treatment of Alcoholism. Oxford, England, Pergamon, 1976

Miller WR, Caddy GR: Abstinence and controlled drinking in the treatment of problem drinkers. J Stud Alcohol 38:986–1003, 1977

Pattison EM, Sobell MB, Sobell LC: Emerging Concepts of Alcohol Dependence. New York, Springer, 1977

Pelletier KR: Holistic Medicine: From Stress to Optimum Health. New York, Delacorte Press/Seymour Lawrence, 1979

Sobell MB, Sobell LC: Behavioral Treatment of Alcohol Problems. New York, Plenum, 1978

Stone GC, Cohen F, Adler NE: Health Psychology. San Francisco, CA, Jossey-Bass, 1979

Index

AANB-to-leucine ratio test, 9
Abstinence controversy, 366–367
Abstinence syndrome
  barbiturates, 162–163
  benzodiazepines, 146–147
  cocaine, 210–216
  glutethimide, 154
  nicotine, 330–331, 334–338
  phencyclidine, 286–288
Abstinence Violation Effect, 385, 390
Acetaldehyde, 29–30
Acetaldehyde addicts test, 9
Acetylcholine
  alcohol effects, 34
Addictive potency of cocaine, 203
Adenosine receptor test, 10
Adolescents
  cocaine abuse, 195–196, 198
  tobacco use, 324, 325
Adoption studies of alcoholism, 20–22
Adrenergic systems
  alcohol effects, 31
Advertising and tobacco use, 325, 326
Affective disorders
  cocaine abuse, 202
  opioid dependence and addiction, 114–115
Affective dysfunction, 345–346
Alanine aminotransferase test, 8
Alcohol
  absorption and distribution, 27–28
  benzodiazepines and, 141–142
  detoxification, 48
  disulfiram-ethanol reaction, 58–59
  metabolism, 28–29
  neurotransmitter and neuroreceptor effects, 31–36
  pharmacokinetics, 22–23
  pharmacology, 27–36
  withdrawal, 365–366
Alcohol abuse. *See* Alcoholism
Alcohol hallucinosis, 11
Alcoholic cardiomyopathy, 69
Alcoholic myopathy, 71

401

Alcoholic personality, 12–14, 15, 17
Alcoholics Anonymous
    advantages, 369–370
    history, 50–51, 361–362
    meetings, 362–363
    membership, 360–361
    philosophy, 362
    Preamble, 360
    problems, 368–369
    psychotherapy and, 53–54, 347–348, 354–355, 366–368
    referral, 370–372
    sponsorship, 364, 366
    treatment outcome, 347–348
    Twelve Steps, 363, 364–365
    See also Alcoholism treatment
Alcoholism
    adoption studies, 20–22
    depression and, 57–58
    diagnosis, 2–11
    "disease" concept, 352, 360
    etiology, 11–27
    opioid dependence and, 114
    prevalence, 1–2
    stages, 3–5
    twin studies, 19–20
    types, 21–22
Alcoholism treatment
    nursing care, 39
    nutritional, 40, 41–43, 48
    pharmacologic, 40–48, 54–63
    postwithdrawal, 49–63
    psychiatric, 49–54
    psychotherapeutic, 348–354
    treatment outcome studies, 51–53
    zimelidine, 33
    See also Alcoholics Anonymous
Alcohol screening tests, 7–10
Alcohol withdrawal syndrome
    criteria for hospitalization, 36, 39
    symptoms, 37–38
    treatment, 36–49, 365–366
    See also Alcoholism treatment
Alexithymia, 346
l-alpha-acetylmethadol. *See* Levomethadyl acetate
Alpha-adrenergic agonists
    alcohol detoxification, 46–47
Alprazolam
    detoxification, 148

Amantadine, 211
Amenorrhea, 70
American Indians
  alcohol elimination rate, 22
Amnesia, 64–65, 153
Amotivational syndrome, 182
Amphetamine
  history of use, 235
  pharmacology, 238–240
  side effects, 240
Amphetamine abuse
  overdose symptoms, 250
  prevalence, 237
  tolerance, 240
Animal studies
  alcoholism, 24
  amphetamine, 239
  phencyclidine, 288
  stimulants, 245
Anorectics, 241–242
Anticholinergics, 273–275
  detoxification, 275–276
  intoxication, 275
Anticonvulsants
  alcohol detoxification, 48
Antidepressants
  alcoholism treatment, 57
  cocaine abuse treatment, 211
Anxiety, 153
  barbiturates as treatment, 156
  marijuana-induced, 182–183
  opioid-induced, 115
  treatment outcomes, 151
Anxiolytics
  absorption, 143
  alcoholism treatment, 55–57
  See also specific drugs
Appetite-suppressants, 241–242
Artane, 274
Ascites, 67
Asians
  alcohol elimination rate, 22–23
Assertiveness training, 219
Athletic performance
  amphetamine effects, 240
Attention-deficit disorder, 14
  cocaine abuse, 202
AVE. *See* Abstinence Violation Effect

"Bad trip," 267
Barbiturates
  alcohol detoxification, 47
  brand and street names, 160
  clinical uses, 165–167
  detoxification, 162–165
  pharmacokinetics, 161–162
  pharmacology, 156–159
  prevalence, 155
  psychological effects, 159–160
  side effects, 165–167
  tolerance, 162
  types, 159
  withdrawal, 163
Basic ego operations, 16–17
Behavioral conditioning
  benzodiazepine use, 145
  cocaine abuse, 202, 218
Benzedrex, 238
Benzedrine inhaler, 235–236
Benzene, 311
Benzodiazepines
  abstinence syndrome, 146–147
  alcohol and, 141–142
  alcoholism treatment, 56
  alcohol withdrawal treatment, 40, 44
  detoxification, 147–153
  diagnosis, 135–137
  dose equivalency of different types, 148
  etiology of dependence, 144–146
  medical consequences of dependence, 152–153
  metabolism, 143–144
  pharmacokinetics, 143
  pharmacology, 140–142
  prevalence, 137–140
  tolerance, 142, 144
  use with other drugs, 139
Benzoylecgonine, 196, 201
Benztropine, 274
Beta-blockers
  alcohol detoxification, 45
  alcoholism treatment, 55
Beta-hexosaminidase test, 9
Biological theories of alcoholism etiology, 19–27
Biomembranes, 30–31
Blood acetate and ethanol test, 9
Blood alcohol levels, 7, 30
  criteria for hospitalization, 39

Blood groups, 24, 27
Blood levels
  alcohol, 7, 30, 39
  cocaine, 200
  nicotine, 328–329
Boston Collaborative Drug Surveillance Program, 138
Brand names
  barbiturates, 160
  stimulants, 234
Bromocriptine, 211, 216
Buprenex
  opioid detoxification, 110–111
Buprenorphine
  opioid detoxification, 110–111
Buspirone
  alcoholism treatment, 55–56

Caffeine, 244–245
CAGE system, 6–7
Calcium
  alcohol effects, 35
Calcium carbimide
  alcoholism treatment, 62–63
Carbamazepine, 151
  alcohol detoxification, 48
Cardiac arrhythmias, 69, 206
Cardiomyopathy, alcoholic, 69
Cardiovascular system
  cocaine effects, 206
  solvent effects, 307–308
Catalase, 29
Central nervous system
  alcohol effects on fetus, 72
  barbiturate effects, 157–158, 161
  caffeine effects, 244–245
  cocaine effects, 207–208
  opioid effects, 99
  solvent effects, 302, 303–304
Central pontine myelinolysis, 65
Cerebrovascular accident
  cocaine-induced, 207
Children
  tobacco use, 324
Chloral hydrate
  alcohol detoxification, 46
Chlormethiazole
  alcohol detoxification, 45–46
Chromatographic assays, 196–197

Cirrhosis, alcoholic, 66–67
Clonazepam, 151
Clonidine, 150
    methadone and, 109
    naltrexone and, 110
    opioid detoxification, 108–110
    tobacco dependence treatment, 335
Cocaine
    intoxication, 203–204
    pharmacology, 199–202
    side effects, 203–204
    tolerance, 200–201
    withdrawal, 210–216
Cocaine abuse
    diagnosis, 195–197
    etiology, 198–199, 202–203
    laboratory tests, 196–197, 201
    medical complications, 204–209
    prevalence, 198–199
    treatment, 214–215, 216–220
    treatment outcome, 218
Cocaine Anonymous, 116–117, 218–219
Codeine
    withdrawal, 106
Cogentin, 274
Cognitive function
    amphetamine effects, 240
    marijuana effects, 181
Color blindness, 27
Coma
    phencyclidine-induced, 288–290
Competitive binding assays, 196–197, 201
Conditioned aversion
    alcoholism treatment, 63
Controlled drinking, 390–391
Corpus callosum degeneration, 65
Correction fluids, 308
Cotinine, 327–328
Cravings and urges, 396–397
Crime and opioid use, 115–116
Cross-cultural studies of alcoholism, 18–19
Cross-tolerance
    alcohol and morphine, 32
    methadone and other opioids, 117
    See also Tolerance

"Deadly nightshade," 274

Death
  barbiturate overdose, 166
  cocaine abuse, 204–206
  solvent abuse, 298
  tobacco dependence, 331–332
Delirium tremens, 11
Delta-receptors, 101–102
Dementia, alcoholic, 65
Dental problems
  cocaine-induced, 209
Depression
  alcohol-induced, 12–13, 57–58
  cocaine-induced, 204, 209–210
"Designer drugs," 237–238, 270–271
Desipramine, 211, 216
  amphetamine abuse treatment, 251
  side effects, 217–218
DET. *See* Diethyltryptamine
Detoxification
  alcohol, 36–49
  anticholinergics, 275–276
  barbiturates, 162–165
  benzodiazepines, 147–153
  glutethimide, 154
  LSD, 268–269
  marijuana, 186
  methadone maintenance, 120–121
  opioid, 108–111
  phencyclidine, 288–291
Diazepam
  LSD detoxification, 268
Diet pills, 241–242
2,5-dimethoxy-4-methylamphetamine, 271, 272–273
  treatment, 273
N,N-dimethyltryptamine, 263, 269
N$_2$N-dimethyltryptamine, 263, 269
Discriminant function analysis, 10
"Disease" concept of alcoholism, 352, 360
Distal renal acidosis, 300
Disulfiram
  contraindications, 61
  dosage, 61–62
  efficacy, 62
  mechanism, 58
  side effects, 58–61
DMT. *See* Dimethyltryptamine
DOM. *See* 2,5-dimethoxy-4-methylamphetamine

Dopaminergic system
  alcohol effects, 33–34
  amphetamine effects, 239
  cocaine effects, 211
Driving impairment, 181
Drug counseling, 347–348
Drug interactions
  barbiturates and central nervous system sedatives, 165–166
  benzodiazepines and alcohol, 141–142
  benzodiazepines and opioids, 150
  benzodiazepines and other drugs, 139
  clonidine and methadone, 109
  lithium and methadone, 115
  nicotine and other drugs, 332
Drug paraphernalia, 102–103
Dry-cleaning fluids, 309
DSM-III-R criteria
  alcoholism, 4–5
  benzodiazepine dependence, 136
  hallucinogenic hallucinosis, 266
  psychoactive substance abuse, 6
  psychoactive substance dependence, 5

"Ecstasy." *See* 3,4-Methylenedioxymethamphetamine
Ego functions, 346
Electrolyte imbalance
  solvent-induced, 301
Emergency rooms
  drugs mentioned most frequently, 157
Endogenous opioids, 100
Environmental factors of opioid addiction and dependence, 103
Enzyme immunoassay for cocaine detection, 196
Erythrocyte enzyme test, 8–9
Esophageal cancer, 68
Ethanol. *See* Alcohol
Ethnic differences
  alcohol elimination rate, 22–23
  alcoholism, 18–19
Ethyl chloride abuse, 311–312
Etiology
  alcoholism, 11–27
  benzodiazepine dependence, 144–145
  cocaine abuse, 198–199, 202–203
  opioid dependence and addiction, 96–98, 102–104
  stimulant abuse, 245–247
  tobacco dependence, 325–326

Families
 alcoholism treatment, 7, 356
 cocaine abuse, 202, 218, 219
 family therapy, 356
 opioid use, 104, 125
Fetal alcohol syndrome, 71–73
 marijuana use, 185
Fetal solvent syndrome, 311
Field dependence, 14
Flashbacks, 267, 268, 269
Fluorocarbons, 298, 299
Fluoxetine as alcoholism treatment, 33
Flushing
 alcohol reaction, 23, 60
 opioid reaction, 99
Folate deficiency, 68
Freud, Sigmund, 15

GABA
 alcohol effects, 31–32
Gas chromatograph-mass spectrometry, 197, 201
Gas-liquid chromatography, 197
Gasoline sniffing, 306
Gastric alcohol dehydrogenase, 28
Gastrointestinal system
 opioid effects, 99
Genetic components of alcohol pharmacokinetics, 22–23
Genetic markers of alcoholism, 24–27
Genetic predisposition
 to alcoholism, 24
 to opioid dependence, 104
Global self-control strategies, 395
Glue sniffing, 304
Glutamate
 alcohol effects, 34–35
Glutethimide, 154
Group therapy, 355–356

Hallucinations
 solvent-induced, 304
Hallucinogens
 major groups, 260
 street names, 262
 See also Phenylalkylamine hallucinogens;
  Tryptamine-related hallucinogens; *specific drugs*
HDL cholesterol test, 10
Hearing
 solvent effects, 303

Hematology
  alcohol effects, 68
  solvent effects, 310–311
Hepatic encephalopathy, 67
Hepatitis, alcoholic, 66
Heroin
  prevalence, 96
  tolerance, 105
  withdrawal, 106
Hexane, 305–306
High-density lipoproteins, 69–70
High-pressure liquid chromatography, 197, 201
Himmelsbach Scale, 107
Histamine
  flushing reaction to alcohol, 23
HIV infection and opioid use, 111–112
Hospitalization
  alcohol detoxification, 36, 39
  cocaine abuse, 217
Hydantoin embryopathy, 311
Hypertension, 68–69
  cocaine-induced, 206
Hypnotics, 155

ICD-9 criteria, 139
Ice, 236
Immunoglobulin test, 9
Individual psychotherapy
  opioid dependence treatment, 124
Indolealkylamines. *See* Tryptamine-related hallucinogens
Infants
  fetal alcohol syndrome, 71–73, 185
  fetal solvent syndrome, 311
  mother's cocaine abuse, 207
Infections
  cocaine-induced, 208
  opioid-induced, 111–112
Inhalants. *See* Solvent abuse; Solvents; *specific chemicals*;
    specific products
Inner control, 347
Interpersonal conflict and relapse, 382–383
Intestinal infarct, 209
Intoxication
  alcohol, 10–11
  amphetamine, 247–248
  anticholinergics, 275
  benzodiazepines, 146
  cocaine, 203–204

glutethimide, 154
LSD, 265–269
marijuana, 180–183
nicotine, 329–331
phencyclidine, 282
Ischemia, 209

Jimsonweed, 274
Jung, Carl
  alcoholism treatment views, 50–51

Kappa receptors, 101
Ketamine, 280
Korsakoff's syndrome, 64

LAAM. *See* Levomethadyl acetate
Labels on products containing solvents, 297
Laboratory tests
  alcohol, 7–10
  cocaine, 196–197, 201
  LSD, 268
  mescaline, 273
  phencyclidine, 281
Late withdrawal syndrome, 48–49
Levomethadyl acetate
  as opioid dependence treatment, 106, 122–123
Life expectancy
  opioid addiction and, 111–112
Lithium
  alcohol detoxification, 45
  methadone and, 115
Liver
  alcohol effects, 66–67
  solvent effects, 308–309
Liver alcohol dehydrogenase, 28–29
Liver enzyme test, 8
Lorazepam
  tolerance, 142
LSD
  intoxication, 268–269
  mechanism, 264–265
  medical complications, 267–268
  psychiatric complications, 261, 267–268
Lymphadenopathy, 112
Lysergic acid diethylamide. *See* LSD

MAO inhibitors
  alcoholism treatment, 56

MAO inhibitors *(cont)*
    alcohol reaction, 59–60
Marchiafava-Bignami disease, 65
Marijuana
    cocaine abuse, 199
    detoxification, 186
    perception effects, 180–181
    pharmacokinetics, 179–180
    pharmacology, 179
    physiologic effects, 184–185
    prevalence, 175–178
    psychiatric complications, 182–183
    tolerance, 183–184
    treatment of dependence, 186
    withdrawal, 183–184
Markers
    alcohol, 25–26
    cigarette smoking, 328
    cocaine use, 201
MDA. *See* Methylenedioxyamphetamine
MDMA. *See* 3,4-Methylenedioxymethamphetamine
Mean corpuscular volume test, 8
Medical complications
    cocaine abuse, 204–209
    LSD use, 267–268
    marijuana use, 196
    stimulant abuse, 249–250
Memory
    marijuana effects, 182
Meperidine
    withdrawal, 106
Mescaline
    laboratory tests, 273
    mechanism, 273
    pharmacokinetics, 272
    prevalence, 270
Methadone
    clonidine and, 109
    mechanism, 117–118
    opioid withdrawal treatment, 106
    side effects, 118
    tolerance, 118
Methadone maintenance programs
    philosophy, 119–120
    regulations, 118–119
    staffing, 118
Methamphetamine
    history of use, 235–236

Methylenedioxyamphetamine, 237–238, 243–244, 271
3,4-Methylenedioxymethamphetamine, 237–238, 243–244
   psychological effects, 272–273
Methylphenidate, 240–241
Microsomal alcohol oxidizing system, 29
Minnesota Multiphasic Personality Inventory, 12–13
MMPI. *See* Minnesota Multiphasic Personality Inventory
Morning glory seeds, 261–262, 269
Morphine withdrawal, 106
Motivation and marijuana, 182
Mu receptors, 101
Mu-receptor
   tolerance, 104–105
Myopathy, alcoholic, 71

Naloxone
   opioid dependence treatment, 121
   withdrawal, 107
Naltrexone
   clonidine and, 110
   opioid dependence treatment, 121–122
   opioid detoxification, 110
Narcissistic issues, 346, 347
Narcolepsy
   amphetamine-induced, 235
Narcotics Anonymous, 116–117, 218–219
National Institute on Alcohol Abuse and Alcoholism, 50–51
National Institute on Drug Abuse National Household Survey on
      Drug Abuse, 96
Negative emotional states and relapse, 382
Neuroleptics
   alcohol detoxification, 47
Neurotransmitter and neuroreceptor effects of alcohol, 31–36
Nicotine
   abstinence syndrome, 334–338
   intoxication, 329–331
   metabolism and excretion, 327–328
   pharmacokinetics, 327
   pharmacology, 326–327
   plasma levels, 328–329
   tolerance, 329
   withdrawal, 330–331, 334–338
   See also Tobacco use and dependence
Nicotine gum, 335–336
Nitrous oxide, 309–310
Nursing care for alcoholism treatment, 39
Nutritional treatment of alcoholism, 40, 48

Object substitute, 346
Opiate systems
    alcohol effects, 32
Opioid antagonists, 121–123
Opioid dependence and addiction
    alcoholism and, 114
    etiology, 96–98, 102–104
    physical effects, 99–102
    prevalence, 96
    treatment, 116–125
    withdrawal, 106
Opioid receptor types, 100–101
Opioid withdrawal syndrome, 106
Oral-dependent personality, 15
Outpatient drug-free programs for opioid dependence treatment, 124
Oxford Movement, 50–51, 361

Paint thinner, 305–306
Pancreatitis, alcoholic, 67–68
Panic disorder
    cocaine-induced, 210
Paraldehyde
    alcohol detoxification, 47–48
Passive-dependent personality, 15
PCP. See Phencyclidine
Pemoline, 243
Pentazocine, 97
Perception
    LSD effects, 266–267
    marijuana effects, 180–181
Peripheral neuropathies, 305–306
Personality disorders and cocaine abuse, 202
Peyote. See Mescaline
Pharmacokinetics
    alcohol, 22–23
    barbiturates, 161–162
    benzodiazepines, 143
    marijuana, 179–180
    nicotine, 327
    phencyclidine, 286, 287
Pharmacology
    alcohol, 27–36
    amphetamine, 238–240
    barbiturates, 156–159
    benzodiazepines, 140–142
    cocaine, 199–202
    marijuana, 179
    nicotine, 326–327
    phencyclidine, 281–285

Phencyclidine
   abstinence syndrome, 286–288
   detoxification, 288–291
   history of use, 279–280
   intoxication, 282
   laboratory tests, 281
   pharmacokinetics, 286, 287
   pharmacology, 281–285
   prevalence, 280–281
   street names, 280
Phenelzine, 219
Phenylalkylamine hallucinogens, 270–273
Phenylthiocarbamide, 27
Phobics Society, 138–139
Phosphatidylethanol synthesis test, 10
Physiologic dependence
   benzodiazepines, 145–146
PIG phenomenon, 393
Platelet MAO test, 10
Positive addictions, 379, 396
Pregnancy
   alcohol use, 71–73
   cigarette smoking, 328
   cocaine use, 205–206
   inhalant abuse, 311
   marijuana use, 185
   opioid use, 112–113
   See also Fetal alcohol syndrome; Fetal solvent syndrome
Prevalence
   alcoholism, 1–2
   amphetamine abuse, 237
   barbiturate abuse, 155
   benzodiazepine abuse, 137–140
   cocaine abuse, 198–199
   marijuana abuse, 175–178
   mescaline abuse, 270
   opioid dependence and addiction, 96
   phencyclidine abuse, 280–281
   psychiatric disorders, 113–114
   solvent abuse, 296–297
   tobacco dependence, 321–325
   tryptamine-related hallucinogen abuse, 261–263
Propane sniffing, 312
Propranolol, 150
Propylhexedrine, 238
Psilocin, 262
Psilocybin, 262–263, 264, 269
Psychiatric complications
   alcoholism, 57–58

Psychiatric complications *(cont)*
    amphetamine abuse, 235, 246
    barbiturates, 159–160
    cocaine abuse, 202, 209–210
    LSD use, 261, 267–268
    marijuana use, 182–183
    opioid dependence, 113–116
    prevalence, 113–114
Psychodynamic factors
    opioid addiction and dependence, 103–104
Psychological dependence
    marijuana, 186
Psychopathic State Inventory, 13
Psychosis
    amphetamine-induced, 236, 247–248
    LSD-induced, 261
    phencyclidine-induced, 285
    stimulant-induced, 247–248
Psychotherapy
    Alcoholics Anonymous and, 347–348, 354–355, 366–368
    alcoholism treatment approaches, 348–354
    family therapy, 356
    group therapy, 355–356
    inpatient treatment for alcoholism and, 348
    psychodynamic formulations, 345–347
    studies, 347–348
    treatment outcome, 347–348
Pulmonary function
    cocaine effects, 208–209
    solvent effects, 307

Radioimmunoassay
    cocaine detection, 196, 201
Receptor-effector coupling
    alcohol effects, 35–36
Relapse
    assessment procedures, 392–393
    coping response in high risk situations, 383–385
    covert antecedents, 385–389
    definition, 380–381
    determinants, 381–385
    intervention strategies, 389–397
    opioid use, 106
    prevention program design, 377–378
    prevention treatment goals and philosophy, 378–380
    psychotherapy and, 348–349
    skill training, 393–394
    See also Treatment outcome

Relaxation training, 151, 219
Renal function
    solvent effects, 299–301
Renal tubular acidosis, 311
Reproductive system
    LSD effects, 268
    marijuana effects, 185
Respiratory function
    alcohol effects, 71
    marijuana effects, 184
    solvent effects, 299
Respiratory tract infections, 71

Schizophrenia and opioid use, 115
Scopolamine, 274–275
Sedative-hypnotics, 155
Sedatives, 156
Seizures
    cocaine-induced, 208
Self-care deficits, 346, 353
Self-control and relapse prevention, 379
Self-esteem, 346
Self-Rating Depression Scale, 13
Serotonin
    alcohol effects, 32–33
Serum aspartate aminotransferase test, 8
Side effects
    amphetamine, 240
    barbiturates, 165–167
    cocaine, 203–204
    desipramine, 217–218
    disulfiram, 58–61
Situational Competency Test, 392
Sleep
    barbiturate effects, 161
    stimulant effects, 248
Smoke-free environments, 337–338
Smokeless tobacco, 328
Snuff, 263
Social factors
    alcoholism, 17–19
    amphetamine abuse, 246
    opioid addiction and dependence, 103
    relapse, 383
Solvent abuse
    death, 298
    medical complications, 299–311
    prevalence, 296–297

Solvent abuse *(cont)*
  treatment, 301, 312
Solvents
  product labelling, 297
  types of products, 298
Sponsorship in Alcoholics Anonymous, 364, 366
Spray paints, 299–300
Stimulant abuse
  etiology, 245–247
  medical complications, 249–250
  treatment outcomes, 250–251
  withdrawal, 249
Stimulants
  brand and street names, 234
  clinical uses, 233
  history of use, 235–236
  See also specific drugs
"Stovetop speed," 238
Street names
  barbiturates, 160
  hallucinogens, 262
  phencyclidine, 280
  stimulants, 234
Succinylcholine, 205
Sudden infant death syndrome
  cocaine abuse, 207
Suffering, 346

Tachycardia, 184
Temperament
  alcoholism and, 13–14
Therapeutic communities for opioid dependence treatment, 123–124
Therapist-patient relationship, 351–352
Therapist's attendance at Alcoholics Anonymous meetings, 372–373
Therapist's role in alcoholism treatment, 351
Thin-layer chromatography, 197, 201
Thyroid function, 71
Tobacco use and dependence
  advertising and, 325, 326
  degree, 334–335
  economic impact, 326
  etiology, 325–326
  prevalence, 321–325
  treatment, 332–338
  treatment outcome, 337
  See also Nicotine
Tolerance
  amphetamine, 240

barbiturates, 162
benzodiazepines, 142, 144
cocaine, 200–201
marijuana, 183–184
methadone, 118
nicotine, 329
opioid, 104–105
See also Cross-tolerance
Tranquilizers, 156
Treatment
alcoholism, 33, 36–63, 359–374
cocaine abuse, 214–215, 216–220
inhalant abuse, 312
LSD intoxication, 268–269
marijuana dependence, 186
opioid dependence, 116–125
solvent abuse, 301
tobacco dependence, 332–338
Treatment outcome
alcoholism, 51–53, 347–348
anxiety disorders, 151
cocaine abuse, 218
opioid dependence and addiction, 98–99, 120
psychotherapy, 347–348
relapse, 397
stimulant abuse, 250–251
tobacco use and dependence, 337
Trihexyphenidyl, 274
Tripelennamine, 97
Tryptamine-related hallucinogens, 260
pharmacokinetics, 263–264
prevalence, 261–263
Twelve Steps of Alcoholics Anonymous, 363, 364–365
Twin studies of alcoholism, 19–20

Urine acidification, 289–290

Vision
solvent effects, 305

Wernicke's encephalopathy, 64
Wernicke's syndrome, 64–65
Wilson, Bill, 361
Withdrawal
alcohol, 36–49, 365–366
barbiturates, 163
benzodiazepines, 146–147
cocaine, 210–216

Withdrawal *(cont)*
    marijuana, 183–184
    nicotine, 330–331, 334–338
    opioids, 105–107
    sedative-hypnotics, 155
    stimulants, 249
Women
    marijuana effects, 185
    opioid effects, 112–113
    See also Pregnancy

Zimelidine
    alcoholism treatment, 33